AF844923

Basal Implantology

Gérard M. Scortecci
Editor

Basal Implantology

Springer

Editor
Gérard M. Scortecci
Nice
France

ISBN 978-3-319-44871-8   ISBN 978-3-319-44873-2 (eBook)
https://doi.org/10.1007/978-3-319-44873-2

© Springer Nature Switzerland AG 2019, corrected publication 2019
This work is subject to copyright. All rights are reserved by the Publisher, whether the whole or part of the material is concerned, specifically the rights of translation, reprinting, reuse of illustrations, recitation, broadcasting, reproduction on microfilms or in any other physical way, and transmission or information storage and retrieval, electronic adaptation, computer software, or by similar or dissimilar methodology now known or hereafter developed.
The use of general descriptive names, registered names, trademarks, service marks, etc. in this publication does not imply, even in the absence of a specific statement, that such names are exempt from the relevant protective laws and regulations and therefore free for general use.
The publisher, the authors and the editors are safe to assume that the advice and information in this book are believed to be true and accurate at the date of publication. Neither the publisher nor the authors or the editors give a warranty, expressed or implied, with respect to the material contained herein or for any errors or omissions that may have been made. The publisher remains neutral with regard to jurisdictional claims in published maps and institutional affiliations.

This Springer imprint is published by the registered company Springer Nature Switzerland AG
The registered company address is: Gewerbestrasse 11, 6330 Cham, Switzerland

Foreword

Basal implantology is both an art and a science. Restoration of the lost dental organ must adequately fulfill the esthetic, phonetic, and functional requirements of the patient and last in a state immune to disease. Multidisciplinary research and clinical trials have played an essential role in the development of state-of-the-art implant systems that satisfy both professional needs and the public's demand for safe, effective therapy that is both affordable and as rapid as possible.

It has been our endeavor to present a sound application of proven principles, placing emphasis on the importance of familiarity with the biological, mechanical, and prosthetic aspects of basal implants and their supporting structures as revealed by analysis of more than three decades of clinical studies, research projects, and experimental investigations.

This manual is a guide to the practical application of biological and mechanical principles in the everyday practice of basal implantology and osseointegration (BIO concept), from single tooth replacements to full arch reconstructions. In particular, it provides an introduction to techniques to improve the future implant bed by activating the patient's own stem cells (application of bone matrix osseotensors several weeks before implant installation) and multicortical osseointegration obtained using specially designed maxillo-mandibular basal Diskimplants®. Used by leading restorative implantologists for more than 30 years, these well-established treatment modalities offer patients an attractive alternative to more invasive procedures. In desperate clinical situations, basal implantology can represent the last chance for an oral invalid to have fixed teeth once again and thus be able to pursue normal personal, professional, and social activities. However, basal implantology is also indicated in less complex cases. For partially edentulous patients with little available bone, laterally inserted Diskimplants® represent a safe and rapid solution. The same is true for patients reluctant to undergo a bone graft procedure when bone anatomy is too shallow or too thin to receive a root-form implant.

Guillaume Odin
ENT and Maxillo-facial Surgery Department
Institut Universitaire de la Face et du Cou
University of Nice-Sophia Antipolis Medical School
Nice, France

Preface

Basal implantology has undergone tremendous growth in recent years correlated with multiple innovations, including the flat implant emergence profile, screw-secured plate-form Diskimplants®, micro-threaded tubero-pterygoid Fractal® implants, and bone matrix osseotensors. CAD/CAM technologies, 3D treatment planning, and digital workflow processes have all contributed to this progression.

As applied sciences, medicine and dentistry are a training ground. Regardless of the implant system selected, the clinician must be prepared both technically and psychologically to manage potential complications and failures. Unexpected reactions or events can occur at any time and surprise even the most experienced teams using the most reliable systems. Hands-on courses and training with mentors are thus essential to develop skill in this particular field.

Of course, more important than the brand of implant is the ability of the professional to make the correct diagnosis and establish an appropriate treatment plan, paying attention to anticipation of potential problems. This may even mean deciding not to use implantology at all. When implants are indicated, patients must be followed up over the long term so that any necessary preventive and curative actions can be taken. While this is no absolute guarantee against failure, it reduces the potential severity and consequences. Should a problem arise, effective solutions exist. For example, screw-retained prostheses on basal implants are easily retrieved. This facilitates verification of individual implants and makes correction of problems easier and less expensive.

Today, all well-trained surgical and prosthodontic teams can incorporate basal implantology in their implant practice to successfully perform oral rehabilitation without more invasive procedures. This book is written to help professionals in this way.

Having followed these simple rules over so many years, I can say that I still enjoy practicing basal implantology as it allows so many oral invalids to once again benefit from fixed teeth.

Nice, France Gérard M. Scortecci

The original version of this book was revised. The correction this book can be found at
https://doi.org/10.1007/978-3-319-44873-2_16

Contents

Contributors

Alexandre-Amir Aalam Private Practice, Los Angeles, CA, USA

Franck Afota Institut Universitaire de la Face et du Cou, Nice, France

Alp Alantar Private Practice, Paris, France

Itzhak Binderman Department of Oral Biology, University of Tel Aviv, Tel Aviv, Israel

Joseph Choukroun SYFAC, Nice, France

Pierre Doglioli Centre de Biotechnologies, Cannes, France

Jean-Marie Donsimoni Centre Médical Europe, Paris, France

Fabio Levratto Laboratoire Levratto, Monaco, Principality of Monaco

Jean-Paul Meningaud Hôpital Henri Mondor, Créteil, France

Carl E. Misch*

Patrick Missika University Paris 7 and Private Practice, Paris, France

Isabelle Morin Laboratoire Arcade, Nice, France

Laurent Morin Laboratoire Arcade, Nice, France

Guillaume Odin ENT and Maxillo-facial Surgery Department, Institut Universitaire de la Face et du Cou, University of Nice-Sophia Antipolis Medical School, Nice, France

Patrick Philip Faculté de Médecine, Département d'Histologie, Unité d'Exploration Fonctionnelle Cellulaire et Tissulaire, Hôpital Pasteur, University of Nice-Sophia Antipolis, Nice, France

---

* Deceased

Charles Savoldelli Institut Universitaire de la Face et du Cou, Nice, France

Gérard M. Scortecci University of Nice-Sophia Antipolis Medical School, Nice, France

New York University, New York, NY, USA

University of Southern California, Los Angeles, CA, USA

Private Practice, Nice, France

Part I

Fundamental Basis

Principles of Basal Implantology

1

Gérard M. Scortecci, Carl E. Misch, and Guillaume Odin

1.1 Definition of Basal Implantology: Dynamic Dental Implant Classification

Endosseous dental implants can be categorized according to their shape, surface characteristics, chemical composition, or the manner in which they are inserted into the jaw. Based on their dynamic mode of insertion, all dental implant systems can be divided into one of two categories (Fig. 1.1):

Axially Inserted Crestal Dental Implants (Root-Forms, Blades, Mini-pins, etc.)

Osteotomy is initiated on the crest of the jaw and proceeds axially (downward in the mandible, upward in the maxilla). The one exception is staple implants. This category includes blades (vertical platform dental implants) and root-form dental implants such as screws and cylinders. The crestal approach allows the surgeon to insert the implant perpendicular to the crest or tilted, i.e., angulated with respect to the bone crest.

C. E. Misch (Deceased)

G. M. Scortecci (✉)
University of Nice-Sophia Antipolis Medical School, Nice, France

New York University, New York, NY, USA

University of Southern California, Los Angeles, CA, USA

Private Practice, Nice, France
e-mail: scortecci@wanadoo.fr

G. Odin
ENT and Maxillo-facial Surgery Department, Institut Universitaire de la Face et du Cou, University of Nice-Sophia Antipolis Medical School, Nice, France
e-mail: odin.g@chu-nice.fr

© Springer Nature Switzerland AG 2019

G. M. Scortecci (ed.), *Basal Implantology*, https://doi.org/10.1007/978-3-319-44873-2_1

Laterally Inserted Basal Dental Implants (Diskimplants®)
(Figs. 1.2, 1.3, and 1.4)

Osteotomy is initiated apically on the basal bone of the buccal or lingual/palatal aspect of the jaw. The entire procedure is performed laterally, at the same initial depth. This category covers all types of Diskimplants® and their clones (cf. "Disk implant," ICOI glossary, 2017).

Basal Implantology

This term refers to the lateral insertion of disk-form implants into basal bone and, more generally, to the anchorage of implants in basal bone (e.g., root-form implants placed in the zygomatic and/or pterygoid process). The range of designs (single-, double-, and triple-disk implants, horizontal plate-form implants secured with osteosynthesis screws, etc.) allows management of the diversity of anatomic situations and bone qualities.

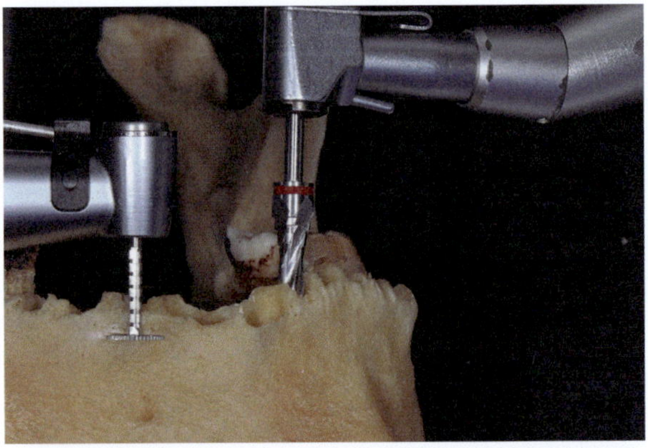

Fig. 1.1 Lateral osteotomy (basal implants) and crestal osteotomy (axial implants)

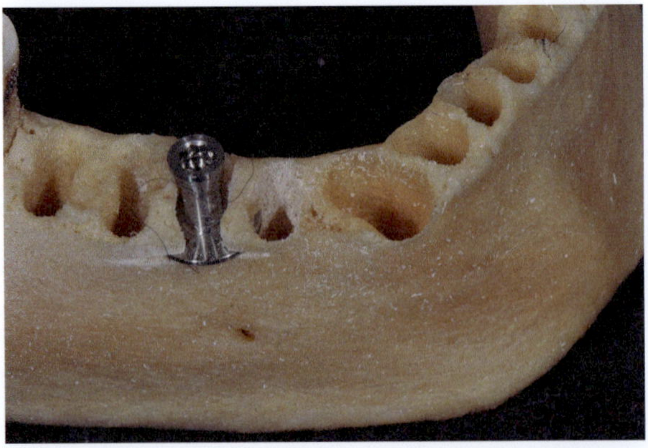

Fig. 1.2 Basal Diskimplant® inserted laterally above the mandibular canal

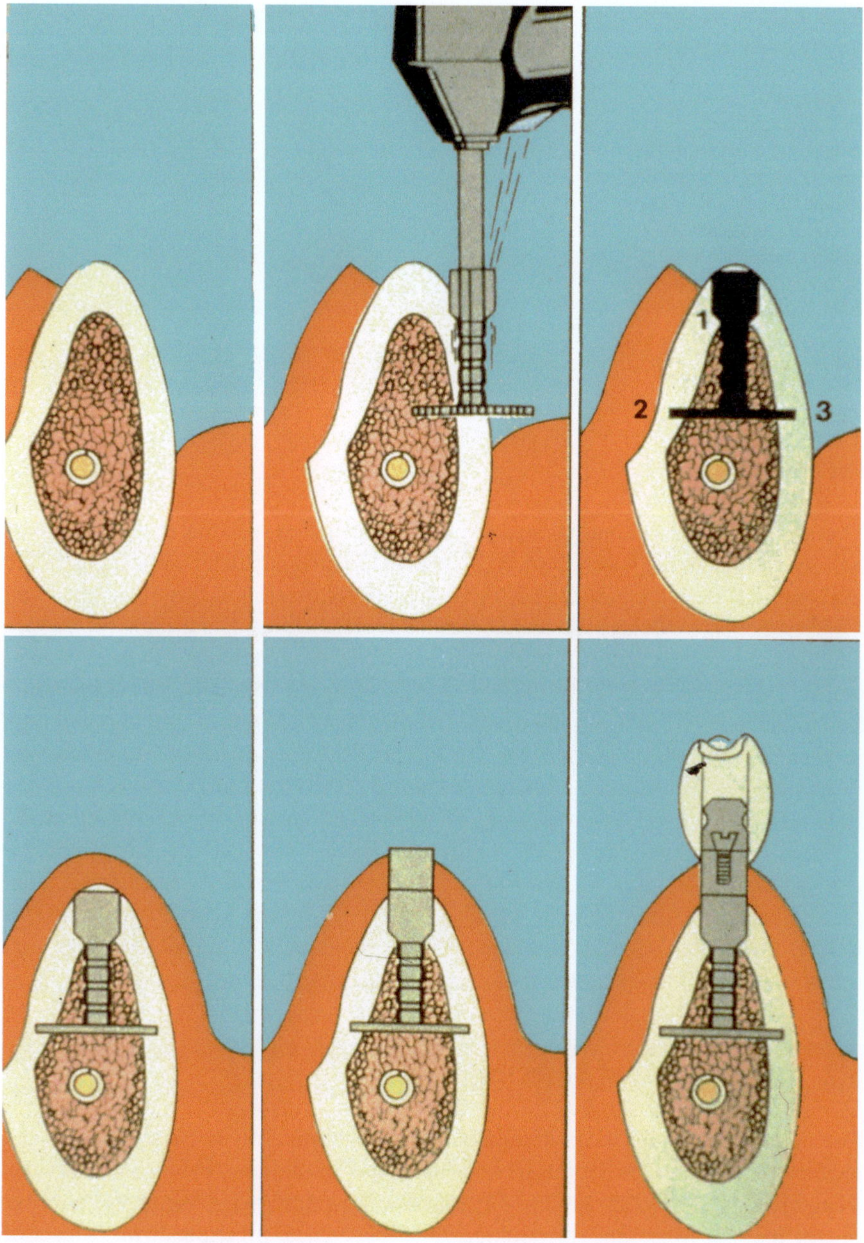

Fig. 1.3 Lateral osteotomy with a titanium cutter; full-thickness flap procedure (submerged protocol; waiting period 4–6 months)

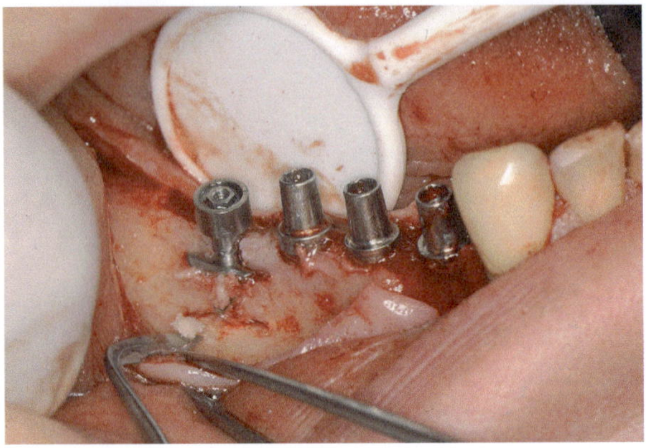

Fig. 1.4 Three root-form implants and one laterally inserted double Diskimplant® (7G2-DDM5) were installed to replace the two missing lower right molars and the missing lower right premolar (immediate loading protocol). The lateral osteotomy was filled in with autologous bone chips from the axial drilling procedure for the root-form implants

Diskimplants®

These laterally inserted basal dental implants are installed such that their wide apical base extends from the buccal cortical plate to the lingual or palatal cortical plate. The Diskimplant® design combines a horizontal platform (similar to blade implants) and a perpendicular cylindrical shaft (equivalent to a root-form dental implant). A specific titanium instrument, called a cutter, is utilized to prepare the "T-shaped" osteotomy. This unique tool "cuts" the bone horizontally and vertically at the same time. Diskimplants® were first presented at the International Congress of Oral Implantology in Munich, Germany on June 13, 1984. The BIO concept (Basal Implants and Osseointegration) was internationally developed at the First European BIO Forum in Paris on Nov. 29, 2001. Over the years, Diskimplants® have undergone various modifications (external threaded shaft, external hexagon, internal thread, Monobloc flat emergence profile, etc.). However, three features have remained unchanged: one-piece fabrication from titanium bars (i.e., true even for the large horizontal plate-form Diskimplants®), a non-modified surface machined *ad modum Brånemark*, and use of one-piece T-shaped titanium cutters for lateral osteotomy.

1.2 Objectives of Basal Implantology

The main objective of basal implantology is restoration of the vital function and characteristic beauty of the masticatory apparatus in difficult or extremely difficult anatomic situations using a minimally invasive procedure based on rational application of biologic, anatomic, physiologic, and mechanical principles with respect of hygiene and esthetic requirements. Straightforward basal implant techniques are generally preferable to invasive high-risk procedures involving long waiting periods. A "root-form implant only" approach, for example, may require prior modification of the bone anatomy using grafting procedures before implant placement is feasible.

As oral implantology is not an emergency procedure, the only candidates for this prosthetically driven technique procedure are physically and mentally fit individuals, preferably non-smokers. Well-controlled ASA 1 to ASA 3 patients may also be suitable implant candidates. Along with general good health, satisfactory oral hygiene and absence of infection are essential.

Basal implants enlarge the scope of implant dentistry without requiring recourse to complex techniques such as distraction, bone splitting, grafting, etc. prior to implant installation. Of course, they can also be used in combination with more invasive procedures (sinus elevation, lateral displacement of the inferior alveolar nerve, calvarial bone graft, iliac bone graft, pedicled fibula bone graft, etc.). Root-form dental implants and basal Diskimplants® can be used separately or in association to provide stable and reliable support for fixed, implant-supported restorations. This is especially useful for immediate functional loading protocols (Figs. 1.5 and 1.6). Laterally inserted Diskimplants® are often indicated whenever root-form implants cannot be installed directly due to insufficient bone volume and/or quality, but they can also be placed in much larger bone volumes if so desired.

Basal implants are always placed in native living bone. Bone grafting and GBR may be performed at the time of installation in order to increase bone volume, but not to provide mechanical anchorage.

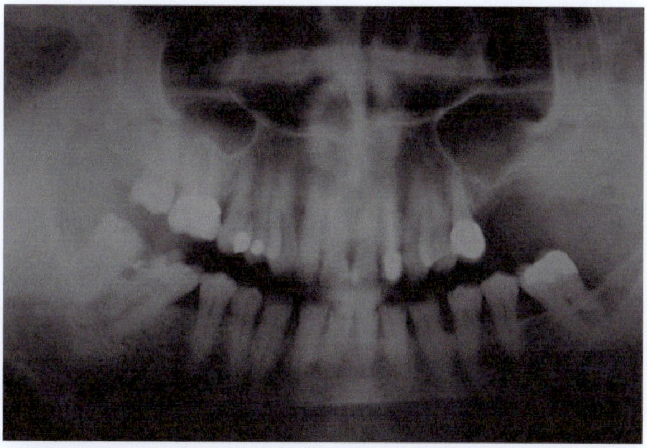

Fig. 1.5 Panoramic radiograph: atrophic posterior upper left maxilla

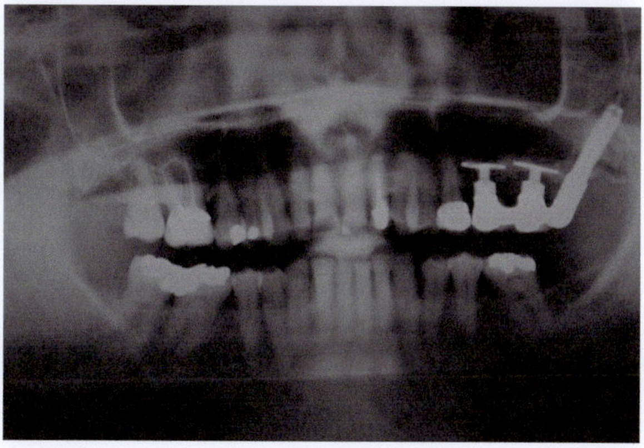

Fig. 1.6 Two monodisk Diskimplants® and a tubero-pterygoid root-form implant. Screw-secured, implant-supported fixed ceramic bridge. No sinus elevation was required

Diskimplants® are particularly indicated in the following cases:

- High, thin bone ridges less than 3 mm thick (Fig. 1.7). Technical reduction of such ridges is unnecessary because the osteotomy starts from the apical portion of the bony implant bed.
- Flat ridges with an available bone height of less than 5 mm (Figs. 1.8, 1.9, and 1.10).
- Extremely atrophic jaws, which can be directly managed with basal implants associated with guided bone regeneration (GBR) and immediately loaded with a highly rigid, screw-secured fixed prosthesis.

The various indications and contraindications for basal implants are developed in more detail in Chap. 6.

The surgeon, prosthodontist, and dental technician must all be trained in the fundamental concepts of basal implantology that differ in many aspects from those

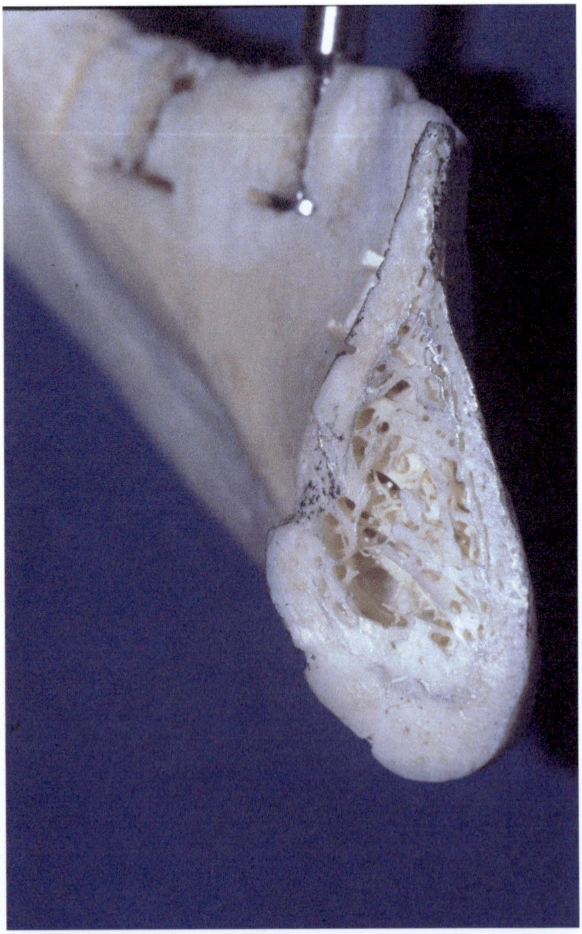

Fig. 1.7 Laterally inserted Diskimplant® placed from the lingual aspect in a high knife ridge (bone thickness at crest level ≤2 mm)

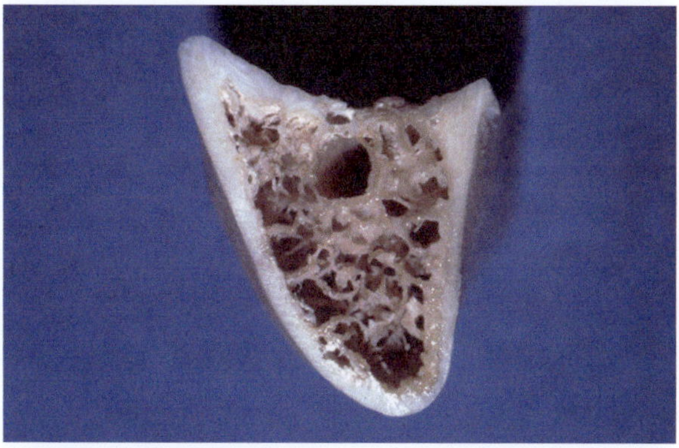

Fig. 1.8 Typical indication for basal implantology in an atrophic posterior mandible with less than 1.5 mm of bone height available above the mandibular nerve. The flat, wide ramus area is an indication for a horizontal plate-form Diskimplant®

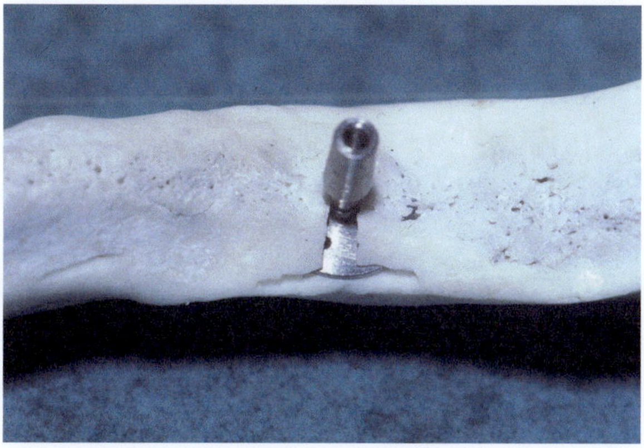

Fig. 1.9 Occlusal view of a posterior lateral osteotomy in a dry mandible at a bone depth of 1.5 mm (disk diameter 9 mm)

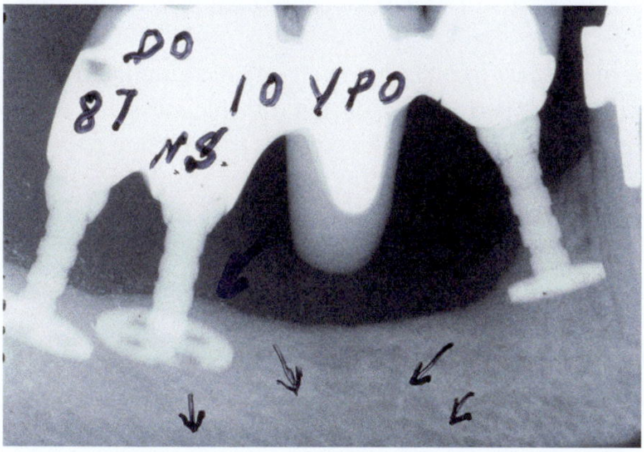

Fig. 1.10 Periapical radiograph after 10 years of function (initial bone height was less than 2 mm). No bone loss. Bone gain visible above the three Diskimplants®. After removal of a failing cobalt-chromium subperiosteal implant, the lateral osteotomy was performed starting on the lingual aspect of the mandible. The final cement-retained bridge was installed after 6 months (delayed loading protocol)

for root-form implants. Mastery of basal implant procedures, which require full-flap elevation, involves a progressive learning curve that is longer than for root-form implants; continual practice and close collaboration with a dental laboratory familiar with the technique are paramount. The surgeon must be familiar with maxillofacial surgical anatomy and be trained in sinus elevation procedures and intraoral bone grafting. Immediate loading protocols for rehabilitation of completely edentulous arches require both surgical skills and prosthodontic expertise; in particular, the surgical team must be able to take the impression and register primary inter-arch occlusion in the operating room at completion of surgery.

1.3 Basic Principles of Basal Implantology

No superstructure can be more enduring than its foundation. Occlusal stress and foundation resistance are reciprocal forces which must be properly balanced to obtain durable functional efficacy. The long-term function of an osseointegrated, cortically anchored basal implant restoration requires establishment of an active bond between the tissues and the Diskimplant®. Thanks to an osseo-adaptative process, the multicortical basal implant is incorporated into the hard and soft tissues, which gradually adapt to their new function through the remodeling process.

Creation and maintenance of this structural and functional bond between biological and non-biological materials mandate precision during the various stages of treatment plus respect of basic principles:

- Adequate treatment planning and presurgical bone matrix activation of the future implant bed with osseotensors to promote stem cell recruitment and improve the blood supply
- Use of an aseptic protocol to avoid contamination and infection of the implant site
- Preservation of the peri-implant blood supply by atraumatic handling of the soft tissues, especially the periosteum, during full-thickness flap elevation and use of a lateral osteotomy procedure under copious irrigation to prevent thermal injury
- Achievement of multicortical support providing absolute primary implant stability in dense living native bone (including pedicular grafts such as fibula grafts), not in bone substitute material or a free bone graft

Respect of Bone Biology: The Importance of Initial Osteogenic Activation

The future recipient bone bed should be activated prior to implant placement using a bone matrix osseotensor in order to reinforce the local blood supply, stimulate bone cell growth, and improve initial bone quality for better osseointegration of the intended basal implant (see Chap. 5 for more details).

Care must be taken not to contaminate the super-clean surface of the basal implant to allow establishment of a reliable primary biological bond and to avoid the risk of peri-implantitis in the future by limiting metal release during mastication. Finally, the body of the basal implant should never be in direct contact with the soft tissues; autologous bone grafts, bone substitute material, and PRF should be used to completely cover any protruding titanium surfaces.

Multicortical Anchorage and Long-Lasting Primary Stability

The wide horizontal platform of the basal implant (disk or other horizontal design) must be installed with multicortical anchorage because absolute primary stability is essential to obtain osseointegration that is maintained over time. The design and dimensions of the implant must permit the connection of prosthetic components in a functionally useful manner to create a fixed prosthesis. The occlusal forces transmitted via the future prosthesis must be properly distributed so as not to exceed the breaking point of the bone and the prosthetic components.

In extremely atrophic jaws, multicortical anchorage of extra-maxillary and extra-mandibular plate-form Diskimplants® using orthopedic screws placed in the major skeletal pillars of the jaws ensures functional stability during mastication over the long term (Figs. 1.11, 1.12, and 1.13).

In high knife ridges (crestal bucco-palatal bone thickness <2 mm), double- or triple-disk basal Diskimplants® can serve as scaffolding for bone substitute material and PRF membranes to increase bone volume at the implant site by guided bone regeneration (GBR) (Figs. 1.14 and 1.15). Thin ridges of this type are not suitable for horizontal plate-form Diskimplants®, which require a wide, flat bone bed for correct installation. Primary basal implant stability is mandatory in both situations.

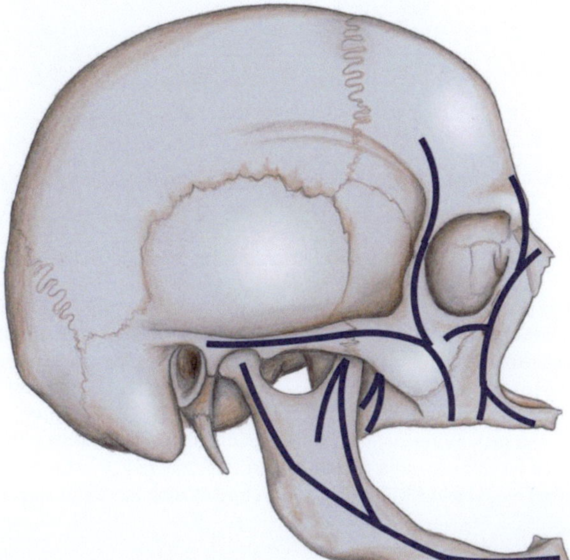

Fig. 1.11 Basal bone in an atrophic jaw; the alveolar bone has completely disappeared. The blue lines show the main bony buttresses for reliable anchorage of basal implants in the maxilla and the mandible

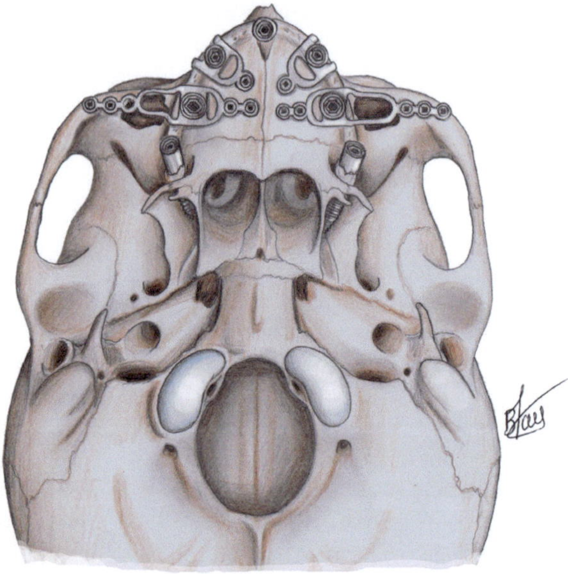

Fig. 1.12 The main areas for installation of horizontal plate-form Diskimplants® in the maxilla. Zygomatic Diskimplants® can be installed such that they span lateral openings in the sinus wall; absolute stability is obtained by firmly screwing them onto the dense malar and palatal bone. They must then be covered by bone substitute material and PRF. Strong distal anchorage is achieved in the tubero-pterygoid area with microthreaded root-form Fractal® implants

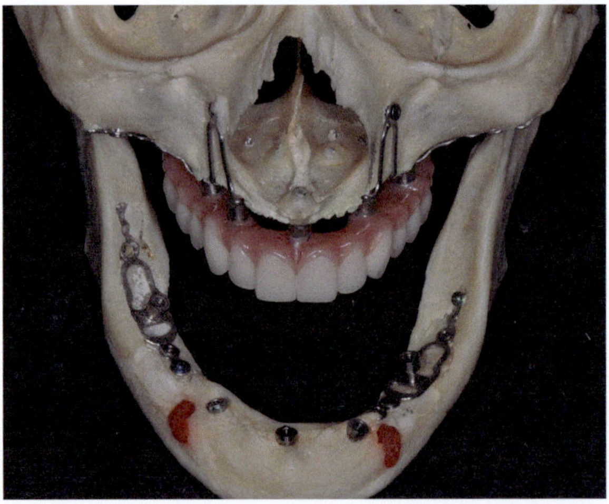

Fig. 1.13 The ramus area offers dense bone for placement of horizontal plate-form Diskimplants®. Sharp crestal soft tissue incisions should be made until the scalpel reaches the bone crest. The plate-form Diskimplant® must fit passively into the bony site prepared by the titanium cutter and is stabilized by mini orthopedic screws (4–6 mm in length). The same technique is used for the canine and zygomatic areas of the upper jaw. A screw-secured, fixed maxillary prosthesis acts as an external orthopedic fixator for the implants. All extra-mandibular portions of the basal implant must be fully covered by bone substitute material (Bio-Oss®, CoreBone®, Dentin Grinder graft, Ivory®, etc.) and PRF membranes before closing the full-thickness flap

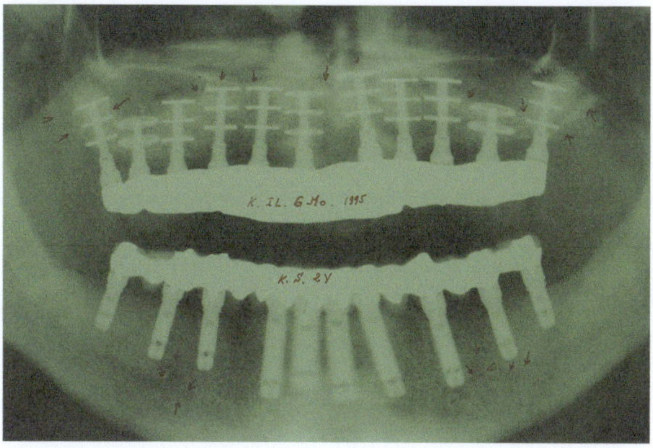

Fig. 1.14 Full-mouth rehabilitation: high maxillary knife ridge (bucco-palatal width <2 mm at crest level) managed with double and triple Diskimplants®. The protruding disk base is covered by bone substitute material for GBR (immediate functional loading protocol). Horizontal plate-form Diskimplants® are not indicated in this anatomic situation. Root-form implants can be installed in the mandible depending on available bone volume and quality

Fig. 1.15 The protruding portion of the Diskimplant® is used as scaffolding for GBR (tent effect) with bone substitute material and PRF (submerged technique for single-tooth replacements) in mandibular knife ridges

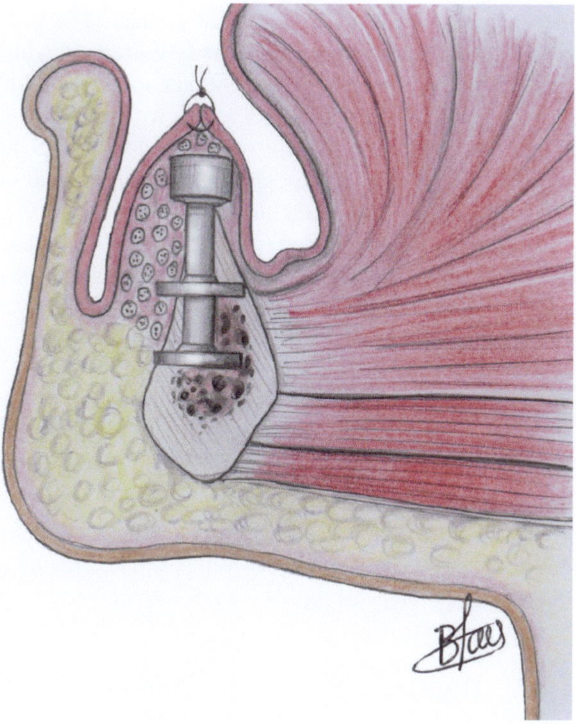

Implant Loading Protocols

Loading protocols vary as a function of the clinical situation:

- Immediate loading of full-arch restorations is possible using a highly rigid, fixed prosthesis that is screw-secured to basal implants with a flat emergence profile (Monobloc emergence).
- Delayed loading of basal implants is recommended for implant management of partial edentulism and single-tooth replacements with difficult occlusal conditions.

Biomechanical, surgical, and prosthetic requirements mandate close collaboration between the surgeon, prosthodontist, and dental laboratory. Passive fit of the final prosthesis is critical for satisfactory mastication and speech. Use of a transitional prosthesis for a period of time allows verification that functional and cosmetic requirements are met.

Maintenance and Follow-Up

3D imaging investigations are necessary for assessment of any biological or mechanical complications at an early stage. The radiological images around the base of a Diskimplant® must always be correlated with clinical findings as they can differ from those seen with conventional root-form implants. For example, minimal radiolucency around the base of a disk without any pain or mobility does not mandate removal. Implant mobility associated with pain, however, is cause for implant removal. Awareness of these differences can prevent unnecessary removal of what is actually a well-integrated implant.

Appropriate maintenance (plaque control) and atraumatic, well-balanced occlusion is essential for long-term success. The gingiva surrounding prosthetic abutments and implant emergences must be kept in a clinically healthy state by appropriate peri-implant soft tissue management and local hygiene. Revision and correction of complications, when necessary, can be achieved in a minimally invasive manner thanks to the easy retrievability of screw-secured, bone-anchored prostheses.

Anticipation of potential problems is also an important factor for the long-term success of basal implant-supported restorations. The knowledge and experience needed to satisfy these requirements cannot be improvised nor can they be acquired without appropriate theoretical and practical training. Coordinated treatment planning, precise execution, careful follow-up, and maintenance over time are the keys to successful, long-lasting fixed basal implant-supported rehabilitations.

1.4 Divisions of Available Bone Anatomy and Bone Density

Divisions of Available Bone (Figs. 1.16, 1.17, 1.18, and 1.19)

Long-term success in implant dentistry requires the evaluation of more than 50 dental criteria, many of which are unique to this discipline [1]. The training and

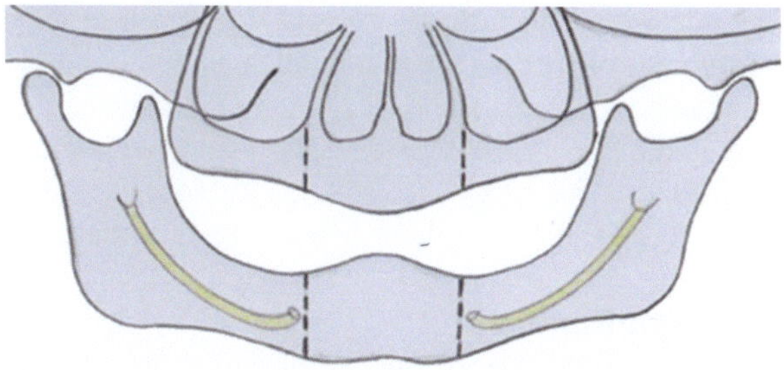

Fig. 1.16 Division A: there is sufficient bone volume for root-form implants. However, volume alone is not sufficient; bone density is more important. In case of low density, even with sufficient volume, it is safer to use basal implants with anchorage of the wide base in the cortical plates

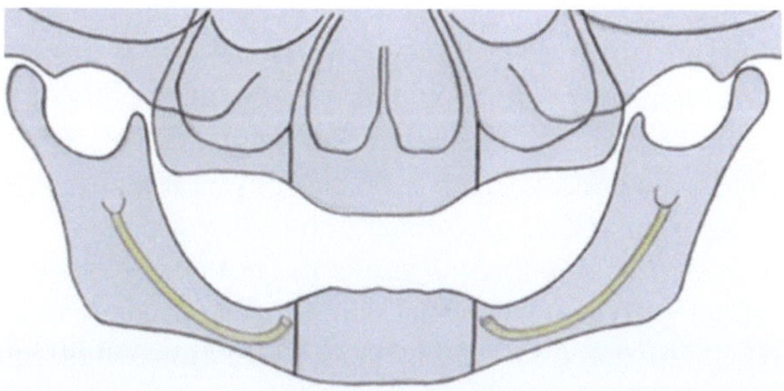

Fig. 1.17 Division B: sufficient bone volume for root-form implants (short implants in the posterior area, sinus elevation, or short implants in the posterior maxilla) or basal implants. Here, again, bone density is more important, and it is safer to place basal implants if low-density bone is detected

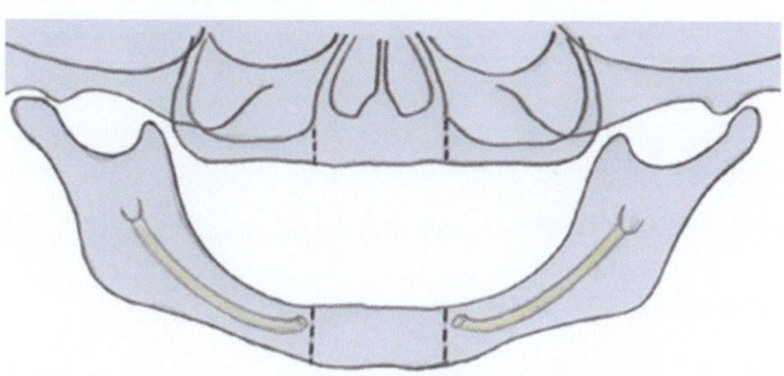

Fig. 1.18 Division C: insufficient bone volume in the posterior sectors (maxilla and mandible). Root-form implants combined with prior bone grafting and/or GBR or basal implantology are indicated

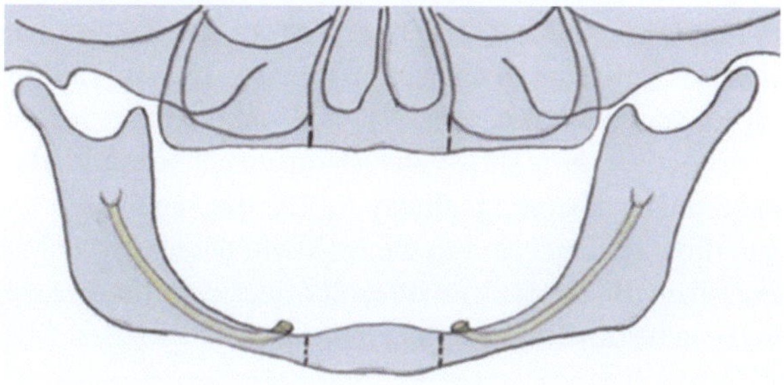

Fig. 1.19 Division D: skeletal basal bone. This situation can be managed either immediately, by basal implantology, or by performing an autologous extraoral bone graft procedure prior to implant placement

experience of the doctor and the volume, density, and shape of the available bone are primary determinants of success for an individual patient. The Misch/Judy classification of available bone (Divisions A, B, C, and D) follows the natural patterns of bone resorption in the jaws. Each division is associated with unique surgical and prosthetic approaches.

Division D (Deficient Bone)

The completely edentulous Division D patient is the most difficult to treat in implant dentistry. Benefits must be weighed carefully against the risks. Although the practitioner and patient often regard this condition as the most dramatic possible, these patients do not usually have oral antral fistulae or deviated facial features prior to treatment. If implant failure occurs, the patient may become a dental cripple, unable to wear any prosthesis. Treatment of the Division D arch requires more training and results in more frequent complications related to grafting, early implant failure, and soft tissue management. Treatment options thus include a more guarded prognosis. When physical and psychological general health, smoking habits, and occlusal conditions are aggravating factors, a wise and safe decision is to not install implants (not even basal implants) and to maintain the patient with a conventional denture. The prudent solution is to educate the patient about the risks of his or her situation when proposing basal implantology and GBR after initial osteogenic preparation with bone matrix osseotensors. The choice to render treatment is the doctor's, not the patient's. Initial bone support must not be compromised if implant failure could result in significantly greater risks.

1.5 Alveolar Bone and Basal Bone (Figs. 1.20 and 1.21)

Characteristic of human jaws, these complementary bony structures are correlated with the presence or the absence of teeth and their periodontal apparatus.

Alveolar Bone

This highly differentiated bony structure is "born with the tooth, develops and functions with the tooth, and progressively disappears after tooth loss." The alveolar bone lies above the basal bone, without any visible anatomical landmarks. Alveolar bone is connected to the teeth by means of the periodontal ligament that has a dense blood supply, lymph vessels, and nerves. The periodontal ligament and related fluids represent a shock-absorbing mechano-hydraulic system. This sophisticated apparatus is also the pathway for the mechanoreceptors involved in proprioception and directly connected to the brain via the trigeminal nerve. Alveolar bone can progressively disappear as the result of periodontal disease, tooth extraction, or trauma and can be drastically reduced in cases of agenesis. Alveolar bone is also capable of

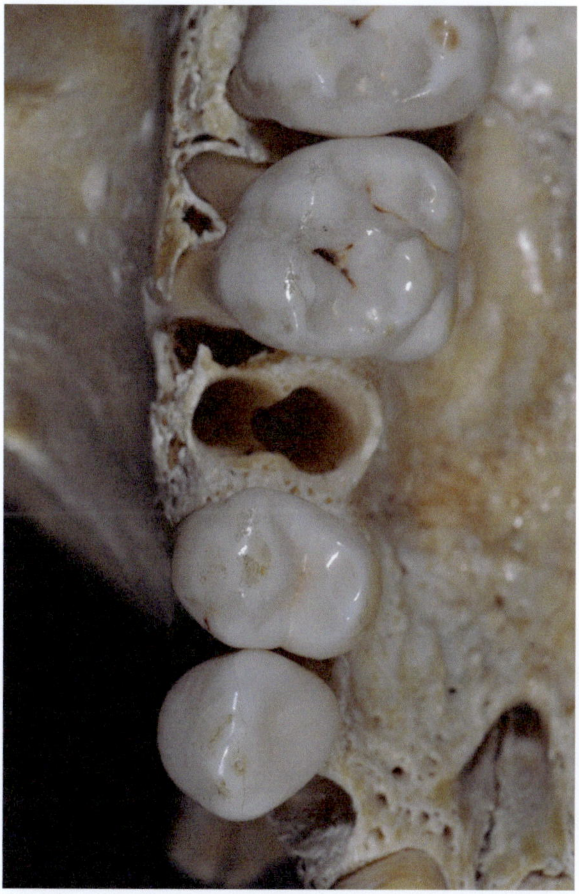

Fig. 1.20 D3 bone is very common in the maxilla. In this situation, a root-form implant can easily be installed in the palatal aspect immediately after extraction of the second upper premolar. If the buccal plate is absent, a double-disk asymmetric Diskimplant® (7 × 5 mm) must be inserted laterally and covered by bone substitute material and PRF membrane (delayed loading 6–7 months)

following the tooth pathway during orthodontic movements, whereas an osseointegrated implant directly anchored in bone remains in place and does not move.

Basal Bone

The skeletal bone that remains after tooth loss and complete resorption of the alveolar crest is termed basal bone. This bone structure has a very low turnover (ten times less than alveolar bone) and is highly sensitive to thermal injury and infection. Besides reduced bone volume and extreme differences in density depending on the sector (D1 in the mandibular mental area versus D4 in the posterior maxilla), basal bone has a limited blood supply. In atrophic jaws, for example, the main source of blood is the inner layer of the periosteum. This explains why maintenance of aseptic conditions during surgery, careful handling of the periosteum, profuse saline irrigation during lateral osteotomy, and primary stability are of paramount importance for bone healing after basal implant installation.

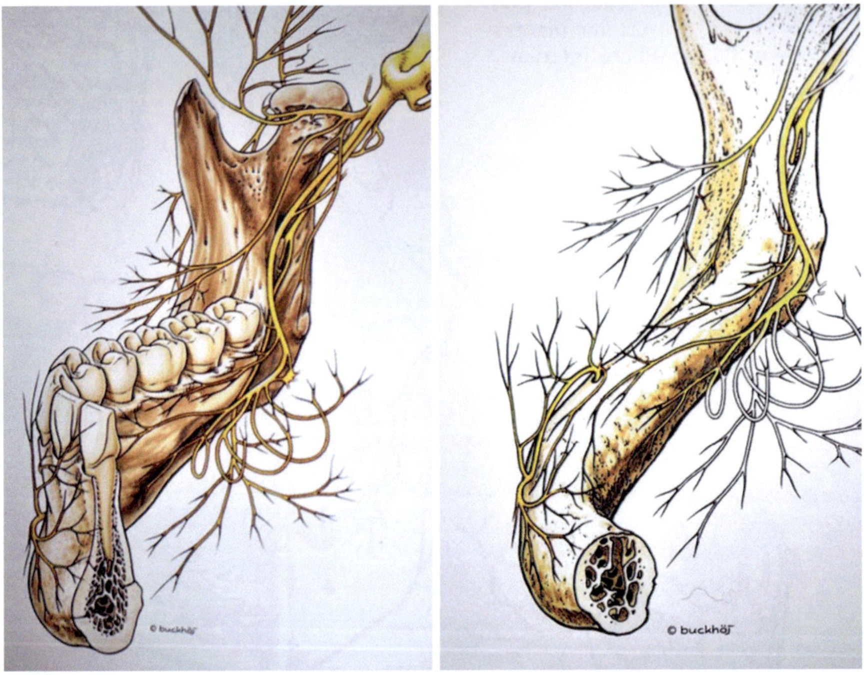

Fig. 1.21 Comparison of alveolar bone and basal bone (from Evers and Haegerstam, 1982)

1.6 Bone Density

Particularly important in implant dentistry, "available bone" describes the external architecture or volume of the edentulous area considered for implants. The internal structure of bone is described in terms of quality or density, which reflect its strength. As stated by Wolff [2]: "Every change in the form and function of bone or of its function alone is followed by certain definite changes in the internal architecture, and equally definite alteration in its external conformation, in accordance with mathematical laws." Bone density may be determined preoperatively by tactile sense using a manual osseotensor, by tactile determination during osteotomy, or, more accurately, by CT scans.

Clinical Evidence Highlighting the Influence of Bone Density on Implantation Success Rates

The anterior mandible has greater bone density than the anterior maxilla. The posterior mandible has poorer bone density than the anterior mandible. The poorest bone quality in the oral environment typically exists in the posterior maxilla and is associated with high failure rates. Jaffin and Berman [3] reported a 44% failure rate when poor density was observed in the maxilla, with the majority of failures noted after second-stage surgery. Of all implant failures in their study sample, 55% occurred in soft bone. The group documented a 35% implant loss in all regions of the mouth when bone density was poor. Engquist et al. [30] also reported a high percentage of clinical failures (78%) in soft bone types.

The Misch Bone Density Classification

The degree of crestal bone loss has also been related to stress and bone density. In 1988, Misch defined four bone density groups independent of the regions of the jaws, based upon macroscopic cortical and trabecular bone characteristics. The regions of the jaws with similar densities were often consistent. A suggested implant design, surgical protocol, healing, treatment plans, and progressive loading time spans have been described for each bone density type. Following this regimen, similar implant survival rates are observed for all bone densities.

The Misch bone density classifications are shown in Tables 1.1 and 1.2. Dense and/or porous cortical bone are found on the outer surfaces of bone and include the crest of an edentulous ridge. Coarse and fine trabecular bone are found within the outer shell of cortical bone and occasionally on the crestal surface of an edentulous residual ridge. These four macroscopic types of bone may be arranged from the densest to the least dense:

1. Dense cortical (Fig. 1.22)
2. Porous cortical (Fig. 1.23)
3. Coarse trabecular (Fig. 1.24)
4. Fine trabecular (Fig. 1.25)

Table 1.1 Misch/Scortecci bone density classification

	Description of bone
D1 bone	Dense cortical bone with very little spongiosa within
D2 bone	Thick dense cortical bone plate and coarse trabecular bone within
D3 bone	Thin cortical bone plate and fine trabecular bone within
D4 bone	Fatty trabecular bone with no cortex
D5 bone	Immature, non-mineralized bone

Table 1.2 Usual anatomic location of bone density types (% occurrence)

	Bone site			
Classification	Anterior maxilla	Posterior	Anterior mandible	Posterior
D1 bone	0	0	8	2
D2 bone	45	5	67	51
D3 bone	65	50	25	46
D4 bone	5	45	0	1

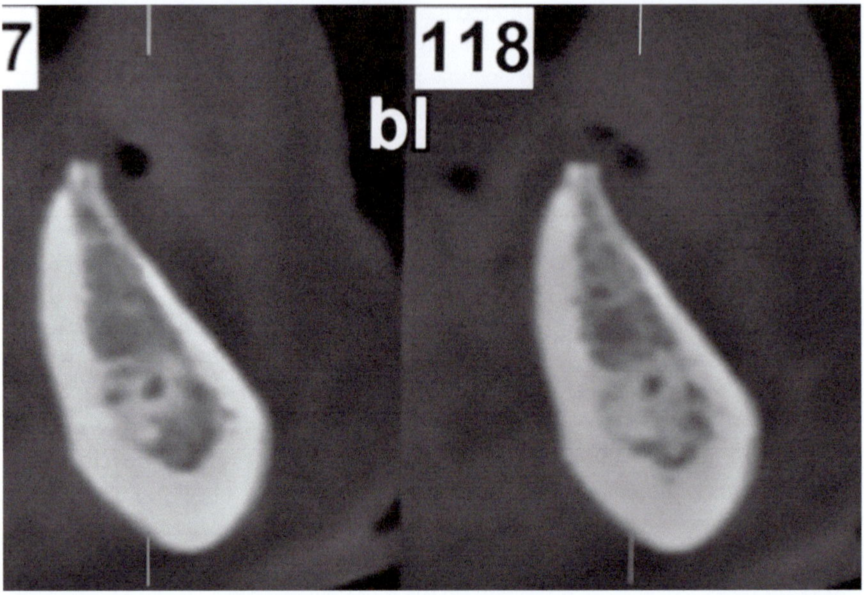

Fig. 1.22 D2 thick cortical bone plate and porous spongiosa

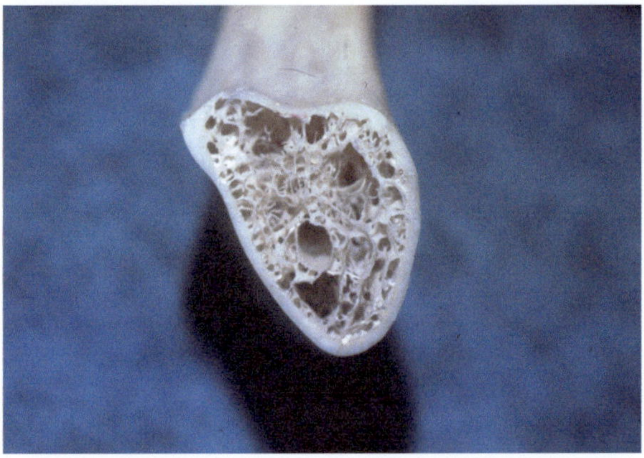

Fig. 1.23 D3 coarse trabecular bone and thin cortical plate

These four macroscopic densities describe and, in combination, establish four categories of bone located in the edentulous areas of the maxilla and mandible. The regional locations of the different densities of cortical bone are more consistent than the locations of trabecular bone, which are highly variable.

The macroscopic description of Misch bone density classification D1 bone is primarily dense cortical bone. D2 bone has dense to thick porous cortical bone on the crest and coarse trabecular bone within. D3 has a thinner porous cortical crest and fine trabecular bone. D4 bone has almost no crestal cortical bone. Almost all of

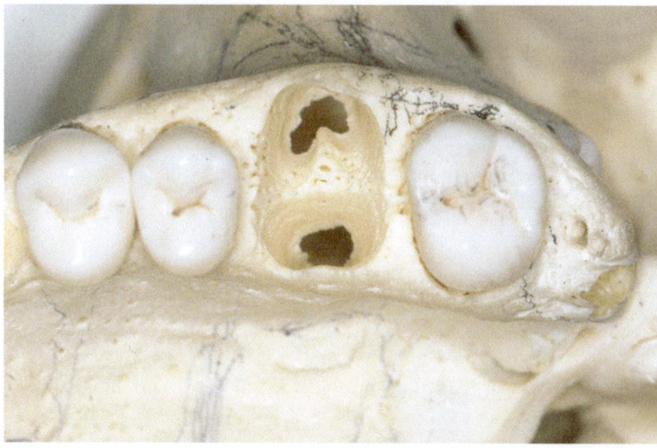

Fig. 1.24 Extraction of the maxillary molars may result in creation of an oro-antral communication. Socket preservation with a bone substitute material is mandatory

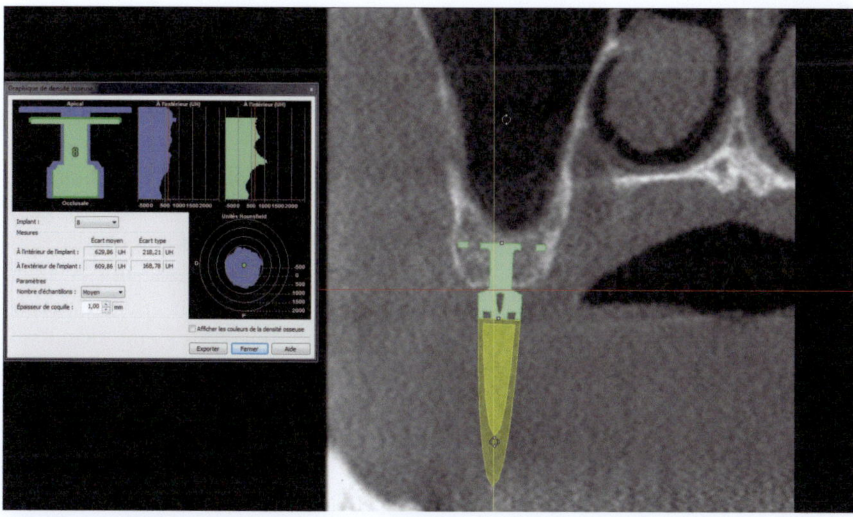

Fig. 1.25 Simulation of a 9-mm-diameter monodisk Diskimplant® placed beneath the sinus; the disk base extends from one cortical plate to the other

the total volume of bone next to the implant is composed of fine trabecular bone. A very soft bone, with incomplete mineralization, may be addressed as D5 bone. This description is usually of immature bone.

Bone Density Determined by Tactile Sense

In order to communicate broadly to the profession relative to the tactile sense of different bone densities, this classification is compared with materials of varying densities. Drilling and placing implants into D1 bone is similar to drilling into oak or maple wood. D2 bone is similar to the tactile sensation of drilling into white pine or spruce. Balsa wood is similar to drilling into D3 bone, and D4 bone is similar to drilling into Styrofoam™. Perception of bone density is similar with manual and rotary osseotensors.

Bone Density by Location

A review of the literature, blended with a post-surgery survey of 200 consecutive completely and partially edentulous patients, found that the location of different bone densities may be superimposed with the different regions of the mouth. D1 bone is almost never observed in the maxilla but may be found in the pterygoid process and the zygoma. In the mandible, D1 bone is observed approximately 8% of the time. D1 bone is observed four times as often in the anterior mandible compared with the posterior mandible (8% versus 2%). As the bone is reduced in volume, especially in the anterior mandible, D1 bone will occur with greater frequency and may reach 25%, whereas D3 will be less and be reduced to under 10%. The edentulous mandible often exhibits an increase in torsion and/or flexure in the anterior segment between the foramina during function. This increased strain causes the bone to increase in density.

Bone density D1 may be encountered in the anterior Division A mandible of a Kennedy Class IV partially edentulous patient with a history of parafunction and recent extractions. It may also be observed when angulation of an anterior implant requires the engagement of the lingual cortical plate in a Division A bone volume.

Bone density D2 is the most common bone density observed in the mandible. The anterior mandible consists of D2 bone two-thirds of the time. More than one-half of patients have D2 bone in the posterior mandible. In the maxilla, D2 bone is found less often than in the mandible. Approximately one-quarter of patients have D2 bone, and this is more likely in the partially edentulous patient's anterior and premolar region rather than in completely edentulous posterior molar areas. Single-tooth or two-tooth partially edentulous spans almost always have D2 bone.

Bone density D3 is very common in the maxilla (Fig. 1.26). More than one-half of patients have D3 bone in the upper arch. The anterior maxilla has D3 bone about 65% of the time, while almost one-half of patients have posterior maxillae with D3 bone (more often in the premolar region). Almost one-half of posterior mandibles also present with D3 bone, whereas approximately 25% of anterior edentulous mandibles have D3 bone.

The softest bone, D4 (Fig. 1.27), is most often found in posterior maxillae (approximately 60%), especially in the molar regions or after a sinus graft augmentation (where almost two-thirds of patients have D4 bone). The anterior maxilla has D4 bone less than 10% of the time, more often after an onlay iliac crest bone graft. The mandible presents with D4 bone in less than 3% of patients. When observed, it is usually Division A bone in a long-term, completely edentulous patient after an osteoplasty removes the crestal bone.

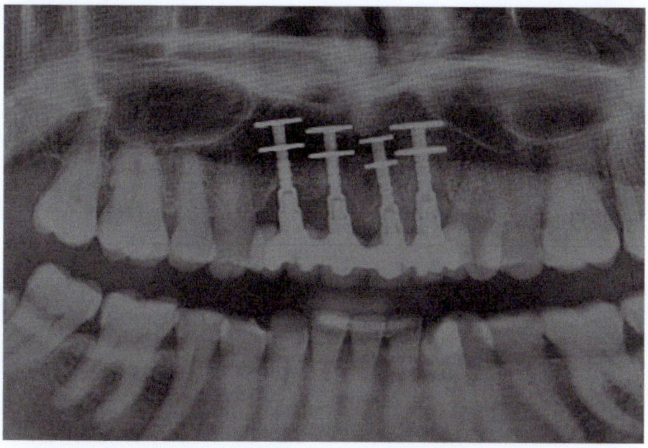

Fig. 1.26 D3 bone in the anterior maxilla. Severe facial trauma resulted in loss of the six upper front teeth along with their anterior buccal plate, leaving a high knife bone ridge. Four double-disk Diskimplants® were placed in 1985. The panoramic radiograph taken in 2016 shows these implants that are still in service after 31 years with no signs of peri-implantitis. A bone gain is visible in many areas

Fig. 1.27 D4 bone in the posterior maxilla

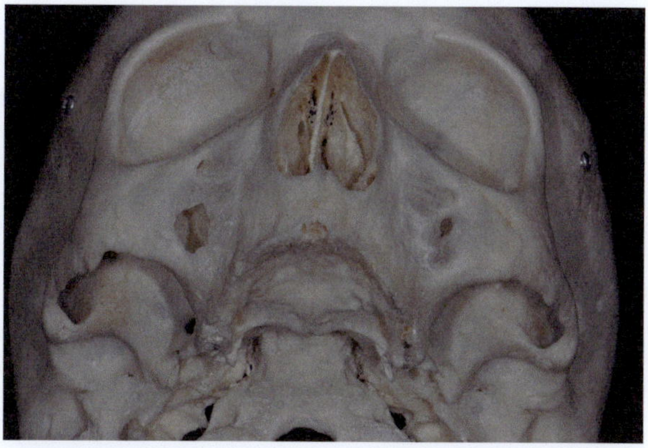

Generalizations for treatment planning can be made prudently, based on location. It is safer to begin by planning for less-dense bone so that the prosthesis is designed with slightly more, rather than less, support. The anterior maxilla is usually treated as D3 bone, the posterior maxilla as D4 bone, the anterior mandible as D2 bone, and the posterior mandible as D3 bone. Bone bed preparation with osseotensors prior to implant installation can dramatically improve initial bone density (see Chap. 5). The use of rotary osseotensors in D1 and D2 bone transforms the bone to active D2 status (i.e., D2 bone with active new bone cells and new blood supply [see Chap. 4]); an 8- to 15-day waiting period must be respected before proceeding with implant installation. Use of manual osseotensors in D3 and D4 bone promotes transformation to active D2 status but requires a longer waiting period (45–60 days) prior to surgery.

Radiographic Bone Density and 3D Anatomic Shape (Figs. 1.28 and 1.29)

Periapical or panoramic radiographs are not helpful for determining bone density because the lateral cortical plates often obscure trabecular bone density and bone shape. Furthermore, such radiographs cannot quantify the subtle changes of D2 to

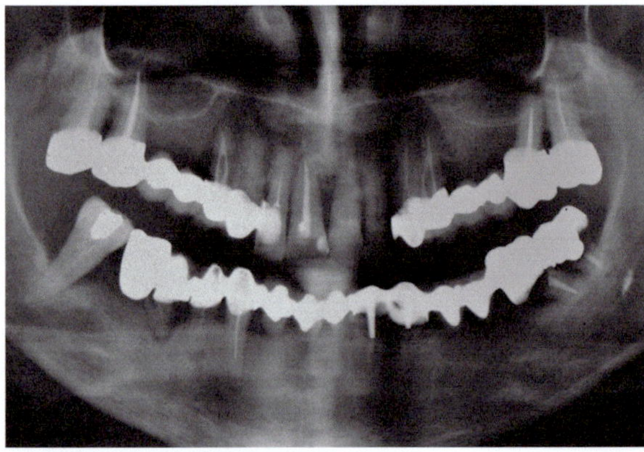

Fig. 1.28 The panoramic view gives the illusion that there is sufficient bone volume

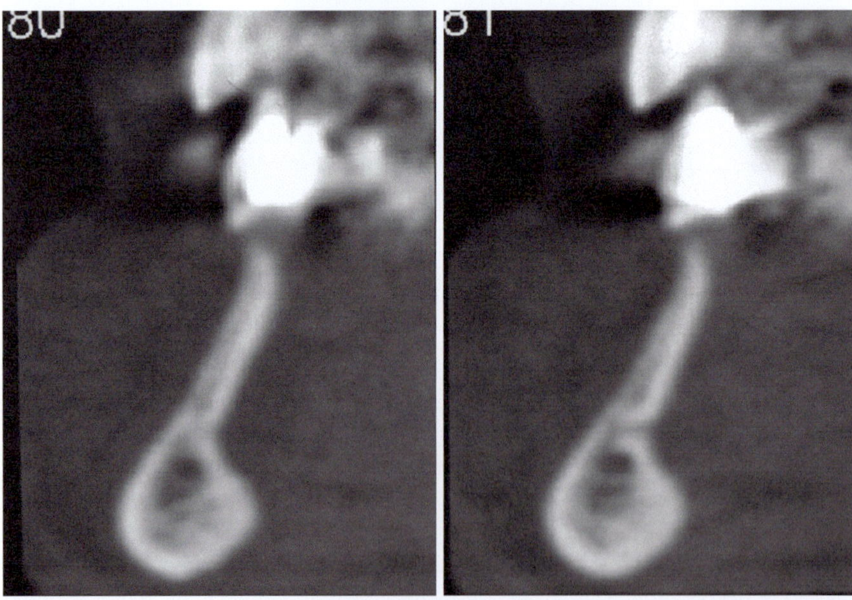

Fig. 1.29 Cone beam CT showing the considerable discrepancy between panoramic radiographs and cone beam CT: high knife ridge with a thickness of less than 3 mm but a bone height of more than 13 mm. Typical high knife ridge (D1 bone) suitable for double Diskimplants®. The remaining natural teeth are maintained by just a thin shell of alveolar bone. Extraction of natural teeth is particularly challenging because as much surrounding bone as possible must be preserved

D3 bone. Bone density and bone anatomy may be determined more precisely using tomographic radiographs, especially computerized tomograms (CT) and cone beam CT. Computed tomography produces axial images of the patient's anatomy, perpendicular to the long axis of the body. In general, the higher the CT number, the denser the tissue. Modern CT scanners and cone beam CT units can resolve objects less than 0.5 mm apart. The Misch bone density classification may be evaluated on CT images by correlation to a range of Hounsfield units: D1 corresponds to values greater than 1250 HU, D2 to 850–1250 HU, D3 to 350–850 HU, D4 less than 150–350 HU, and D5 bone less than 150 HU. The very soft bone observed after some bone grafts may be 100–300 HU.

Bone density is determined clinically using CT determination, as follows:

D1: >1250 Hounsfield units
D2: 850–1250 Hounsfield units
D3: 350–850 Hounsfield units
D4: <350 Hounsfield units

Evaluation of Bone Density During Lifetime

Bone density and bone anatomy (Fig. 1.30) are implant treatment plan modifiers in several ways: they influence not only pre-surgery bone management, selection of root-form and/or basal implants, implant dimensions, design, surface condition, number, the implant loading protocol, but also prosthetic choices (Figs. 1.31, 1.32, and 1.33). Consideration must be paid to the hormonal changes that occur in post-menopausal patients as considerable decreases in bone density can occur rapidly starting around the ages of 49–53 years. This is why multiple sites of initial cortical implant anchorage are so important.

A decrease in bone density is accompanied by a decrease in the strength of the bone. Reduction of the incidence of microfractures requires reduction of the strain

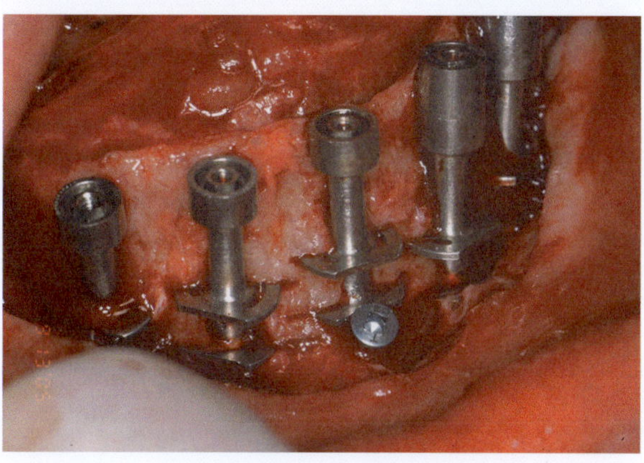

Fig. 1.30 After tooth loss, the residual high knife ridge (buccal-lingual width <2 mm) is managed with double-disk Diskimplants®. The protruding disk base is then covered with bone substitute material and PRF (immediate loading protocol). Mini orthopedic screws are placed at the base of the disk in order to guarantee primary stability

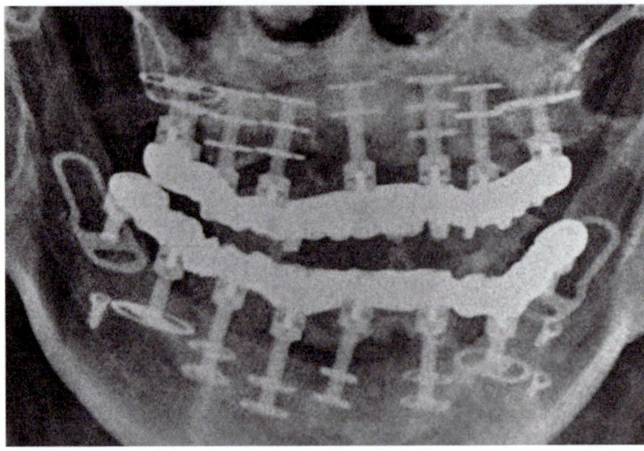

Fig. 1.31 Full-mouth rehabilitation with basal implants (immediate loading 48 h post-op): this patient suffered multiple maxillary and mandibular fractures in an automobile accident (panoramic view after 13 years of function)

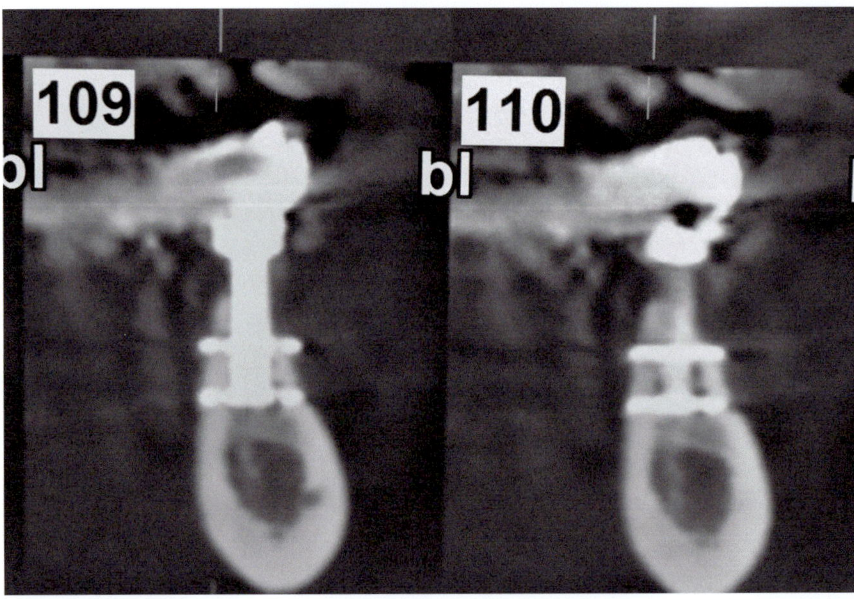

Fig. 1.32 Multicortical anchorage of double Diskimplants® above the mandibular nerve in a high knife ridge (D1 bone) after 13 years of function (same patient as Fig. 1.30)

applied to the bone. As strain is directly related to stress, the stress placed on the implant system should also be reduced as the bone density decreases. Stress is equal to the force divided by the functional area over which it is applied, such that S = F/A.

One way that biomechanical loads on implants may be reduced is by prosthesis design. For example, cantilever length may be shortened or eliminated, narrower occlusal tables designed and offset loads minimized, all of which reduce the amount of load. Night guards and acrylic occlusal surfaces distribute and dissipate

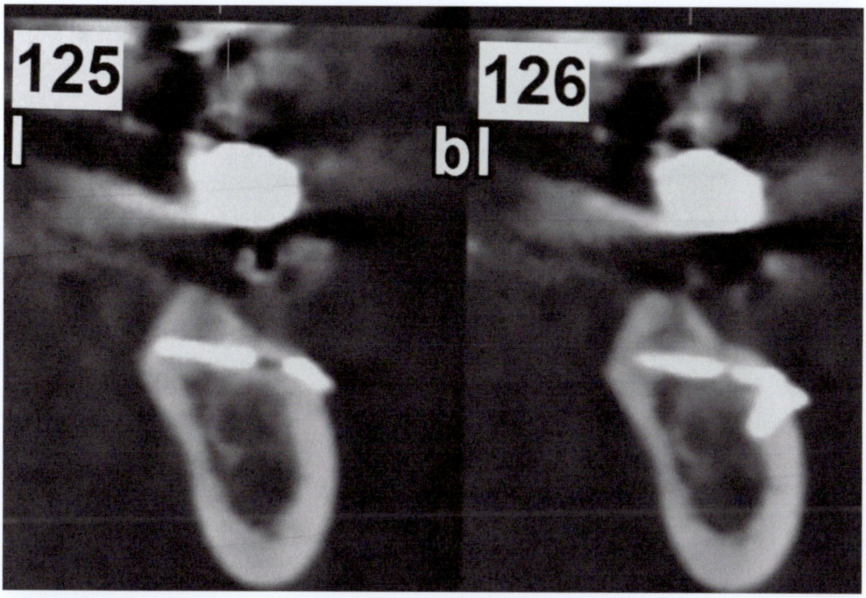

Fig. 1.33 Tricortical support of a 9-mm monodisk Diskimplant® placed 2 mm above the mandibular nerve in the flat bone ridge of this atrophic mandible (same patient as Figs. 1.37 and 1.38). A buccal orthopedic screw was placed at the base of the Diskimplant® to increase initial stability

parafunctional forces on an implant system. As the bone density decreases, these prosthetic factors become more important.

Stress may also be reduced by increasing the functional area over which the force is applied. Increasing the number of basal implants is an excellent way to reduce stress by increasing the functional loading area.

The width of the base of a Diskimplant® firmly anchored in the buccal and palatal or lingual cortical bone plate decreases stress by increasing the surface area. For every 0.5 mm increase in width, the surface area increases between 10% and 15%. Wider basal implants should be used in D4 bone compared with D1 or D2 bone.

Progressive Bone Loading

Progressive bone loading provides for a gradual increase in occlusal loads, separated by a time interval to allow the bone to accommodate. The softer the bone, the more important progressive loading. This can be achieved with a highly rigid CoCr/titanium/acrylic resin restoration screw-secured to basal implants instead of a ceramic bridge.

1.7 Surgical Anatomy Considerations (Figs. 1.34, 1.35, 1.36, 1.37, 1.38, and 1.39)

Basal implantology is applicable in a variety of clinical situations, from single-tooth replacement to full arch reconstructions. Even for oral invalids with moderately or severely atrophic jaws, the technique represents a unique means to restore fixed teeth without painful, time-consuming, expensive, and invasive preimplant bone grafting.

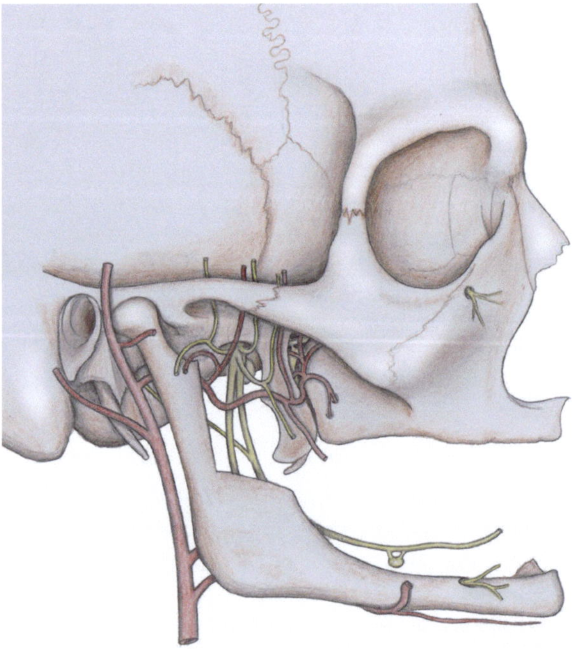

Fig. 1.34 Important anatomic landmarks: surgical anatomy showing critical areas to be avoided– Mandible: lingual and mandibular nerves and the submental artery– Maxilla and tubero-pterygoid area: maxillary artery and infraorbital nerve

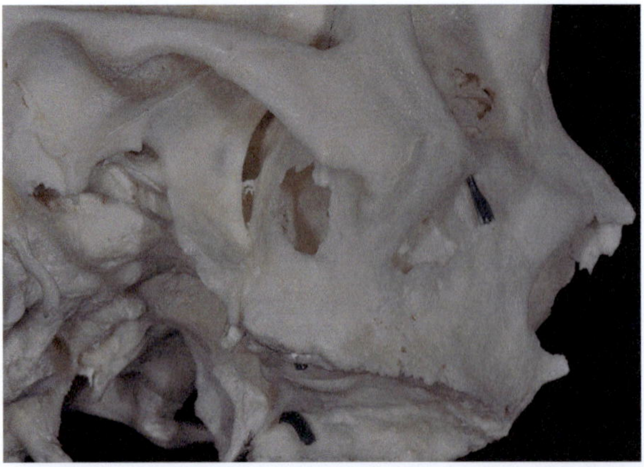

Fig. 1.35 Maxillary sinus area: very soft bone, if any ("eggshell-thin" bone). Use of a bone matrix osseotensor is mandatory (cf. Chap. 4)

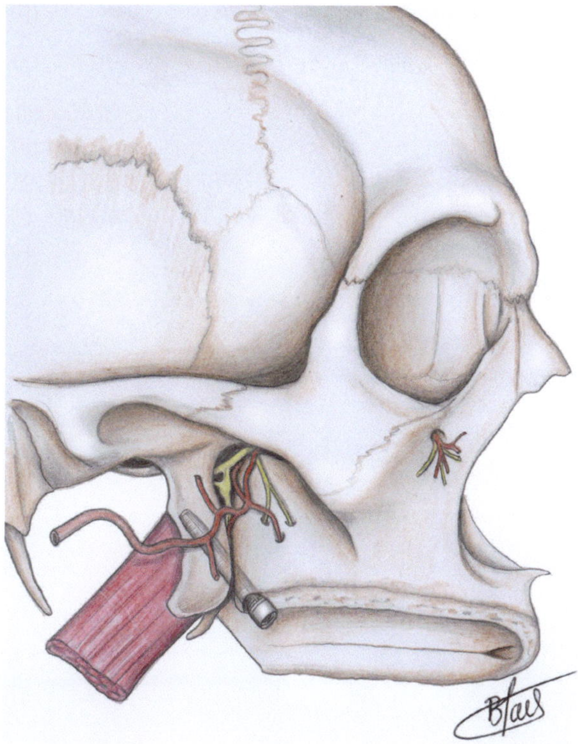

Fig. 1.36 Maxilla: the dense bones of the nasal floor, zygoma, and canine pillar area are suitable for basal implants screw-secured with osteosynthesis screws (length 4, 5 or 6 mm). Lateral view of the tubero-pterygoid area: this long root-form implant engages the dense bone of the pterygoid process

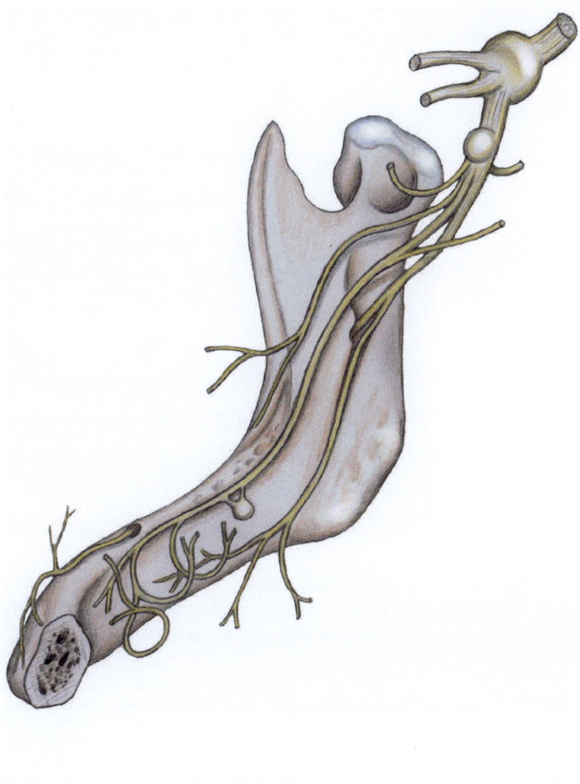

Fig. 1.37 Atrophic mandible: dense D1 bone in the mental area. The mandibular nerve foramen opens out on the crest. Lingual and mandibular nerves are critical structures that must be protected during surgery

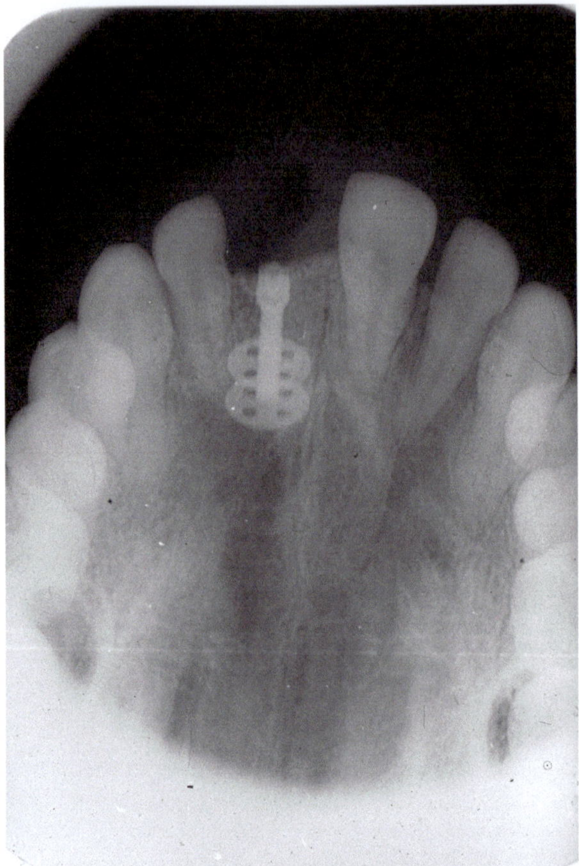

Fig. 1.38 Missing central incisor with complete loss of the buccal plate replaced by a double Diskimplant®

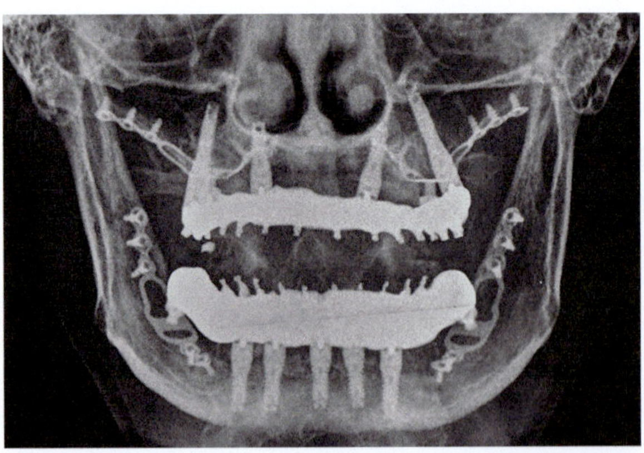

Fig. 1.39 Front view of a basal rehabilitation of an atrophic maxilla and mandible using an immediate loading protocol. Root-form implants were combined with plate-form Diskimplants®. The basal implants were screwed onto the zygomatic process and the trigone area using 5 mm long orthopedic screws. Radiographic status after 2 years of service (2015–2017)

Atrophic Maxilla

The limits of maxillary sinus buccal landmarks are easily identified because basal implantology is a full-flap procedure. Atraumatic elevation of the periosteum by gently separating the tissues using a gauze pad avoids injury to the inner layer of the periosteum and inadvertent penetration of the sinus through the fragile eggshell-thin lateral wall. The bottom and the vertical borders of the nasal fossae must be delineated during flap elevation. The entire bony structure must be visualized before starting osteotomy. Where applicable, the infraorbital foramen must be exposed; the infraorbital nerve remains in the full-thickness buccal flap.

Sharp crestal soft tissue incisions should be made until the scalpel reaches the bone crest. During osteotomy, the soft tissues and nerves should be protected by holding them with a large, rigid plastic suction tube maintained firmly against the buccal bony plate. In the tubero-pterygoid area, full-thickness buccal and palatal mucoperiosteal flaps are elevated using the same approach. Major and minor palatal arteries must remain in the full-thickness palatal flap. This can be obtained by remaining in close contact with the palatal bone during flap elevation. Use the gauze separation technique and a flap retractor.

Atrophic Mandible

Two critical anatomic elements must be avoided during basal implant installation: the lingual nerve and the mandibular nerve. A sharp crestal incision should always be made in the middle of the remaining attached gingiva. The scalpel must be in contact with the bony crest.

The full-thickness flap must be elevated from the lingual side first, always keeping close contact with the bony wall. The gauze separation technique is recommended to avoid damaging the periosteum or mandibular nerve. This technique also eliminates the risk of injuring the lingual nerve because this structure remains inside the lingual flap. This is important because the lingual nerve cannot be visualized on CT scans or cone beam CT exams. The procedure is then repeated from the buccal aspect in order to identify the mental foramen. As for the atrophic maxilla, critical soft tissue structures can be easily protected during rotary osteotomy by holding a large plastic suction tube firmly against the bony plate.

Conflict of interest statement Gérard M. Scortecci is the inventor of the Diskimplant and holder of several associated patents that are exploited by the Victory company. He is an unpaid consultant to this firm and a minority shareholder in the company. No money was received from any of the companies mentioned in the book or from any of the companies whose products are mentioned.

Recommended Reading

1. Misch CE. Density of bone: effect on treatment plans, surgical approach, healing and progressive bone loading. Int J Oral Implant. 1990;6:23–31.
2. Wolff J. Das Gesetz der Transformation der Knochen. Berlin: A Hirschwald; 1892. (English translation published in 1986 by Springer-Verlag).
3. Jaffin RA, Berman CL. The excessive loss of Brånemark fixtures in type IV bone: a 5-year analysis. J Periodontol. 1991;62:2–4.
4. Adell R, Lekholm U, Brånemark PI. Surgical procedures. In: Brånemark PI, Zarb GA, Albrektsson T, editors. Tissue-integrated prostheses: osseointegration in clinical dentistry. Chicago: Quintessence; 1985. p. 211–32.
5. Adell R, Lekholm U, Rockler B, Brånemark PI. A 15-year study of osseointegrated implants in the treatment of the edentulous jaw. Int J Oral Surg. 1981;6:387–99.
6. Albrektsson T, Zarb G, Worthington P, Eriksson RA. The long-term efficacy of currently used dental implants: a review and proposed criteria of success. Int J Oral Maxillofac Implants. 1986;1:11–25.
7. Aras E, Sönmez M, Zora M, Basarir M, Kurtulmus H. The use of prefabricated titanium tissue abutments for the construction of a maxillary subperiosteal implant. J Oral Implantol. 2005;31(5):255–8.
8. Atalay B, Doganay O, Saracoglu BK, Bultan O, Hafiz G. Clinical evaluation of zygomatic implant-supported fixed and removable prosthesis. J Craniofac Surg. 2017;28(1):185–9.
9. Atwood DA. Reduction of residual ridges: a major oral disease entity. J Prosthet Dent. 1971;26:266–79.
10. Balshi TJ, Wolfinger GJ, Slauch RW, Balshi SF. Brånemark system implant lengths in the pterygomaxillary region: a retrospective comparison. Implant Dent. 2013;22(6):610–2.
11. Becktor JP, Isaksson S, Abrahamsson P, Sennerby L. Evaluation of 31 zygomatic implants and 74 regular dental implants used in 16 patients for prosthetic reconstruction of the atrophic maxilla with cross-arch fixed bridges. Clin Implant Dent Relat Res. 2005;7(3):159–65.
12. Berg H, Carlsson GE, Helkimo M. Changes in shape of posterior parts of upper jaws after extraction of teeth and prosthetic treatment. J Prosthet Dent. 1975;34(3):262–8.
13. Bidez M, Misch CE. Three-dimensional finite element analysis of bone volume and density. Alabama: University of Alabama School of Biomechanical Engineering; 1992.
14. Bidez M, Misch CE. Force transfer in implant dentistry: basic concepts and principles. J Oral Implantol. 1992;18:264–74.
15. Bocklage R. Advanced alveolar crest atrophy: an alternative treatment technique for maxilla and mandible. Implant Dent. 2001;10(1):30–5.
16. Bothe RT, Beaton LE, Davenport HA. Reaction of bone to multiple metallic implants. Surg Gynecol Obstet. 1940;71:592–602.
17. Brånemark PI. Osseointegration and its experimental background. J Prosthet Dent. 1983;50:399–410.
18. Brunski JB. Influence of biomechanical factors at the bone-biomaterial interface. In: Davies JE, editor. The bone-biomaterial interface. Toronto: University of Toronto Press; 1991. p. 391–404.
19. Candel-Marti E, Carrillo-Garcia C, Penarrocha-Oltra D, Penarrocha-Diago M. Rehabilitation of atrophic posterior maxilla with zygomatic implants: review. J Oral Implantol. 2012;38(5):653–7.
20. Claffey N, Bashara H, O'Reilly P, Polyzois I. Evaluation of new bone formation and osseointegration around subperiosteal titanium implants with histometry and nanoindentation. Int J Oral Maxillofac Implants. 2015;30(5):1004–10.
21. Curi MM, Cardoso CL, Ribeiro Kde C. Retrospective study of pterygoid implants in the atrophic posterior maxilla: implant and prosthesis survival rates up to 3 years. Int J Oral Maxillofac Implants. 2015;30(2):378–83.
22. Davo R. Zygomatic implants placed with a two-stage procedure: a 5-year retrospective study. Eur J Oral Implantol. 2009;2(2):115–24.

23. Del Fabbro M, Ceresoli V. The fate of marginal bone around axial vs. tilted implants: a systematic review. Eur J Oral Implantol. 2014;7(suppl 2):S171–89.
24. Doms P. The tissue response to endosteal blade implants. Microradiography and tetracycline markings. Oral Implantol. 1974;4:470–4.
25. Doms P, Scortecci GM. Nouvelles solutions thérapeutiques en prothèse – racines artificielles en titane pur. Implantologie Orale. 1985;18:6.
26. Dorland's Illustrated Medical Dictionary. Saunders: Philadelphia; 1994. 28th edn.
27. Dos Santos PL, Silva GH, da Silva Pereira FR, da Silva RD, Campos ML, Mattos TB, Gulinelli JL. Zygomatic implant subjected to immediate loading for atrophic maxilla rehabilitation. J Craniofac Surg. 2016;27(8):e734–7.
28. Doundoulakis JH. Surface analysis of titanium after sterilization: role in implant-tissue interface and bioadhesion. J Prosthet Dent. 1987;58:471–8.
29. English CE. Implants. Part III: an overview. CDA J. 1988;16:34–8.
30. Engquist B, Bergendal T, Kallus T, Linden U. A retrospective multicenter evaluation of osseointegrated implants supporting overdentures. Int J Oral Maxillofac Implants. 1988;3(2):129–34.
31. European Directive 93/42. Journal officiel des Communautés Européennes. Directive 93/42/CEE du 14-06-1993 relative aux dispositifs médicaux (43 pages including the annexes).
32. Frost MH. Mechanical adaptation. Frost's mechanostat theory. In: Martin RB, Burr DB, editors. Structure, function and adaptation of compact bone. New York: Raven Press; 1989. p. 179–81.
33. Glauser R, Ruhstaller P, Windisch S, Zembic A, Lundgren A, Gottlow J, Hämmerle CH. Immediate occlusal loading of Brånemark system TiUnite implants placed predominantly in soft bone: 4-year results of a prospective clinical study. Clin Implant Dent Relat Res. 2005;7(suppl 1):S52–9.
34. Goiato MC, Pellizzer EP, Moreno A, Gennari-Filho H, dos Santos DM, Santiago JF Jr, dos Santos EG. Implants in the zygomatic bone for maxillary prosthetic rehabilitation: a systematic review. Int J Oral Maxillofac Surg. 2014;43(6):748–57.
35. Jokstad A, Sanz M, Ogawa T, Bassi F, Levin L, Wennerberg A, Romanos GE. A systematic review of the role of implant design in the rehabilitation of the edentulous maxilla. Int J Oral Maxillofac Implants. 2016;31(suppl):s43–99.
36. Leventhal GS. Titanium, a metal for surgery. J Bone Joint Surg Am. 1951;33-A(2):473–4.
37. Loperfido C, Masquida J, Lozada JL. Severe mandibular atrophy treated with a subperiosteal implant and simultaneous graft with rhBMP-2 and mineralized allograft: a case report. J Oral Implantol. 2014;40(6):707–13.
38. Manski RJ, Brown E. Dental coverage of adults ages 21–64, United States, 1997 and 2007. Agency for Healthcare Research and Quality, Statistical Brief #295, 2010.
39. Manski RJ, Moeller JF, Chen H, St Clair PA, Schimmel J, Pepper JV. Wealth effect and dental care utilization in the United States. J Public Health Dent. 2012;72:179–89.
40. Marx RE. Oral and intravenous bisphosphonate-induced osteonecrosis of the jaws. Hanover Park: Quintessence Books; 2007.
41. Minichetti JC. Analysis of HA-coated subperiosteal implants. J Oral Implantol. 2003;29(3):111–6.
42. Misch CE. Contemporary implant dentistry. St. Louis, MO: Mosby Elsevier; 2008.
43. Misch CE. Laterally inserted dental implant assembly and method for securing a dental prosthesis. 2009. US patent US20100297584.
44. Misch CE, Judy KWM. Classification of partially edentulous arches for implant dentistry. Int J Oral Implant. 1987;4:7–12.
45. Misch CM, Misch CE, Resnik RR, Ismail YH. Reconstruction of maxillary alveolar defects with symphysis grafts for dental implants: a preliminary procedural report. Int J Oral Maxillofac Implants. 1992;3(7):360–6.
46. Moore DJ, Hansen PA. A descriptive 18-year retrospective review of subperiosteal implants for patients with severely atrophied edentulous mandibles. J Prosthet Dent. 2004;92(2):145–50.
47. Mraiwa N, Jacobs R, van Steenberghe D, Quirynen M. Clinical assessment and surgical implications of anatomic challenges in the anterior mandible. Clin Implant Dent Relat Res. 2003;5(4):219–25.

48. Nair C, Bharathi S, Jawade R, Jain M. Basal implants – a panacea for atrophic ridges. J Dent Sci Oral Rehab. 2013;Jan–Mar:1–4.
49. Nordquist WD, Krutchkoff DJ. The custom endosteal implant (CEI): histology and case report of a retrieved maxillary custom osseous-integrated implant nine years in service. J Oral Implantol. 2014;40(2):195–201.
50. Penarrocha M, Carrillo C, Boronat A, Penarrocha M. Retrospective study of 68 implants placed in the pterygomaxillary region using drills and osteotomes. Int J Oral Maxillofac Implants. 2009;24(4):720–6.
51. Rams TE, Bakin BE, Roberts TW, Molzan AK. Microbiological aspects of human mandibular subperiosteal dental implants. J Oral Implantol. 2013;39(6):714–22.
52. Resnik RR, Misch CE. Avoiding mandibular nerve impairment, Part 3. Management of neurosensory impairments after dental implant surgery. Dent Today. 2015;34(2):122–5.
53. Roberts RA. Types, uses and evaluation of the plate-form implant. J Oral Implantol. 1996;22(2):111–8.
54. Rodriguez X, Rambla F, De Marcos Lopez L, Mendez V, Vela X, Jimenez Garcia J. Anatomical study of the pterygomaxillary area for implant placement: cone beam computed tomographic scanning in 100 patients. Int J Oral Maxillofac Implants. 2014;29(5):1049–52.
55. Rodriguez X, Lucas-Taulé E, Elnayef B, Altuna P, Gargallo-Albiol J, Penarrocha-Diago M, Hernandez-Alfaro F. Anatomical and radiological approach to pterygoid implants: a cross-sectional study of 202 cone beam computed tomography examinations. Int J Oral Maxillofac Surg. 2016;45(5):636–40.
56. Scortecci G, Meyere P, Zattara H, Doms P. Intra-oral applications in small bone volumes. Patient selection and long-term results. In: Laney W, Tolman D, editors. Tissue integration in oral, orthopedic and maxillofacial reconstruction. Philadelphia, PA: Quintessence; 1990. p. 350–5.
57. Scortecci GM, Misch CE, Benner KU, editors. Implants and restorative dentistry. London: Martin Dunitz; 2001.
58. Suzuki M, Mine Y, Shimoo Y, Yamamoto M, Kaketa A, Kasahara M, Serikawa M, Rhee S, Matsubayashi T, Matsunaga S, Abe S. Regional anatomical observation of morphology of greater palatine canal and surrounding structures. Bull Tokyo Dent Coll. 2016;57(4):223–31.
59. US Department of Health and Human Services. Oral health in America: a report of the surgeon general-executive summary. Rockville MD: US Dept of Health and Human Services, National Institute of Dental and Craniofacial Research, National Institutes of Health; 2000.
60. Wical KE, Swoope CC. Studies of residual ridge resorption. Part I: use of panoramic radiographs for evaluation and classification of mandibular resorption. J Prosthet Dent. 1974;32(1):7–12.
61. Yadav RS, Sangur R, Mahajan T, Rajanikant AV, Singh N, Singh R. An alternative to conventional dental implants: basal implants. Rama Univ J Dent Sci. 2015;2(2):22–8.
62. Zarb G, Lekholm U. Patient selection and preparation. In: Brånemark PI, Zarb G, Albrektsson T, editors. Tissue-integrated protheses. Chicago: Quintessence; 1985. p. 199–209.

Biological Aspects

2

Gérard M. Scortecci, Pierre Doglioli, Patrick Philip, and Itzhak Binderman

2.1 Basal Implants and Osseointegration (Fig. 2.1)

Considerable attention is currently directed at determination of the optimum surface characteristics and the degree of super cleanness required for titanium basal implants, because these parameters influence early osseointegration and long-term results under functional and/or possible parafunctional masticatory forces. This is especially important with basal implants as they are placed in small bone volumes. In extreme situations, minute metal wear particles released at the bone interface from modified, rough titanium surfaces can compromise initial osseointegration by promoting peri-implantitis over time [1]. The principles of osseointegration, discovered by P-I Brånemark, were defined on the basis of this original state of surface, and implants with these surface characteristics offer the largest long-term follow-up results in human jaws.

G. M. Scortecci (✉)
University of Nice-Sophia Antipolis Medical School, Nice, France

New York University, New York, NY, USA

University of Southern California, Los Angeles, CA, USA

Private Practice, Nice, France
e-mail: scortecci@wanadoo.fr

P. Doglioli
Centre de Biotechnologies, Cannes, France
e-mail: pierredoglioli@wanadoo.fr

P. Philip
Faculté de Médecine, Département d'Histologie, Unité d'Exploration Fonctionnelle Cellulaire et Tissulaire, Hôpital Pasteur, University of Nice-Sophia Antipolis, Nice, France
e-mail: pjmphilip@aol.com

I. Binderman
Department of Oral Biology, University of Tel Aviv, Tel Aviv, Israel

© Springer Nature Switzerland AG 2019

G. M. Scortecci (ed.), *Basal Implantology*, https://doi.org/10.1007/978-3-319-44873-2_2

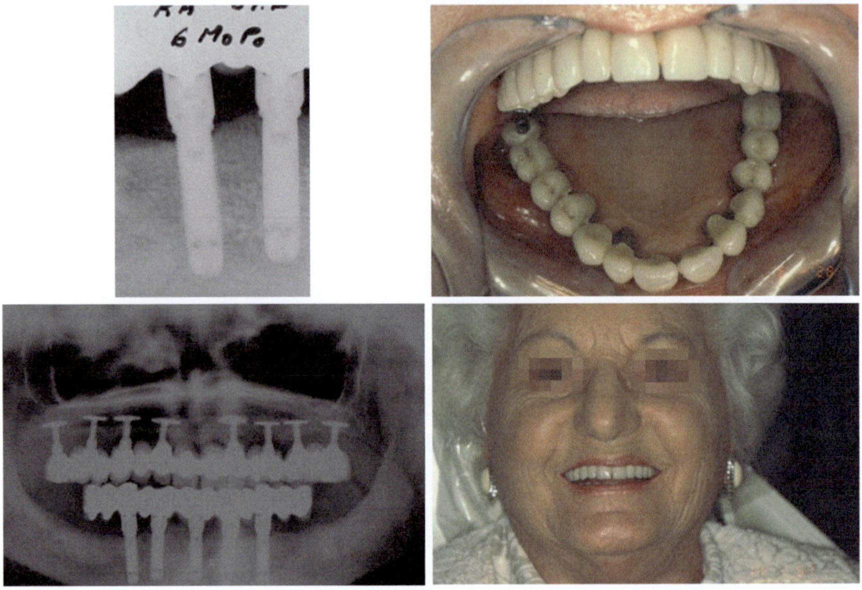

Fig. 2.1 Full rehabilitation of an atrophic maxilla with eight basal Diskimplants® in 1984 (patient aged 77 years). Root-form implants were placed in the lower jaw when the patient was 86 years old (submerged protocol). Panoramic view in 2007 with the bridge still in place: no peri-implantitis is visible after 23 years of service (patient aged 100 years). These titanium implants had a non-modified, *ad modum Brånemark* state of surface

2.2 Titanium as a Biomaterial

Selected Properties

The proven high biocompatibility of titanium as an implant material is related to the properties of its surface oxide. For decades, titanium oxide powder has been used in pharmacology as a baby powder (talc). In air or water, titanium quickly forms an oxide thickness of 3–5 nm at room temperature. Titanium can form several oxides of different stoichiometries: TiO, Ti_2O_3, and TiO_2. TiO_2, the most common, can have three different crystal structures but can also be amorphous. As TiO_2 is very resistant to chemical attack, titanium is one of the most corrosion-resistant metals, particularly in the chemical environment with which we are concerned in the mouth. This is one contributing factor to its high biocompatibility. This property is also shared with several other metals such as tantalum, aluminum, and zirconium, which, respectively, form TaO_2, Al_2O_3, and ZrO_2 on their surfaces.

Another unique physical property of TiO_2 is its high dielectric constant, which can range from 50 to 170, depending on crystal structure. The high value of this constant would result in considerably stronger van der Waal's bonds on TiO_2 than on other oxides, a fact that may be important for interface biochemistry. Like many other transition metal oxides, TiO_2 is catalytically active for a number of inorganic and organic chemical reactions, which also may influence interface chemistry. Finally, the metal titanium itself is a material of more than sufficient strength for most clinical applications and especially for the long-lasting function of basal implant-supported rehabilitations.

2.3 Surface Characteristics of Titanium Diskimplants®

Early, non-modified *ad modum Brånemark* titanium fixtures have been in service for more than 50 years. Very few cases of peri-implantitis have been reported in the literature with this super clean titanium finish. In fact, the term peri-implantitis was never even mentioned in Brånemark's 1985 book *Tissue-Integrated Prostheses*. From the very beginning, Diskimplant® basal implants have been manufactured from bars of wrought titanium with this very same non-modified, super clean surface (i.e., without any surface contaminants); this is still true today. At an ultra-microscopic level, the microgrooves on the machined titanium surface are beneficial because they significantly increase the contact surface between the implant and the bone.

Surface Roughness

The impact of the surface roughness of titanium implants differs as a function of the geometric dimensions involved. From a mechanical standpoint, rough or porous surfaces (approx. 100 μm or more) may sometimes be advantageous because they increase the surface area in contact with the bone and provide immediate stability. According to many publications, this effect is especially notable early on, at implant installation, and at later stages, when high torque values are required if implant removal proves necessary. However, if metal ion dissolution occurs, especially during long-term function, a very rough or porous surface can be a disadvantage, because the total exposed area, and thus the amount of dissolved metal ions, will be greater.

Whereas rough surfaces have been associated with bone loss [1], this complication has rarely been reported with perfectly smooth dental pins without any form of macroscopically visible mechanical retention. For example, removal of unthreaded, non-modified straight tantalum pins (Scialom implants) can prove difficult, even with strong pliers. In some cases, and particularly in type I bone in the mandible, an osseointegrated Scialom pin must be cut at the crestal level and left in place.

Effect of Corrosion and Wear Particles on Living Tissues

Corrosion is not a problem with titanium implants so long as the dense passivation layer of titanium oxide on the non-modified machined metal surface remains intact. A single scratch has no consequences since the oxide layer regenerates in an electrolyte environment within a short time. In contrast, implant instability causes constant rubbing of root-form implants and basal disks against cortical bone. The oxide layer is destroyed with each loading cycle and does not have a chance to regenerate, resulting in a continuing corrosion process.

Differences in the mechanical properties of implants and bone always lead to a minute degree of relative motion between the two, with the possibility of fretting between the implant and bone surfaces and subsequent release of corrosion products over longer periods. Fretting of titanium implants results in a grayish staining of the surrounding tissues but causes no adverse tissue reactions. Modified implant surfaces such as rough and/or coated titanium surfaces (TPS, SLA, TioBlast, HA) cause increased fretting with the bone tissue in case of primary implant instability and are subject to alterations over time, especially in type I bone. Use of an approach based on slightly smaller osteotomy dimensions than those of the intended implant permits achievement of immediate implant/bone stability without need for a rough surface.

In orthopedic surgery, metal release from total hip prostheses may contribute to bone loss by osteolysis. The effects of titanium, cobalt, and chromium debris on human osteoblast-like cells inhibit the synthesis of type I collagen. Wear particles from implants are deposited in peri-implant tissues in which they are phagocytosed by mononuclear and multinuclear macrophage-like cells. Wang et al. [2] demonstrated that osteoclasts are capable of phagocytosing particles of titanium while remaining fully functional, hormone-responsive, bone remodeling cells. In contrast, osteoblasts are affected by titanium particles. The biosynthesis of both type I and type III collagen was decreased in cells that had been contaminated with titanium particles, but neither their viability nor proliferation was affected [3]. Titanium particles smaller than 3 μm suppressed expression of the gene that codes for collagen. This phenomenon was related to the size, but not the composition, of the particles. Polymeric particles of the same dimensions cause the same damage.

Finally, the deleterious effects of wear particles are not limited to metals. The March 2017 FDA update on mammary prostheses described a dramatic rise in peri-implant pathologies when soft silicone prostheses were replaced by rough versions, due essentially to release of polymer particles during body movement.

2.4 **Peri-implantitis** (Figs. 2.2 and 2.3)

The clinical success of dental implants, like orthopedic implants, is based on absolute initial stability in dense living bone and an uncontaminated environment. Rough titanium surfaces drastically increase metal release during function, leading to a high level of macrophage activity. Extensive in vitro studies have shown that macrophages can be activated by polymeric or metallic particles and can show bone-resorbing activity [3]. Fibroblasts stimulated by debris play an important role in peri-implant osteolysis because they enhance metalloproteinase synthesis. This is the beginning of the peri-implantitis process. Titanium particles can also migrate to other parts of the body (lungs, lymph nodes) and may provoke allergic reactions.

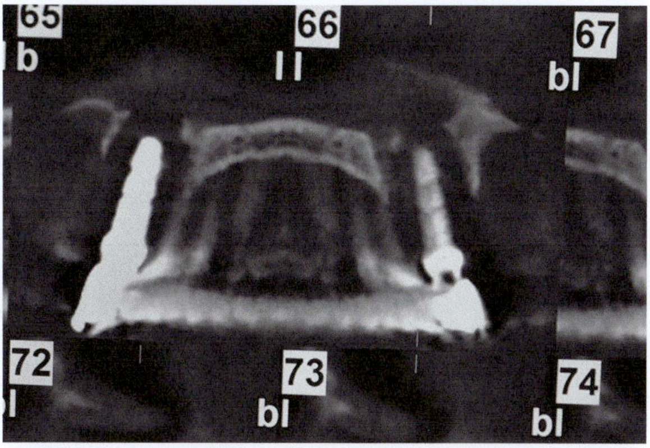

Fig. 2.2 Severe peri-implantitis and an oroantral communication developed after 8 years of function around these immediately loaded, root-form titanium implants with a modified surface state

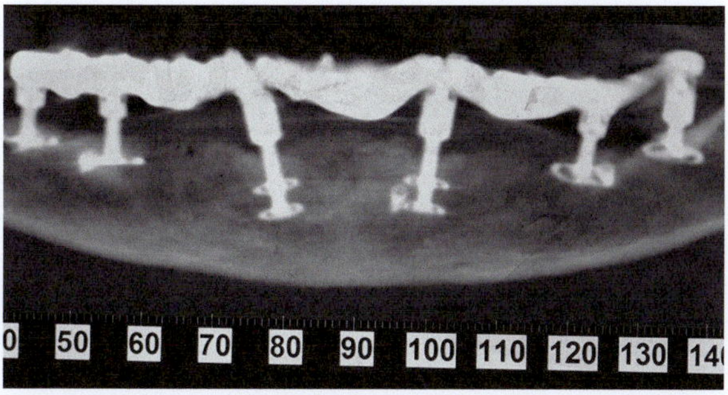

Fig. 2.3 Cone beam CT of basal implants with a non-modified surface state after 14 years of service (2003–2017). Immediate loading procedure

In vivo, excessive quantities of metallic debris released during function and/or parafunction can be toxic. Decreased bone formation by osteoblasts and the bone-resorbing activity of osteoclasts can both disturb the bone remodeling process and result in osteolysis. In vivo, the interfacial membrane provides access for particulate matter caused by wear to the peri-implant space and influences bone resorption. Osteoblast function is altered by exposure to debris from wear. Friction during function between the titanium implant and bone is critical with rough surfaces. The posterior mandible is particularly susceptible to this phenomenon, especially in the second premolar and first molar sectors [4]. The peri-implant soft tissue membrane contains fibroblasts, macrophages, and foreign-body giant cells associated with particulate wear debris. In 1997, Haynes and coworkers suggested that bone loss around orthopedic replacement prostheses may be related to the activation of mononuclear phagocytes (MNP). Particle-activated mononuclear phagocytes may thus alter the balance between bone formation and resorption by a number of mechanisms.

Recent research has shown that debris activates macrophage activity. There are two types of macrophages. Macrophage type 1 is dedicated to catabolic activity, inflammatory response, and phagocytosis of debris. If there is too much debris, macrophage type 1 activity can become more aggressive, leading to pathologic activity because type 1 macrophages remain too long in too great a quantity. At this point, type 2 macrophages cannot be produced in sufficient amounts; in the end, the inflammatory process (which is enhanced by bacterial activity) starts to destroy the implant environment. With non-modified surfaces, there is very little release of metallic particles. In this situation, type 1 macrophages are rapidly replaced by type 2 anabolic macrophage activity that promotes stem cells for formation of new blood vessels. This favorable environment is less susceptible to be destroyed by bacterial activity.

In addition to bone resorption, the implant body may be exposed, and calculus may form on the surface of the titanium; these are the characteristic features of peri-implantitis. Interestingly, one of the most common chairside treatments for peri-implantitis is removal of the rough surface of a modified titanium implant using burs, followed by polishing to try to obtain a smooth, clean surface very similar to the non-modified *ad modum Brånemark* surface.

Peri-implantitis has been extensively described around dental implants with the more recent and, for a time, very popular modified (rough) surfaces. In contrast, non-modified, machined titanium dental implants free of contaminating overlayers, coatings, or sand-blasting appear to offer the surface characteristics least susceptible to release wear particulate debris during long-term function. This could explain the low incidence of peri-implantitis observed around Diskimplants® machined *ad modum Brånemark* after more than 30 years of continual clinical use. This is particularly relevant because the original machined titanium Brånemark implants have been successful in clinical use for more than 50 years. Today, these implants offer the longest documented surface state for a material implanted in human jaws. Interestingly, IMZ implants and the first Straumann plasma-sprayed hollow cylinder titanium implants are no longer on the market, having been replaced by implants with surfaces that are not as rough.

2.5 Human Jaw Cell Cultures: In Vitro Studies (Figs. 2.4, 2.5, 2.6, 2.7, and 2.8)

Specific Biocompatibility, Cytotoxicity, Mutagenicity

In 1991, cytotoxicity, mutagenicity, and specific biocompatibility assays were conducted using human jaw osteoblasts, fibroblasts, and epithelial cell cultures to determine their reactions to machined *ad modum Brånemark* titanium disks identical to the finished titanium surface of Diskimplants®. Such multiparametric analyses on pertinent biological samples accurately reflect the biological interactions between a given cell type (osteoblasts) and biomaterials that are widely used in oral implantology and are equivalent to those encountered in clinical practice. The absence of cytotoxicity or mutagenicity in cultures of gingival cells (epithelium and connective tissue) and bone cells (osteoblasts) confirmed the biocompatibility of this non-modified, machined titanium surface and the importance of metal surface characteristics. Precautions are thus essential when handling dental implants to avoid contamination.

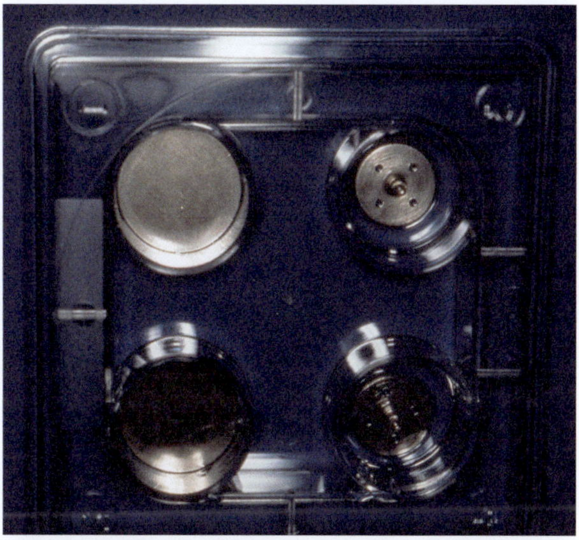

Fig. 2.4 Tissue culture of cells from human jaws grown on titanium disks with modified and non-modified surface states

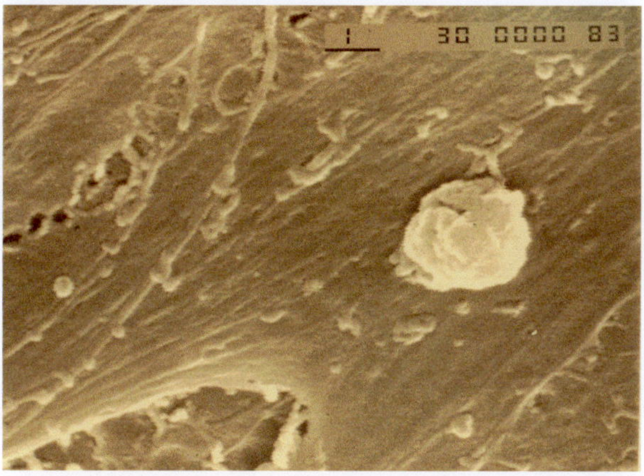

Fig. 2.5 Cell culture of osteoblasts from human jaws: growth is visible as attachment of the cell pseudopods to the titanium disks with a non-modified surface (courtesy Prof. P. Doglioli)

Fig. 2.6 Osteoblasts are well-aligned, perpendicular to the non-modified titanium surface of the Diskimplant®

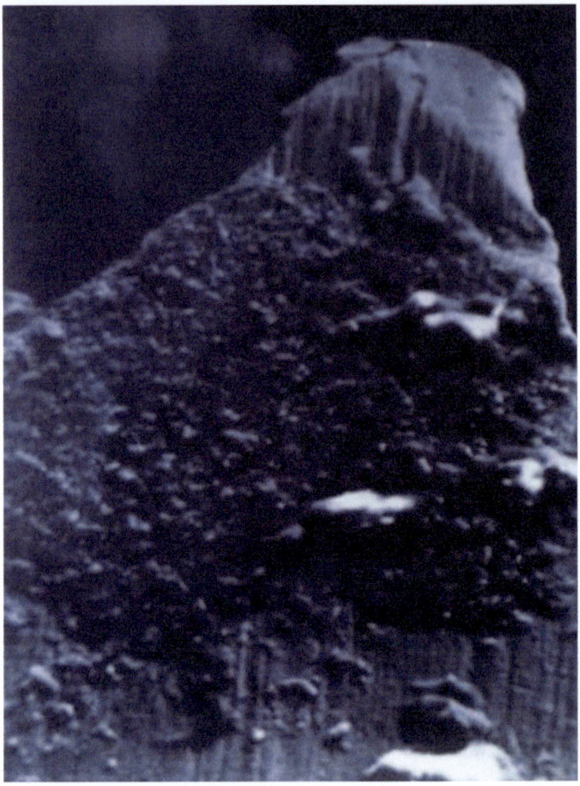

Fig. 2.7 Contaminated titanium surface

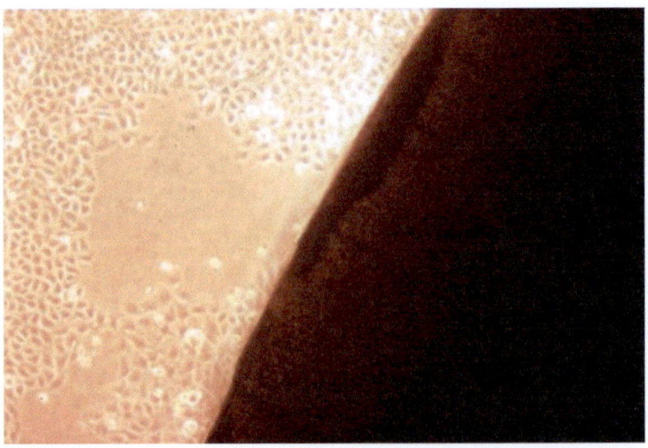

Fig. 2.8 Cell culture: growth of gingival epithelium is disorganized on the contaminated titanium surface. Hemidesmosomes cannot attach to the rough surface of the disk

Spectrofluorometric Analysis of Specific Biocompatibility

Using a spectrofluorometric technique that facilitates determination of osteocalcin and type I collagen expression in the presence and absence of biomaterials, human osteoblast cultures were grown on titanium disks with a modified rough surface, titanium disks coated with hydroxyapatite and non-modified, *ad modum Brånemark*-machined titanium disks with a surface identical to that of Diskimplants® [5]. Alkaline phosphatase activity and osteocalcin expression on the hydroxyapatite disks and the modified titanium disks were always lower than on the non-modified titanium disks.

2.6 Animal Studies (Figs. 2.9, 2.10, 2.11, 2.12, 2.13, and 2.14)

Starting in 1983, animal studies on Diskimplants® were conducted at the University of Marseilles, France, at Boston University, USA, and at the Catholic University of Louvain, Belgium. Block sections of all animals were sent to the Department of Histology, University of Louvain for histological analysis.

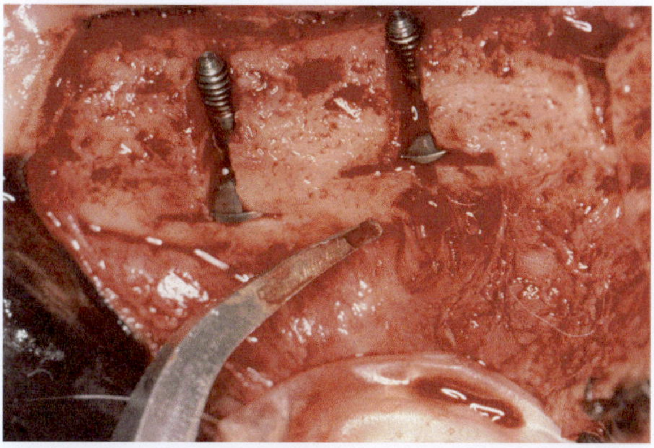

Fig. 2.9 Lateral T-shaped osteotomy with a titanium cutter (dog mandible). The solid, one-piece cutter allows preparation of the vertical and horizontal osteotomies in a single operation thanks to the teeth on the disk base and shaft. Insertion of the Diskimplant® base close to the periosteum

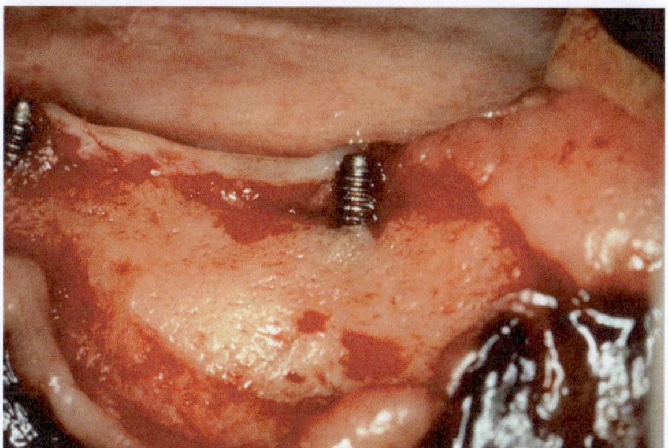

Fig. 2.10 Reentry 3 months later revealed complete reconstruction of the lateral T-shaped osteotomy, thanks to the osteogenic effect of the inner layer of the uninjured, full-thickness periosteal flap (submerged Diskimplants®). No bone substitute material was used

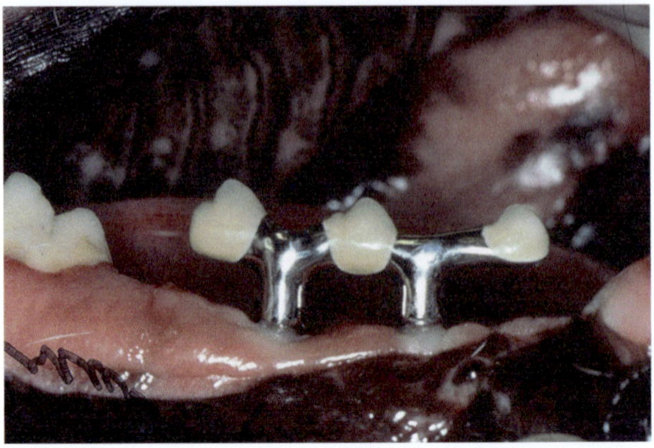

Fig. 2.11 At 3 months, functional fixed teeth with two cantilevers (one on each side) were screw-secured to the Diskimplants® and left in service for 6 months before a block section was obtained for microscope examination

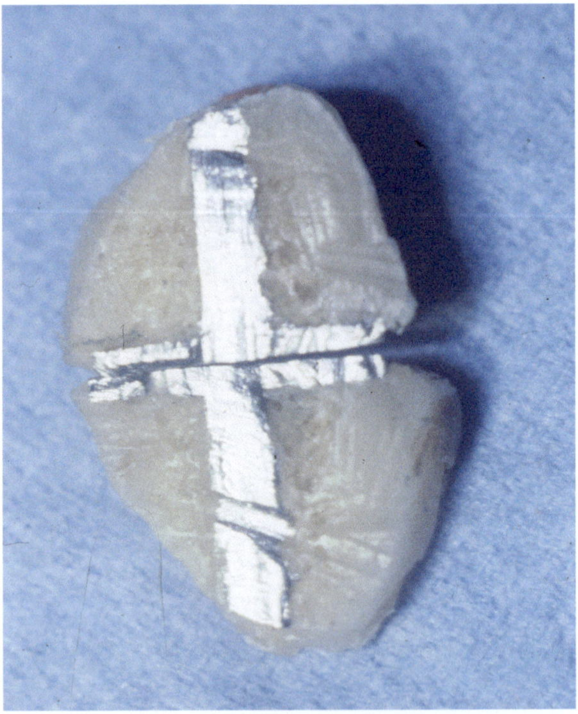

Fig. 2.12 A block section of a functionally loaded Diskimplant® was obtained after 6 months. This macroscopic view shows the intimate contact between the titanium and the bone; there is no soft tissue at the interface. It was impossible to separate the Diskimplant® from the bone; the cortical and cancellous areas were completely reconstructed and had remained stable under function

1983–1985: Studies on Beagle Dogs (University of Marseilles, France)

Two series of experiments were conducted on six beagle dogs for gross analysis of corticalization, defined by Scortecci [6] as osseointegration within the cortical bone. No bone substitute material and/or membrane was used to close the lateral T-shaped osteoincision after implant placement.

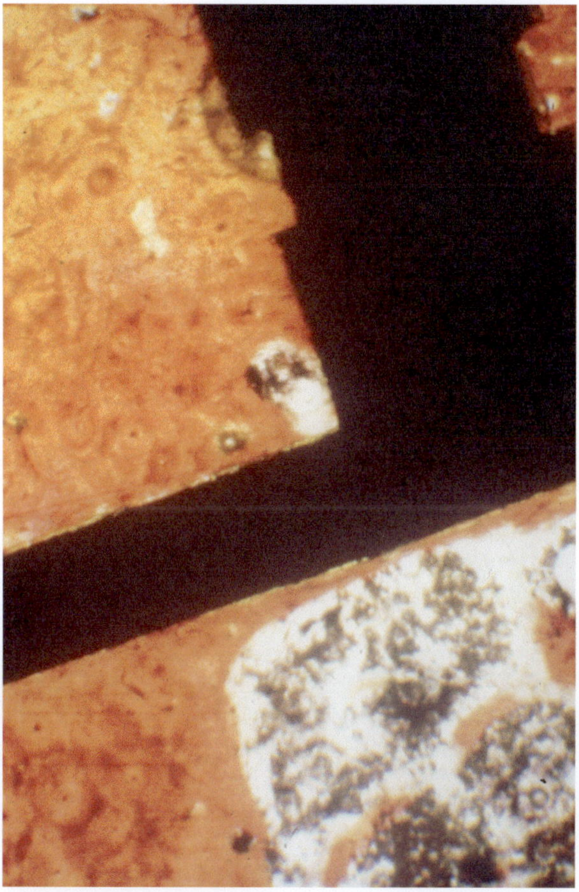

Fig. 2.13 Microradiograph showing complete osseointegration of the Diskimplant®

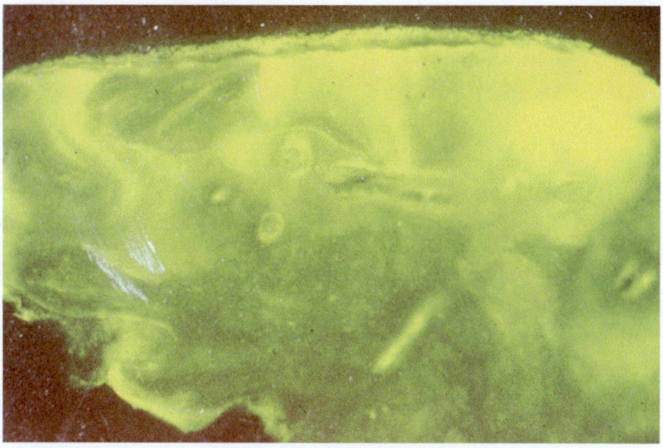

Fig. 2.14 Tetracycline labeling demonstrated living bone at the titanium Diskimplant® interface, attesting to osseointegration of the functional basal implant

Specific aims included investigation of:

- Potential pathological effects (cytotoxicity, genotoxicity, sensitization), acute inflammatory response, or allergic reactions (mucositis, bone destruction)
- Whether normal bone tissue reforms after lateral osteotomy and has the same gross appearance as cortical bone
- Whether renewal of this bone occurs after implant loading with functional teeth (dynamic study by labeling with tetracycline)
- The clinical appearance of the soft issues surrounding the Diskimplant® emergence (irritation, inflammation, pus, etc.)
- Possible Diskimplant® rejection.

Light microscopy studies were also conducted at the Faculty of Medicine, Department of Histology, Louvain, Belgium, by Professor Dhem and coworkers (see [7, 8]). Block sections obtained from two beagle dogs sacrificed 6 months after implant installation with functional teeth were radiographed, and sections were prepared for microscope examination. Microradiographs revealed intimate contact between the bone and the titanium implant, without any intermediate fibrous tissue. Fluorescence investigations (UV) allowed dynamic evaluation of the newly formed bone in intimate contact with the implant; no intermediary fibrous tissue was observed around any of the implants. The histological aspect of the bone tissue was healthy, without any pathological signs.

Conclusion: The non-modified titanium surface of the Diskimplants® did not elicit any allergic or inflammatory reactions, and osseointegration of these basal implants was maintained with function over time.

1986–1987: Studies on Mongrel Dogs (Boston University, USA; G. Scortecci and D. Nathanson)

A study at Boston University (Department of Biomaterials, Henry M. Goldman School of Graduate Dentistry) was conducted by Prof. D. Nathanson, Dept. Chairman, in collaboration with Dr. Z. Mazjoub. A total of twelve Diskimplants® (four per animal) were placed in three mongrel dogs using a high-speed drill, with and without spray. Examination of bone biopsies revealed clinical osseointegration of all of the implants. At gross analysis, the titanium implants appeared integrated in the cortical bone at all points. After labeling with tetracycline, bone sections containing the implants were obtained from one dog prior to loading with a restoration. Microradiograph and histological analysis at the University of Louvain revealed healthy bone tissue, osseointegration, and corticalization.

2.7 Other Histological Studies

Several studies of BOI implants (a clone of Diskimplants®) were conducted in 2003 by Dr. Stefan Ihde (Switzerland), Dr. Zora Aleksic (Belgrade, Serbia and Montenegro), and Pr. Dr. Vitonius S. Konstantinovic (Serbia and Montenegro) [9].

Most of the histological specimens analyzed were obtained from experiments on dogs, but there were also two human specimens that had been obtained fortuitously. In these particular specimens, total bone height above the implant disk ranged from 2 to 3 mm. Macroscopic and microscopic examination revealed complete osseointegration of the entire surface of the implants.

2.8 Human Block Sections (Figs. 2.15, 2.16, 2.17, and 2.18)

1984: Human Block Section of a Laterally Inserted, Immediately Loaded T3D Titanium Basal Implant for Single-Tooth Replacement After 9 Years of Function (University of Louvain, Belgium)

The T3D implant, marketed in the USA by Oraltronics (NYC, NY) from 1974 to 1984, was the substantially equivalent precursor of the present-day Diskimplant®. In 1984, a block section of a free-standing, laterally inserted T3D implant used to replace a maxillary central incisor became available for study 9 years after immediate functional loading in 1975. All of the patient's remaining natural teeth (including the implant) had to be extracted prior to radiotherapy. An injection of tetracycline was administered 6 weeks before implant removal. Microradiography and tetracycline labeling confirmed that osseointegration had been achieved with the immediate loading protocol, as previously demonstrated in animal research.

2012: Block Sections of a Human Cadaver with Upper and Lower Jaws Fully Implanted with Diskimplants® Obtained After 24 Years of Functional Loading (1988–2012) (University of Nice-Sophia Antipolis, France; G. Odin, P. Hofman)

By chance, during an anatomic workshop conducted at the University of Nice Medical School in 2012, both the upper and lower jaws of a cadaver were found to have been rehabilitated with Diskimplants®. A search of our archives revealed that the patient had been operated on 24 years earlier by one of the authors.

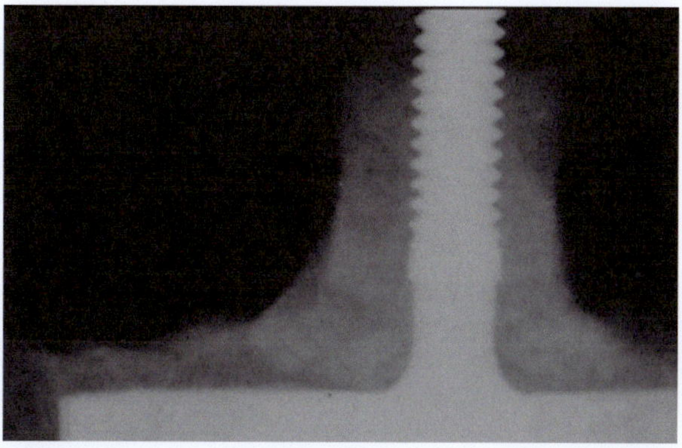

Fig. 2.15 Radiograph of a human block section containing an osseointegrated T3D basal implant that had been placed 9 years earlier for single-tooth replacement (although the immediate loading protocol was successful in this case, it is not recommended for single-tooth replacements). Block section obtained in 1986 prior to radiotherapy

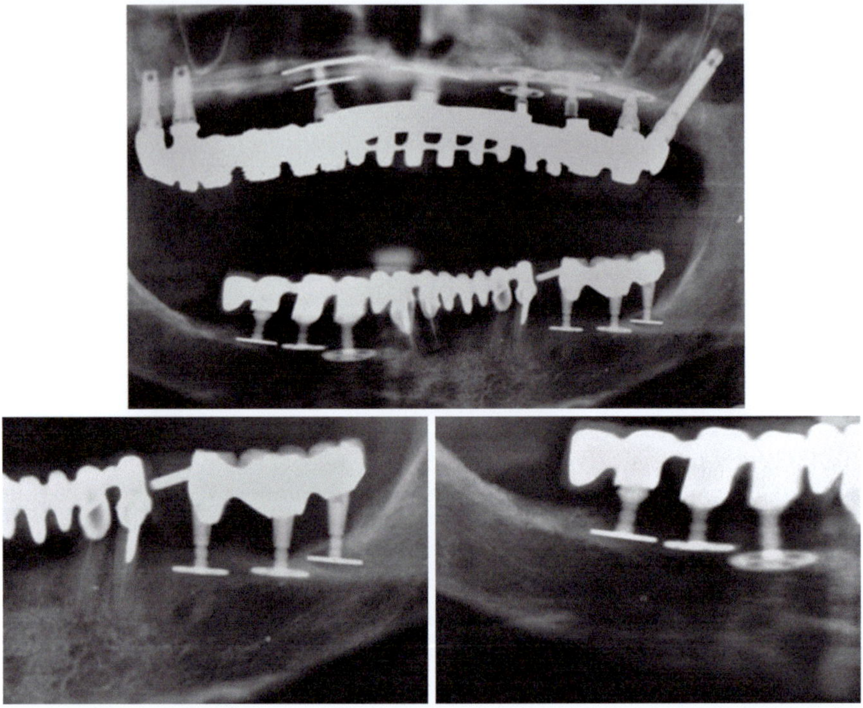

Fig. 2.16 Postmortem panoramic view of the full mouth, implant- and tooth-supported rehabilitation. The Diskimplants® in the mandible had been in function for 24 years (1988–2012). The bone height above the basal disks varied from 0.8 to 2.7 mm

First-generation Diskimplants® had been placed in 1988; root-form implants had been installed in 1991 and in 2005. Radiological and histological examination revealed extraordinary long-term functional integration of the Diskimplants® in a bone of height less than 3 mm in the mandible and in the eggshell-thin maxilla (bone thickness 0.5–2 mm). This example confirms the long-term functional validity of the BIO concept (basal implants and osseointegration).

2.9 Effect of Temperature on Bone Tissue During High-Speed Osteotomy (Figs. 2.19, 2.20, and 2.21)

Albrektsson [10] and Eriksson et al. [11, 12] published several studies demonstrating that heating to 47 °C for 1 min significantly reduces the amount of bone that grows into a porous implant, whereas heating to 42 °C for 1 min causes no demonstrable reduction in bone formation. Since lateral osteotomy with a cutter causes minimal operative trauma without thermal bone injury, this procedure is compatible with osseointegration, even in small bone volumes. Micro channels along the cutter shaft ensure continuous and profuse irrigation of the bone site during the osteotomy. Cooling takes place instantly, as demonstrated by in vivo measurement using electronic thermal

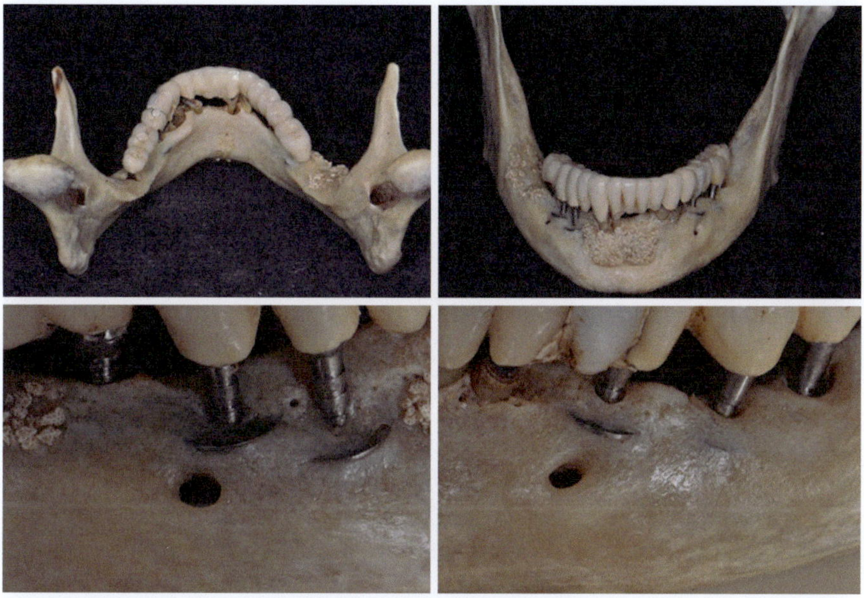

Fig. 2.17 Postmortem macroscopic view of the mandible. Some disks are partially covered by bone, while others are completely embedded in the bone

Fig. 2.18 Osseointegrated root-form implant between the pterygoid processes (same postmortem specimen) after 24 years of service (1988–2012)

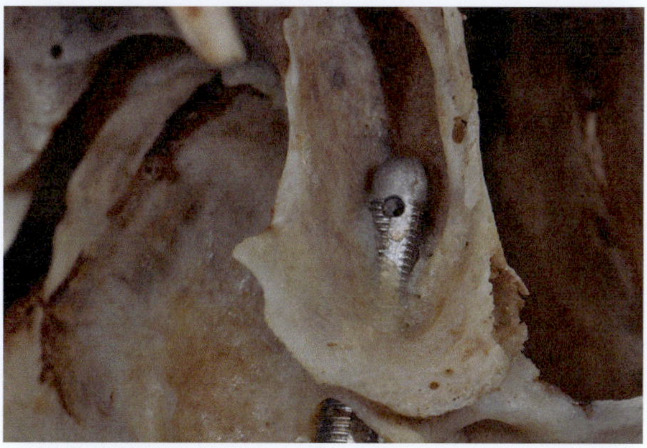

transducers (Digitem No. 3995, Germany) with an accuracy of 0.1 °C (with a water spray at 18 °C, drilling occurs between 26 °C and 28 °C). As reported by Peyton [13], Scortecci and coworkers [14, 15], and Lyer et al. [16, 17], a high-speed turbine with abundant water cooling generates less heat than other rotary instruments.

In addition to facilitating evacuation of the water spray, the lateral bone window created by the cutter used for Diskimplant® placement allows the escape of air, preventing accumulation in the tissues [18]. Placement of a rigid plastic surgical suction tube against the osteotomy site is an additional safety measure. The lateral osteotomy technique has been used routinely for over 35 years without any report of emphysema. Use of cutters is detailed in Chap. 8.

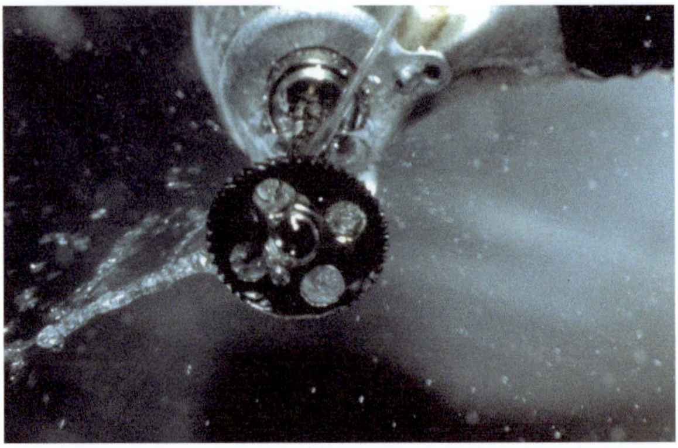

Fig. 2.19 High-speed osteotomy is performed under copious irrigation. The water "adheres" to the base and shaft of the cutter due to the force of suction during high-speed rotation

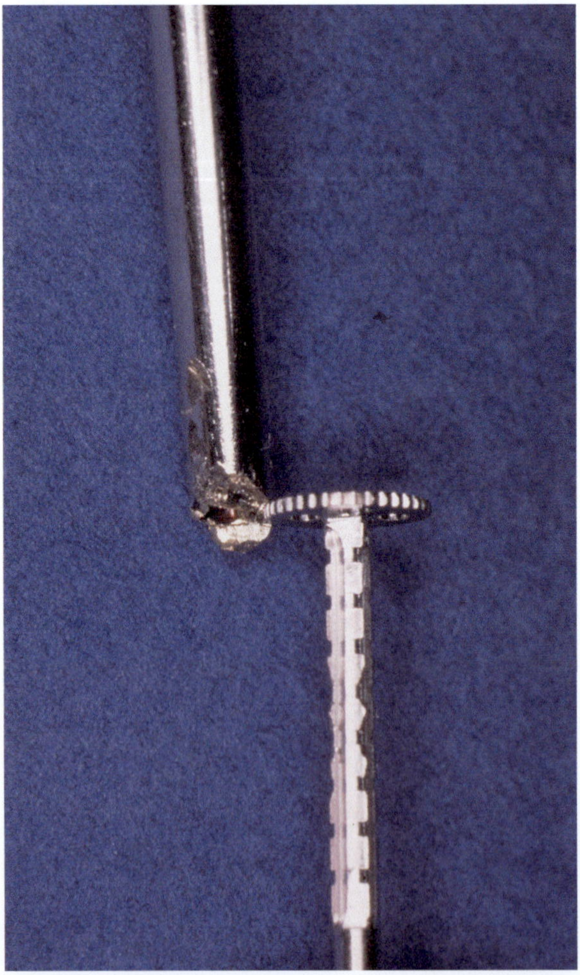

Fig. 2.20 The metal thermal probe, which has the same hardness as high-density type 1 bone (worst-case scenario), is ground by the titanium cutter during the osteotomy procedure under copious irrigation

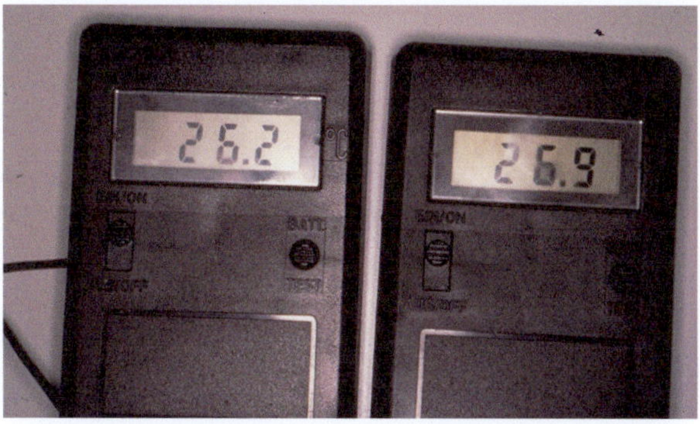

Fig. 2.21 Both electronic thermometers show a temperature of 26 °C under copious irrigation (worst-case scenario). There is no risk of thermal injury despite the very high speed (> 120,000 rpm). Initial water temperature 22 °C

Conflict of interest statement Gérard M. Scortecci is the inventor of the Diskimplant and holder of several associated patents that are exploited by the Victory company. He is an unpaid consultant to this firm and a minority shareholder in the company. No money was received from any of the companies mentioned in the book or from any of the companies whose products are mentioned.

Recommended Reading

1. Jordana F, Susbielles L, Colat-Parros J. Periimplantitis and implant body roughness: a systematic review of literature. Implant Dent. 2018;27(6):672–81.
2. Wang JY, Wicklund BH, Gustilo RB, Tsukayama DT. Prosthetic metals interfere with the functions of human osteoblast cells in vitro. Clin Orthop Relat Res. 1997;339:216–26.
3. Yao J, Szabo GCS, Jacobs JJ, Kuettner KE, Glant TT. Suppression of osteoblast function by titanium particles. J Bone Joint Surg. 1997;1:229–31.
4. Resnik RR, Misch CE. Avoiding complications in oral implantology. St. Louis, MO: Elsevier; 2017. p. 784–91.
5. Doglioli P, Scortecci G. Characterization of endosteal osteoblasts isolated from human maxilla and mandible: an experimental system for biocompatibility tests. Cytotechnology. 1991;7:39–48.
6. Scortecci GM. The Diskimplant: a self-positioning pure titanium implant. Proceedings of the 7th World Congress of Oral Implantology, Munich, FRG (June); 1984.
7. Scortecci G. L'implant Dentaire Tricortical. PhD thesis, University of Aix-Marseilles, France; 1988.
8. Scortecci GM. Etude comparative de l'échauffement lors du fraisage de l'os. Ind Dent. 1988;21:34–7.
9. Ihde S. Principles of BOI. Clinical, scientific, and practical guidelines to 4-D dental implantology. Heidelberg: Springer; 2005.
10. Albrektsson T. Bone tissue response. Tissue integrated prostheses. London: Mosby; 1985. p. 1361.
11. Eriksson RA, Albrektsson T. The effect of heat on bone regeneration. An experimental study. J Oral Maxillofac Surg. 1984;42:701–11.
12. Eriksson RA, Albrektsson T. Thermal injury to bone. A vital microscopic description of heat effects. Int J Oral Surg. 1982;11:115.
13. Peyton FA. Effectiveness of water coolants with rotary cutting instruments. J Am Dent Assoc. 1958;56(5):664–75.
14. Scortecci G, Zattara H, Meyere P, Doms P. Diskimplant System: intraoral applications in small bone values. Patient selection and long-term results. In: Laney W, Tolman D, editors. Tissue integration in oral, orthopedic and maxillofacial reconstruction. Chicago: Quintessence; 1990. p. 350–5.

15. Scortecci GM, Misch CE, Benner KU, editors. Implants and restorative dentistry. London: Martin Dunitz; 2001.
16. Lyer S, Weiss C, Mehta A. Effects of drill speed on heat production and quality of bone formation in dental implant osteotomies. Part I: Relationship between drill speed and heat production. Int J Prosthodont. 1997;10(5):411–5.
17. Lyer S, Weiss C, Mehta A. Effects of drill speed on heat production and the rate and quality of bone formation in dental implant osteotomies. Part II: relationship between drill speed and healing. Int J Prosthodont. 1997;10(6):536–40.
18. Scortecci GM, Doms P. Le Diskimplant. Actual Odontostom. 1987;159:521–38.
19. Albrektsson T. Brånemark System Info. 1999;5(1).
20. Albrektsson T. A nuanced perspective on peri-implantitis. Implant. 2016;17, 2/2016.
21. Baldi D, Menini M, Pera F, Ravera G, Pera P. Plaque accumulation on exposed titanium surfaces and peri-implant tissue behavior. A preliminary 1-year clinical study. Int J Prosthodont. 2009;22(5):447–55.
22. de Waal YC, Eijsbouts HV, Winkel EG, van Winkelhoff AJ. Microbial characteristics of peri-implantitis: a case-control study. J Periodontol. 2016;26:1–13.
23. Esposito M, Ardebili Y, Worthington HV. Interventions for replacing missing teeth: different types of dental implants. Cochrane Database Syst Rev. 2014;22(7):CD003815.
24. Itic J, Bessade J. Réflexions sur les péri-implantites. Alpha Omega News. 2016:28–29.
25. Ivanoff CJ, Sennerby L, Lekholm U. Influence of mono- and bicortical anchorage on the integration of titanium implants. A study in the rabbit tibia. Int J Oral Maxillofac Surg. 1996;25:229–35.
26. Jaffin RA, Berman CL. The excessive loss of Brånemark fixtures in Type IV bone; a 5-year analysis. J Periodontol. 1991;62:2–4.
27. Juillet JM. Three-dimensional implants – development and evaluation. Oral Implantol. 1974;4:101–4.
28. Kasemo B. Biocompatibility of titanium implants: surface science aspects. J Prosthet Dent. 1983;49:832.
29. Lekholm U. Cortical stabilization. In: Lindhe J, editor. Clinical periodontology and implant dentistry. Copenhagen: Munksgaard; 1998. p. 892–902.
30. Michel MC, Veyret D, Pantaloni J, Martin R. Analyse comparative par éléments finis d'implants odontologiques avec et sans appui cortical. Le Chirurgien-Dentiste de France. 1990;510:83–9.
31. National Institute of Health Consensus Development Conference statement on dental implants. Bethesda, MD: NIH; 1988.
32. Peixoto CD, Almas K. The implant surface characteristics and peri-implantitis. An evidence-based update. Odontostomatol Trop. 2016;39(153):23–35.
33. Rodriguez Y, Baena R, Arciola CR, Selan L, Battaglia R, Imbriani M, Rizzo S, Bisai L. Evaluation of bacterial adhesion on machined titanium, Osseotite and Nanotite discs. Int J Artif Organs. 2012;35(10):754–61. https://doi.org/10.5301/ijao.5000143.
34. Schroeder A, van de Zypen E, Stich H, Sutter F. The reactions of bone, connective tissues and epithelium to endosteal implants with titanium plasma-sprayed surfaces. J Maxillofac Surg. 1981;9:15–25.
35. Scortecci GM. Immediate function of cortically anchored disk-design implants without bone augmentation in moderately to severely resorbed completely edentulous maxillae. J Oral Implantol. 1999;25(2):70–9.
36. Scortecci G, Modschiedler T. Ostéointegration et mise en function immediate. 15 ans de recherche et d'application clinique dans le traitement du maxillaire. Implantologie. 1997;24:28–32.
37. Scortecci G, Misch CE, Benner KU. Implants and restorative dentistry. London: Martin Dunitz; 2001.
38. Turkyilmaz I, Tözüm TF. 30-year outcomes of dental implants supporting mandibular fixed dental prostheses: A retrospective review of 4 cases. Implant Dent. 2015;24(5):620–4.
39. Zetterqvist L, Feldman S, Rotter B, Vincenzi G, Wennström JL, Chierico A, Stach RM, Kenealy JN. A prospective, multicenter, randomized-controlled 5-year study of hybrid and fully etched implants for the incidence of peri-implantitis. J Periodontol. 2010;81(4):493–501.

Biomechanics

3

Guillaume Odin and Gérard M. Scortecci

3.1 Mechanical Evaluation of Titanium Basal Implants: Fatigue Testing

The fracture of osseointegrated dental implants is always a serious problem. Such fractures are difficult to manage physically, psychologically, and financially for the patient as well as the practitioner. Besides the implant, associated prosthetic components and the attached artificial teeth may also be involved. Basal implants must thus always be safely installed in the major bony buttresses of the jaws in order to properly absorb mechanical stress during masticatory function (Fig. 3.1).

Early Mechanical Tests

A dedicated test machine for investigation of the mechanical properties of dental implants prior to clinical use was developed by Victory (Nice, France) as early as 1996 (Fig. 3.2). As it could reproduce critical situations (in molar and premolar areas) and difficult mechanical conditions such as type I bone, the practical information provided was immediately applicable. In worst-case situations, two forces F1 and F2 (range

G. Odin
ENT and Maxillo-facial Surgery Department, Institut Universitaire de la Face et du Cou, University of Nice-Sophia Antipolis Medical School, Nice, France
e-mail: odin.g@chu-nice.fr

G. M. Scortecci (✉)
University of Nice-Sophia Antipolis Medical School, Nice, France

New York University, New York, NY, USA

University of Southern California, Los Angeles, CA, USA

Private Practice, Nice, France
e-mail: scortecci@wanadoo.fr

© Springer Nature Switzerland AG 2019

G. M. Scortecci (ed.), *Basal Implantology*, https://doi.org/10.1007/978-3-319-44873-2_3

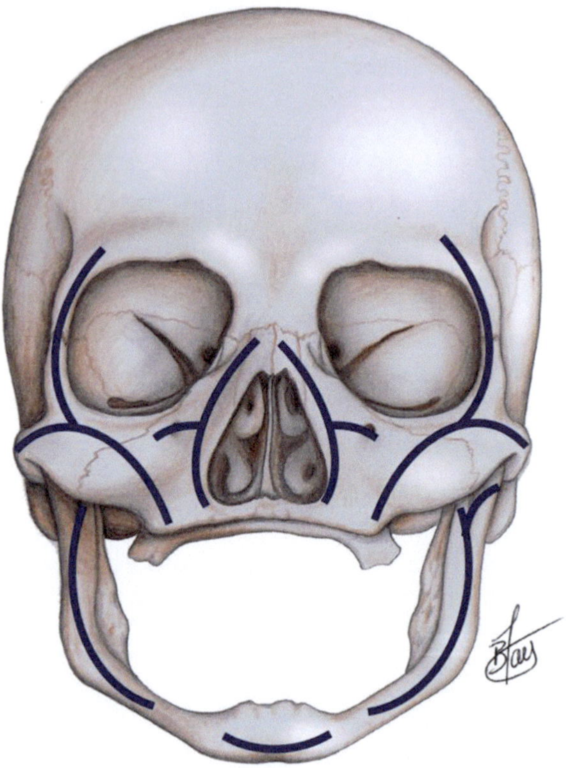

Fig. 3.1 Major maxillomandibular bony buttresses for anchorage of basal implants in severely atrophic jaws

100–400 N at various angles from 0 to 35°) were applied at a distance of 12 mm from the bone level (4 mm transgingival abutment plus 8 mm of tooth height, which is the average height of a human premolar). The system was thermocycled at 37 °C (NaCl 9 g/l), in agreement with oral temperatures. Titanium root-form implants with a diameter of 3.75 mm, the most common type in clinical practice, were selected for calibration purposes. The number of cycles selected as a criterion of resistance (five million) corresponded to a functional lifetime of over 10 years, the recognized desirable duration of an implant at the time (ISO/TC 106/SC8/WG4 N21 ISO/WD 14801, Tokyo, 1995).

Test Protocol

The titanium Diskimplant® was laterally inserted into an Altuglas® support, which has a density similar to that of type D1 bone (Misch classification), and thus corresponds to the worst-case scenario from a mechanical standpoint. A stainless steel cap on a titanium abutment was used to reach a height of 4 mm above the top of the flat Monobloc emergence profile. Secured by a gold screw and Loctite® glue (Henkel), this cap had two inclined surfaces so that the loads were applied perpendicular to their surface. The loads were applied at an angle of 35° with respect to the main axis of the implant by two jacks functioning in alternating manner (distance between the tips of the jacks 6 mm). The frequency was initially set at 0.5 Hz, and the displacement of the cap at point A was measured for 100, 200, 300, and 400 N using a mechanical comparison device. A total of 100 cycles were completed before the load was modified. The same protocol was repeated at frequencies of 1 Hz, 1.5 Hz, 2 Hz, and 2.5 Hz.

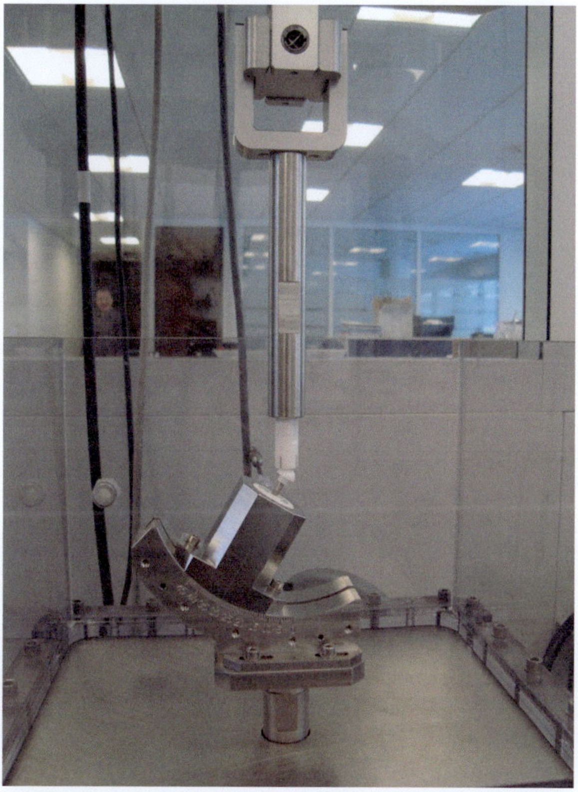

Fig. 3.2 Fatigue testing machine for dental implants (courtesy Hervé Richard, Anthogyr)

Results

Neither the titanium abutment nor the gold screw loosened at any time during testing. This was true for all amplitudes and all loads. As soon as the frequency exceeded 1.5 Hz, the total amplitude of displacement was no longer effective, meaning that we were no longer correctly reproducing the natural model, which has a lower frequency. Below 1.5 Hz, the model appeared to be suitable. The amplitude of displacement was closely correlated with the load applied.

3.2 Finite Element Analysis (Figs. 3.3, 3.4, 3.5, 3.6, 3.7, 3.8, 3.9 and 3.10)

One measure of the success of basal dental implants is their length of service. Long-term results are influenced by the risks of infection, tolerance of the implant material, and distribution of the occlusal forces applied to the implant and surrounding bone. The first two parameters have been extensively evaluated in microbiologic and histologic studies as well as investigations on biomaterials. Stress estimates for systems composed of an implant and adjacent structures were originally calculated by photoelastic stress analysis [1]. Today, increasing use is made of computerized techniques such as finite element analysis (FEA) [2].

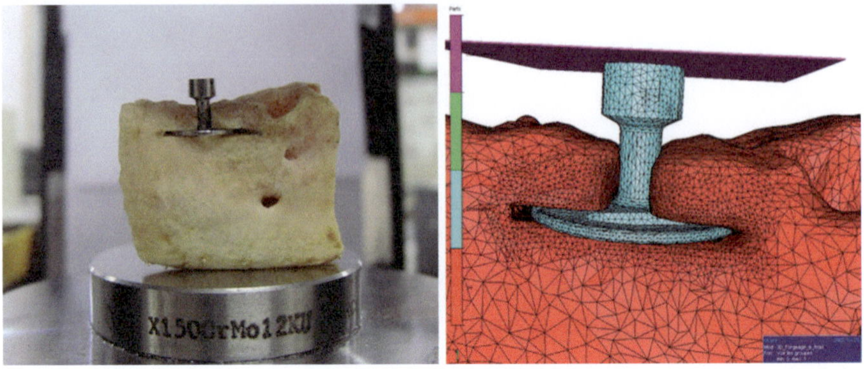

Fig. 3.3 Finite element analysis: Diskimplant® placed at a bone depth of 2 mm (courtesy Prof. G. Odin)

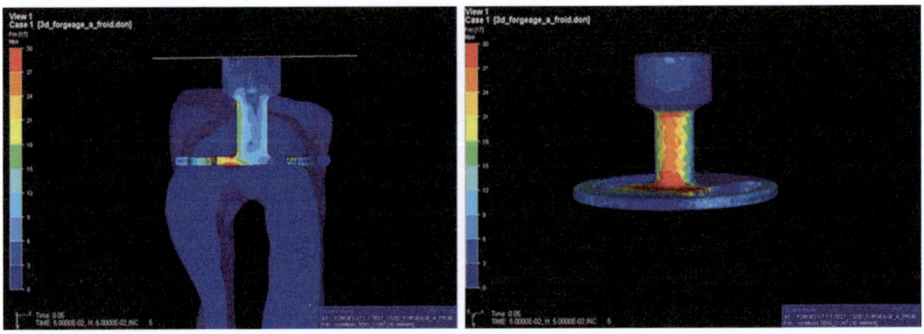

Fig. 3.4 Finite element analysis: monodisk (base diameter 9 mm, shaft diameter 2.35 mm); tricortical anchorage above the mandibular canal (courtesy Prof. G. Odin)

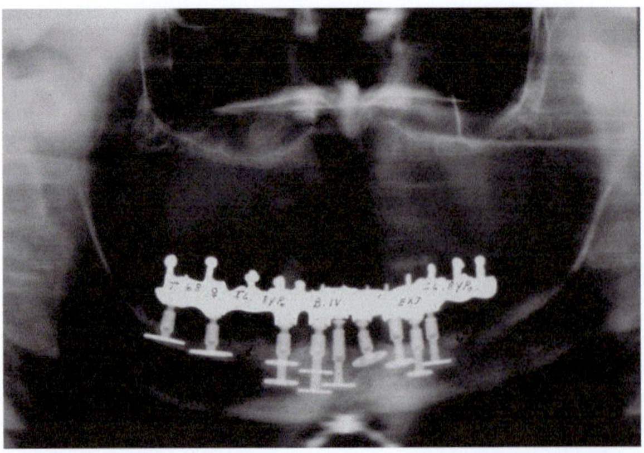

Fig. 3.5 Diskimplant® installed 1.5 mm above the right mandibular canal; 1.2–1.8 mm of bone above the disk (base diameter 9 mm)

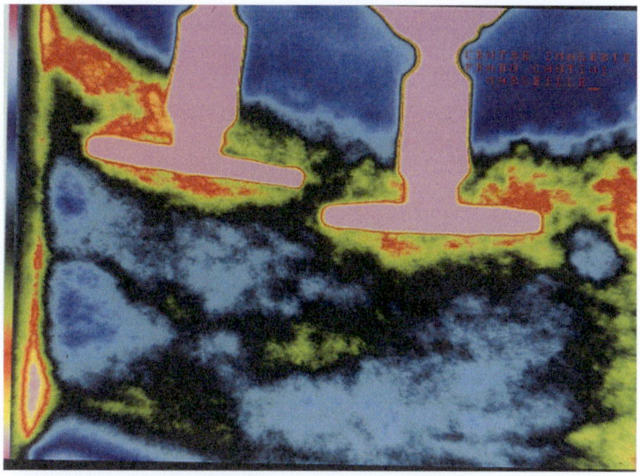

Fig. 3.6 Dense bone around the base of functionally loaded Diskimplants®. The yellow area reveals the dramatic increase in bone density compared to the less dense spongiosa, seen in blue

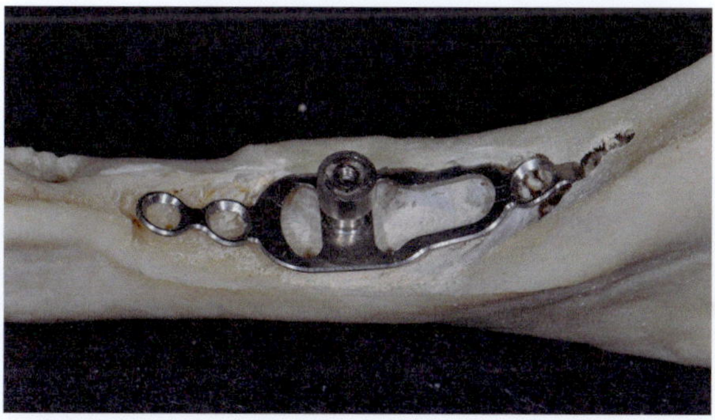

Fig. 3.7 Horizontal plate-form Diskimplant®. The base extends from the buccal cortical plate to the lingual wall. The distance from the mandibular canal is 1.5 mm. The basal implant must be completely covered by bone substitute material and PRF membranes before the full flap is sutured. Whenever possible, a notch should be prepared for the implant in the bone using a titanium cutter or a piezotome

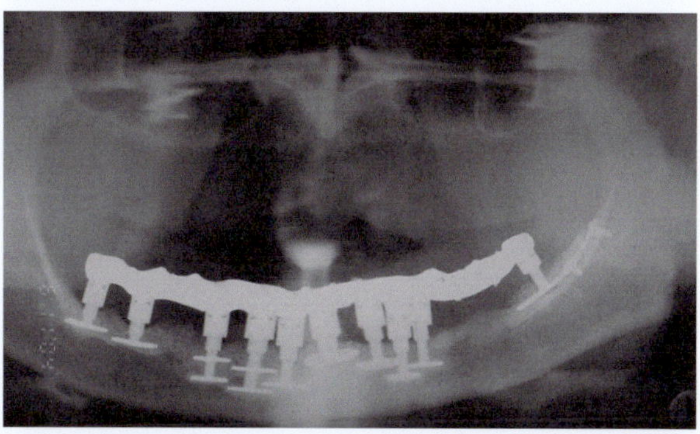

Fig. 3.8 After 15 years of function (1986–2001) (Fig. 3.5), an additional plate-form Diskimplant® was installed in the posterior left mandible to avoid a cantilever. A bone gain of 1.5 mm occurred above the basal implant (panoramic view 2016). Machined *ad modum Brånemark* surface. No sign of peri-implantitis

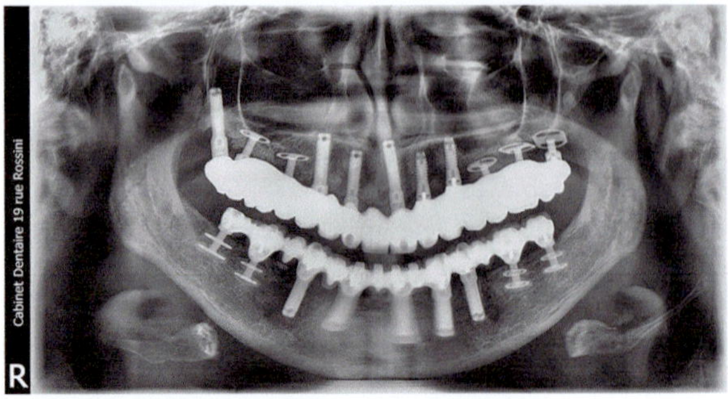

Fig. 3.9 Distal intracortical anchorage in an atrophic knife ridge mandible with two double Diskimplants® on each side. There is no need for cantilevers and mechanical problems with prosthetic components are avoided (panoramic view after 14 years)

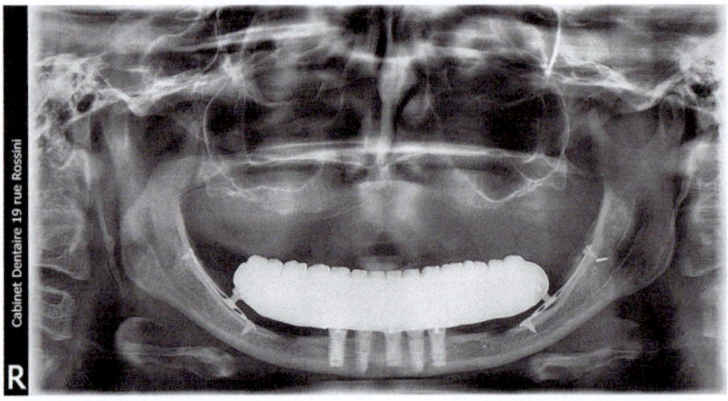

Fig. 3.10 Atrophic posterior mandible (flat shallow ridge) equipped with wide, screw-secured horizontal plate-form Diskimplants®. Five root-form implants were installed between the two foramina (immediate functional loading protocol). Final fixed, screw-secured Zirkonzahn bridge. Panoramic view after 15 years of service (2002–2017)

The distribution of mechanical stress during function of a Diskimplant® differs from that occurring with axially inserted, root-form implants. Comparison of stress distribution by large diameter root-form implants and Diskimplants® (measured along their long axis) has revealed that stress is dissipated more evenly along basal implants. The large horizontal base of the Diskimplant® constitutes the largest bone-anchored diameter and works mainly in compression, as shown by finite element analysis. This geometric design undergoes less dramatic change in stress magnitude along its long axis than a root-form implant. It thus offers better structural stability and transfers stress more evenly to surrounding bone. The cortical support provided by Diskimplants® and horizontal plate-form Diskimplants® also eliminates the zones of deformation seen around root-form implants due to shear stress. The basal implant must be firmly locked in the bone bed in order to neutralize any rotational moment during the healing phase.

3.3 The Stability Principle and Multicortical Anchorage

A proper balance of function and stability in dense living native bone is essential for successful basal implant integration. Primary stability, in particular, is a recognized requirement for the development of a mineralized versus a non-mineralized tissue in areas of mandibular bone fracture [3]. The importance of intracortical stability is highlighted by the fact that instability and/or overload often lead to post-implantation fibrosis (instead of osseointegration) and various complications.

Implant designs providing greater primary stability may thus reduce micromotion to such a degree that bone regeneration is possible even with early loading. A case in point is the disk form implant which offers a geometry compatible with immediate functional loading of full arch restorations, even in extremely resorbed jaws. The major maxillomandibular buttresses of the facial skeleton offer suitable sites of firm anchorage for these purpose-designed basal implants.

Because basal implants are indicated for cases where bone volume is critical and bone density can be unfavorable, intracortical stability is a major determinant of the quality of bone healing. Cortical bone is highly resistant and keeps almost the same structure throughout life, whereas cancellous bone is more sensitive to physiological and biological changes. Dramatic alveolar bone loss can occur around implants due to hormonal changes, especially in menopausal women. In osteoporotic situations, even basal bone may resorb drastically, leading to spontaneous fracture of the mandible. Modifications in bone density during lifetime may partially explain the late loss of osseointegration with root-form implants. They may also contribute to the development of peri-implantitis around root-form implants anchored primarily in cancellous bone or, to a great extent, in bone substitute material. Such implants are also subject to late loss of osseointegration, after 8–10 years of service, due to fatigue microfracture of the spongiosa.

Distal Intracortical Anchorage in Atrophic Jaws

Conventional root-form implants, designed for use in types I, II, III, and IV bone, can be installed when there is a minimum bone height of 8 mm and a bone width of 6 mm. Other clinical situations are better managed with single, double, or triple disk Diskimplants® and plate-form Diskimplants®. The base of the Diskimplant® must engage both cortical plates (buccolingual/palatal); placement in a single cortical plate or in the middle of fragile type IV spongiosa is insufficient. Other means to increase initial, reliable long-lasting stability in basal bone includes stabilization with orthopedic screws and the use of double-disk Diskimplants® and screw-secured plate-form Diskimplants®.

In the maxilla, Diskimplants® or pterygoid Fractal® implants can be placed in the tubero-pterygoid area to obtain the desired distal cortical support. Distal anchorage in the molar sector of the atrophic mandible is safely provided by single- or double-disk Diskimplants® or wide (33 × 9 mm or 43 × 9 mm) screw-secured, plate-form Diskimplants®. Distal anchorage avoids the need for a cantilever, thereby reducing fatigue of the bone-anchored assembly.

3.4 Number of Basal Implants Required (Figs. 3.11, 3.12 and 3.13)

Reliance on root-form implants alone may necessitate prior bone grafting and/or GBR in areas of bone resorption. In totally edentulous patients, unfavorable bone density and/or geometry in the posterior jaw areas may result in compromises in

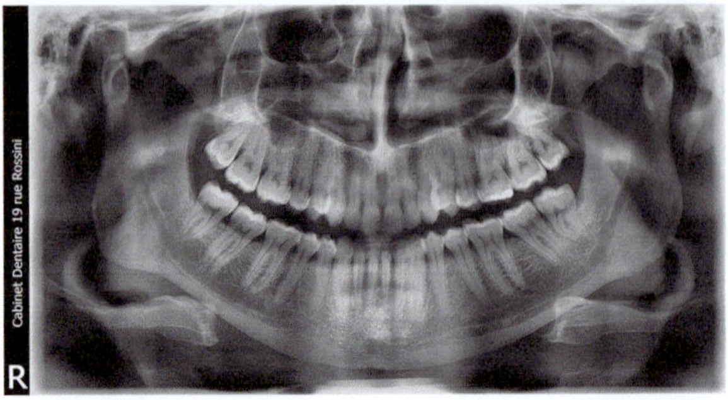

Fig. 3.11 Complete set of natural teeth, including wisdom teeth. As a result of natural selection, molars have more roots to be able to withstand the high masticatory forces in the posterior sectors

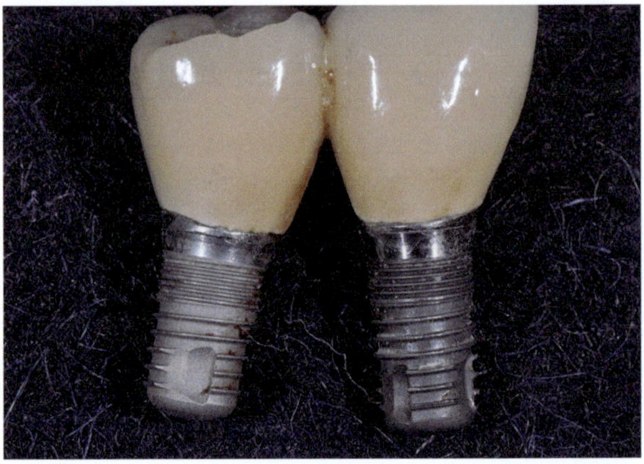

Fig. 3.12 After a 5-year period of clinical success, these two short implants (diameter 4.2 mm, height 6 mm) lost their initial osseointegration in the mandibular molar sector

treatment planning, such as placement of a minimal number of root-form implants solely in the premaxilla and/or mental area and fabrication of a bridge with a distal cantilever. This, in turn, can lead to metal fatigue and subsequent fracture after 4–5 years of service. In other instances, a technically complex and time-consuming bone graft procedure might be needed prior to root-form implant installation.

Including wisdom teeth, the upper jaw has a total of 30 roots, while the lower jaw has 24 roots that support masticatory function over lifetime. Each maxillary molar is "equipped" with three roots as the result of natural selection over millions of years, yet certain clinicians, owing to the paucity of residual alveolar bone, still attempt to manage this mechanically demanding sector with wide, short, or even ultra-short (5 or 6 mm in height) root-form implants. Almost all implant candidates can recover a normal occlusal relationship in the molar area, thanks to strong, distal basal implant support in dense bone as opposed to a reduced prosthetic device with a cantilever.

In the extremely resorbed edentulous mandible and maxilla, the size, location, number, and shape of basal implants plus the design of the corresponding highly rigid, screw-secured fixed prosthesis are fundamental in achieving predictable, reproducible, and durable results as a function of the patient's age and physical condition, including muscle tone. For the completely edentulous maxilla, six to ten implants are usually sufficient for an immediate loading protocol. For the mandible,

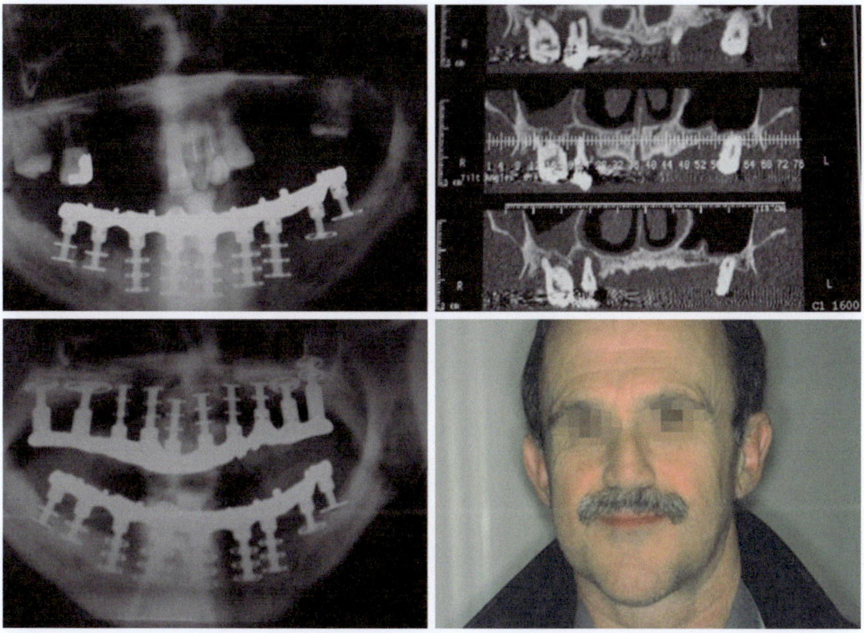

Fig. 3.13 Atrophic maxilla and mandible: high knife ridges. Buccal-lingual/palatal bone thickness ≤ 3 mm. Immediate loading protocol (handicapped patient). No cantilever was used. Panoramic view after 21 years of service (1995–2016). The number of basal implants installed is related to the number of natural roots present in the area

five to nine implants are required for immediate loading (use of a small cantilever or no cantilever at all depends on the number of implants placed).

Important hormonal changes appear in women over age 50, a possible consequence being severe alveolar bone loss. Even well-osseointegrated root-form implants 8–11 mm long can be lost, and great care should thus be taken when considering ultra-short implants. Installation of an adequate number of cortically anchored basal implants, respecting the principle of absolute intracortical stability, remains the guiding policy for implant treatments designed for long-term success (≥10 years).

Severely Atrophic, Completely Edentulous Jaws: An Indication for Immediate Loading

Use of a removable full denture by a patient during the healing phase for submerged basal implants is the main cause of primary implant loss before osseointegration can occur. This is understandable because stress is placed on each implant individually during chewing, clenching, speaking, etc. In contrast, a highly rigid, screw-secured-to-implant fixed bridge prevents micromovements, primary loss of osseointegration, early infection, bone loss, etc. In some situations, a bone gain is observed.

In highly atrophic, eggshell-thin maxillae, a temporary transpalatal bar connected to the fixed, screw-secured basal implant prosthesis provides immediate cross-arch stabilization and reduces stress on the underlying bone. This bar can be removed after 6–12 months (Figs. 3.17, 3.18, 3.19 and 3.20). The passive fit of the implant-supported prosthesis and atraumatic occlusal conditions help maintain osseointegration of the implant during function, with very little, if any, bone loss over time. Interestingly, increased bone density and even increased bone volume have been observed after years of function in atrophic mandibles managed with fixed, basal implant-supported prostheses [4].

Rigid External Fixation: An Orthopedic Concept (Figs. 3.14, 3.15, 3.16 and 3.17)

For completely edentulous atrophic jaws treated by basal implants placed immediately in function, the occlusal section of the prosthetic appliance and the cortically anchored implant material are of equal importance in maintaining an accurate and functional inter-arch relationship (i.e., occlusion between the upper and lower teeth). Postoperative occlusal stability must be guaranteed during function by means of a fixed, rigidly splinted-to-implant prosthesis and well-balanced tooth-to-tooth relationships. This rigid appliance serves a purpose similar to external fixation in orthopedic surgery: it protects the implants from micromovements during the

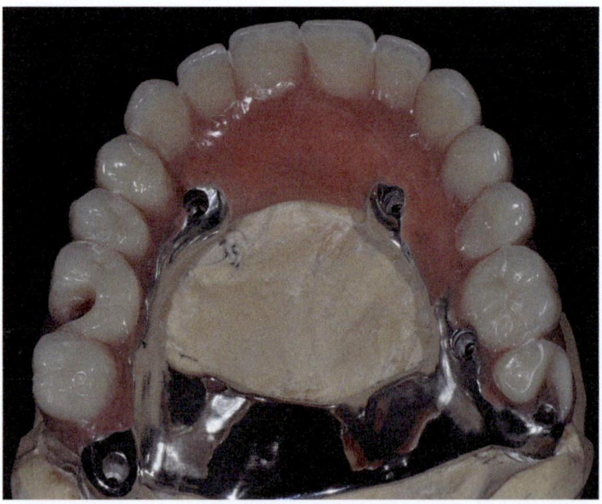

Fig. 3.14 Atrophic eggshell maxilla. After losing eight maxillary root-form implants, this patient wore a removable full denture for 2 years. Because her maxilla was totally flat, large amounts of denture adhesive cream were required to hold the appliance in place. After osteogenic preparation 60 days prior to surgery, four basal implants and two pterygoid implants were placed and connected together with a highly rigid, chromium-cobalt/titanium framework. Cross-arch stabilization was obtained with a solid transpalatal bar (no added parts or welds)

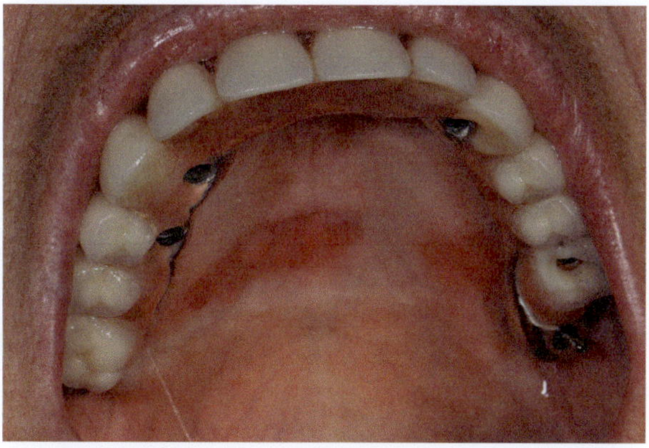

Fig. 3.15 Intraoral view of the highly rigid, fixed prosthesis screw-secured to basal implants. After each implant was checked individually, the smooth, one-piece palatal bar was removed 1-year postop (same patient as Fig. 3.14)

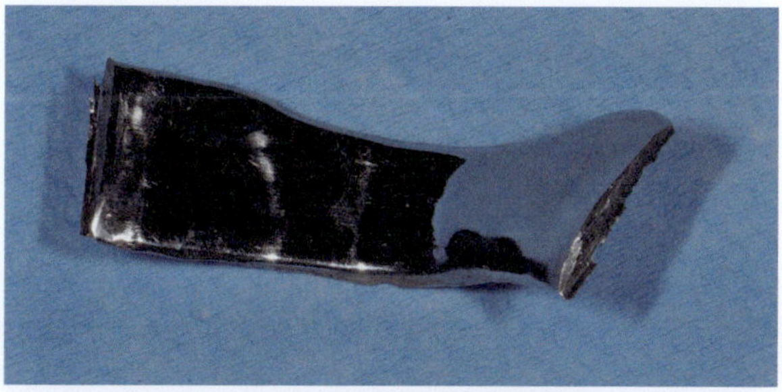

Fig. 3.16 The transpalatal bar (0.6 mm thick, width ≥ 10 mm) must extend from molar to molar

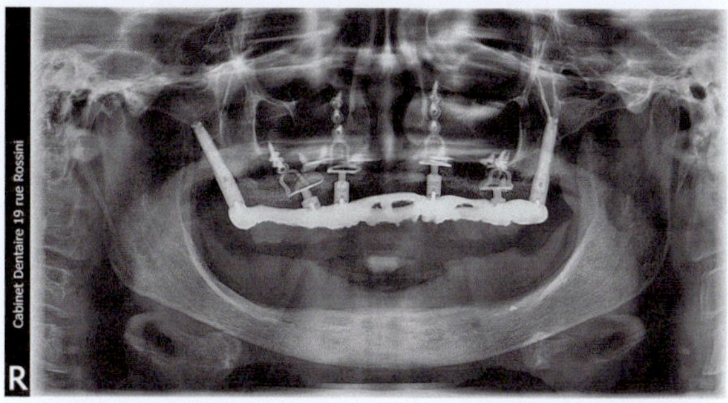

Fig. 3.17 Panoramic view 4 years postop, after removal of the transpalatal bar (same patient as Figs. 3.14, 3.15 and 3.16)

osseointegration process, thereby facilitating bone reconstruction while preventing displacement and allows the patient to rapidly return to a normal lifestyle.

Partial Edentulism: A Two-Stage Procedure Remains the Safest Option (Figs. 3.18, 3.19 and 3.20)

For single-tooth replacements and Kennedy class I and II situations, the most reliable procedure for Diskimplant® success is to leave the implants submerged under

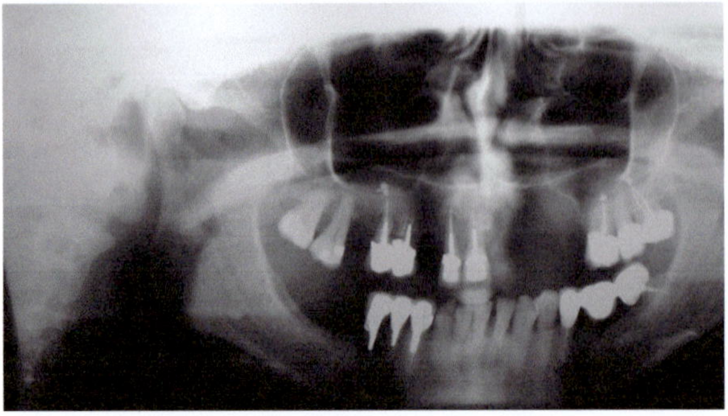

Fig. 3.18 Panoramic view in 1991. Treatment planning for partial edentulism must be mechanically oriented because remaining natural teeth affected by ongoing periodontal disease may be lost over time. This patient wore removable upper and lower dentures

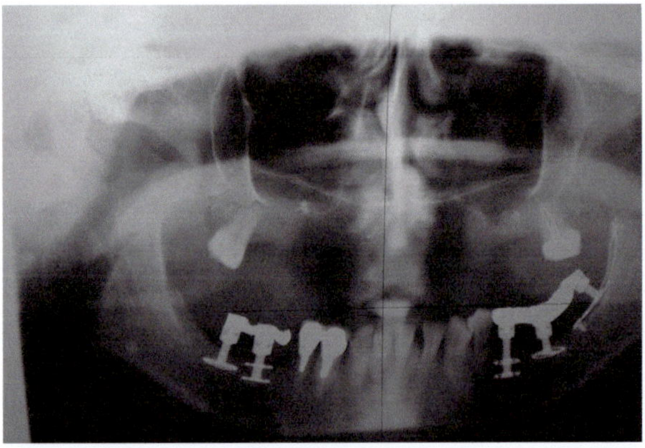

Fig. 3.19 In 1992, the second lower right premolar fractured. A monodisk Diskimplant® and a double-disk Diskimplant® were installed in the molar area when the fractured tooth was removed. Delayed loading procedure. In 2000, the lower left posterior teeth had to be extracted; a double-disk, a single-disk, and a plate-form Diskimplant® were installed (immediate loading procedure). Many maxillary teeth had become loose and were also extracted. An immediate, partial removable denture was fabricated (same patient as Fig. 3.18)

the periosteum for 6 months and let the tissues heal without functional loading. Immediate functional loading is only possible in selected cases where occlusal conditions are favorable.

3.5 Flat Emergence Profile and Passive Fit (Figs. 3.21, 3.22, 3.23, 3.24 and 3.25)

When anatomic conditions prevent parallel installation of implants, various types of abutments can be used to finalize the prosthetic project: commercial or personalized angulated abutments, UCLA abutments, Monobloc flat emergence transgingival abutment, etc. Direct prosthetic connection to implants with a flat emergence profile widens the possibilities for management of problems due to undesirable angulation

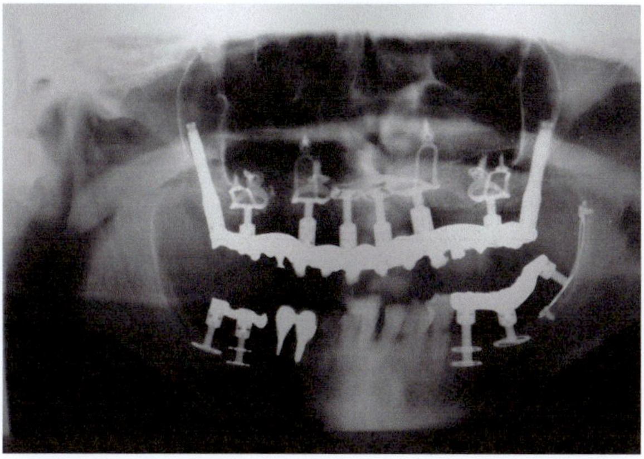

Fig. 3.20 After 6 months, in February 2001, the patient requested fixed implant-supported teeth in the upper jaw. Six basal implants and two pterygoid root-form implants were installed, and an immediate, screw-secured prosthesis was placed. Panoramic view showing the 45° difference in angulation between the pterygoid root-form implant (Fractal, Victory, France) and the zygomatic basal implant managed thanks to the flat Monobloc emergence profile. Panoramic status 16 years postop (March 2017) (same patient as Figs. 3.18 and 3.19)

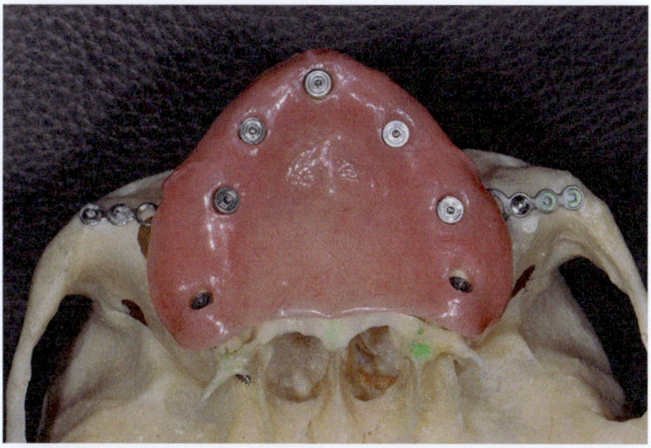

Fig. 3.21 Dry atrophic maxilla. Note the considerable difference in angulation between the basal Diskimplant® and the root-form pterygoid implant, both featuring the same Monobloc flat emergence profile

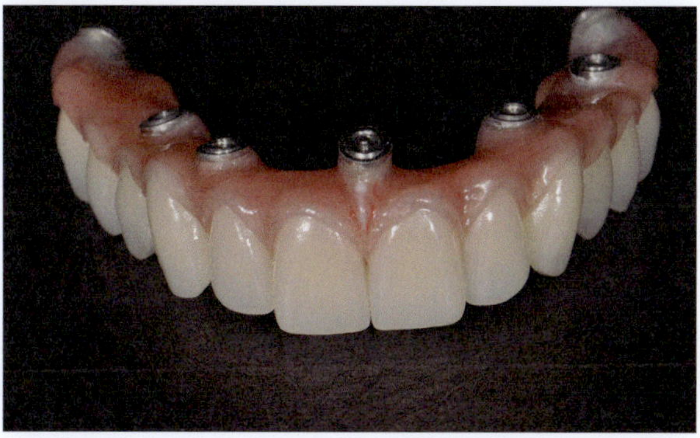

Fig. 3.22 Maxillary prosthesis with machined flat titanium copings to be screw-secured onto implants with a Monobloc flat emergence profile

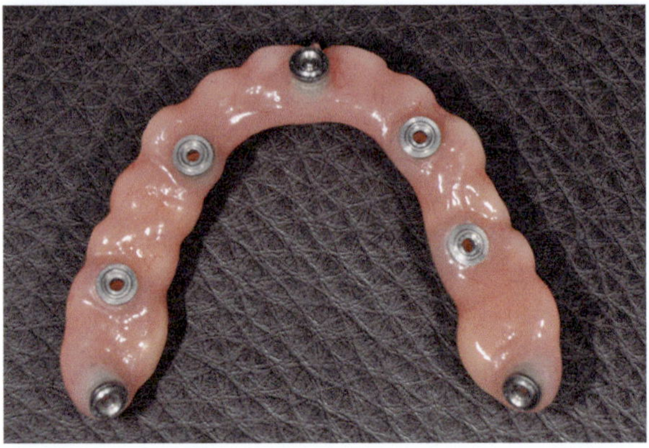

Fig. 3.23 Internal view of the flat connecting components

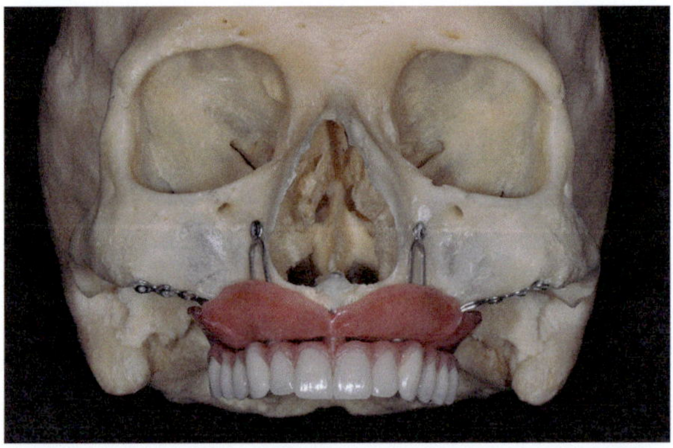

Fig. 3.24 Prosthesis in place: compression forces are transmitted to the main basal pillars of the atrophic maxilla

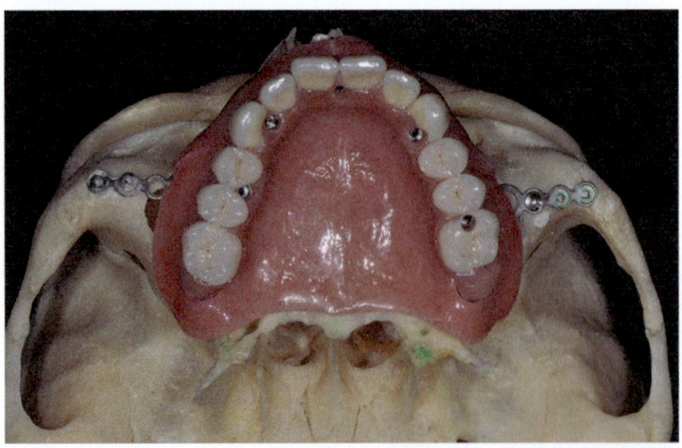

Fig. 3.25 Occlusal view of the prosthesis screw-secured to the extramaxillary zygomatic Diskimplant®

(Table 3.1). First introduced by Victory (Nice, France) in 2000, the Monobloc flat emergence profile characteristic of Diskimplants® facilitates impression taking regardless of implant angulation, allows easy access for maintenance, and ensures improved stress distribution during function. This profile serves as a reliable base

Table 3.1 Prosthetic possibilities for various types of abutments

	Angle correction (degrees)			Passive fit (%)			Compression stress (%)			Shear stress (%)		
	0–15°	0–30°	0–90°	70%	85%	100%	30	70	90	70	30	10
Flat Monobloc connection			X			X			X			X
Angulated abutment	X			X			X			X		
Multiunit		X			X			X			X	

for the connection of a Monobloc transgingival abutment or a hex abutment post for cemented restorations. Passive fit of the prosthesis, which must be checked radiologically after placement of the prosthesis, is facilitated for screw-retained single-tooth restorations by use of a transparent occlusal guide. A positioning screw compatible with the Monobloc emergence thread (M1.4) is helpful to position a multiunit bridge while retaining screws are placed. More recently, firms such as Anthogyr (2016) and Nobel Biocare (2017) have introduced similar emergence profile designs.

Conflict of interest statement Gérard M. Scortecci is the inventor of the Diskimplant and holder of several associated patents that are exploited by the Victory company. He is an unpaid consultant to this firm and a minority shareholder in the company. No money was received from any of the companies mentioned in the book or from any of the companies whose products are mentioned.

Recommended Reading

1. Michel M, Veyret D, Pantaloni J, Martin R. Analyse comparative par éléments finis d'implants odontologiques avec et sans appui cortical. Chirurgien-Dentiste de France. 1990;510:83–9.
2. Odin G, Savoldelli C, Bouchard P, Tillier Y. Determination of Young's modulus of mandibular bone using inverse analysis. Med Eng Phys. 2010;32(6):630–7.
3. Speissl B, editor. Internal fixation of the mandible. Berlin: Springer; 1989.
4. Scortecci G. L'implant tricortical: Intégration Biologique, Recherche Fondamentale et Applications Cliniques. PhD thesis. University of Marseilles, France; 1988.
5. Albrektsson T. The interface zone of inorganic implants in vivo. Titanium implants in bone. Ann Biomed Eng. 1983;11:1–27.
6. Balshi TJ. An analysis and management of fractured implants: a clinical report. Int J Oral Maxillofac Impl. 1996;11:660–6.
7. Borak L, Marcian P, Floran Z, Bartakova S. Biomechanical study of disk implants. Part I. Eng Mech. 2010;17(1):49–60.
8. Branemark PI, Hansson BO, Adell R. Osseointegrated implants in the treatment of the edentulous jaw. Experience from a 10-year study period. Scand J Plast Reconstr Surg. 1977;16:1–132.
9. Cassetta M, Di Mambro A, Giansanti M, Brandetti G. The survival of Morse cone-connection implants with platform switch. Int J Oral Maxillofac Implants. 2016;31(5):1031–9.
10. Idhe S. Principles of BIO. Berlin: Springer; 2004.
11. Jaffin RA, Berman CL. The excessive loss of Brånemark fixtures in type IV bone: a 5-year analysis. J Periodontol. 1991;62:2–4.
12. Kasemo B. Biocompatibility of titanium implants: surface science aspects. J Prosthet Dent. 1983;49(6):832.

13. Marcian P, Florian Z, Borak L, Krpalek D, Valasek J. Biomechanical study of disk implants, part I and part II. Eng Mech. 2010;17(2):111–21.
14. Odin G. Modélisation numérique de l'os mandibulaire appliquée à l'implantologie dentaire et maxillo-faciale. Modélisation et simulation. Thesis. Ecole Nationale Supérieure des Mines de Paris; 2008.
15. Pantaloni J, et al. Biomechanics. In: Scortecci G, Misch CE, Benner U, editors. Implants and restorative dentistry. London: Martin Dunitz; 2001.
16. Savoldelli C, Tillier Y, Bouchard PO, Odin G. Apport de la méthode des éléments finis en chirurgie maxillofaciale. Rev Stomatol Chir Maxillofac. 2009;110(1):27–33.
17. Scortecci G. Le Diskimplant. Implantol Oral. 1984;16:26–32.
18. Scortecci G, Misch CE, Benner KU. Implants and restorative dentistry. London: Martin Dunitz; 2001.
19. Scortecci G, Modschiedler T. Ostéointégration et mise en fonction immédiate: 15 ans de recherche et d'application clinique dans le traitement du maxillaire totalement édenté. Implantodontie. 1997;24:1–28.
20. Scortecci G, Meyere P, Zattara H, Doms P. Intra-oral applications in small bone volumes. Patient selection and long-term results. In: Laney W, Tolman D, editors. Tissue integration in Oral, Orthopedic and Maxillofacial Reconstruction. Chicago: Quintessence; 1990. p. 350–5.
21. Seckinger RJ. A three-dimensional finite element stress analysis in and around the ISIS endosseous dental implant. MS thesis. University of Pittsburgh School of Dental Medicine, USA; 1989.
22. Sennerby L. On the bone tissue response to titanium implants. PhD thesis. Gothenborg, Sweden; 1991.
23. Tillier Y. De la caractérisation mécanique du comportement des matériaux à la modélisation biomécanique par éléments finis; Applications à la simulation chirurgicale et au développement de dispositifs médicaux. Matériaux. Ecole Nationale Supérieure des Mines de Paris; 2013.
24. Tillier Y, Paccini M, Durand-Réville JL. Three-dimensional finite element simulation of surgery: from material forming to biomechanics. ESAFORM Bull. 2004;4(1). ISBN: 1294 12-6222.

Evidence-Based Basal Implantology

4

Gérard M. Scortecci and Guillaume Odin

4.1 Diskimplants®: Continuous Improvement from 1984 to the Present

The first generation of laterally inserted, tricortical artificial titanium dental roots was patented and commercialized in 1984 under the name Diskimplants® [1, 2]. The T3D precursor basal implant of 1974 was not tricortical because the horizontal base remained essentially in the spongiosa. Based on computerized analysis of implant geometries and their indications as a function of bone density, volume, and anatomy plus the mechanical and biological properties of titanium, Diskimplants® are designed to achieve primary multicortical support even in very small bone volumes and weak bone densities not directly accessible to root-form implants. The basic concept is achievement of bi-cortical buccolingual (or palatal) anchorage in addition to crestal anchorage [2–71].

At the outset, the titanium cutter (osteotome) used for lateral osteotomy was left in place to serve as the implant. The slightly larger, identically shaped first-generation Diskimplant® with an external thread was developed soon afterward. The system and results of initial applications were first officially presented at the World Implantology Congress in Munich, Germany, in June 1984 [1]. Double and triple

G. M. Scortecci (✉)
University of Nice-Sophia Antipolis Medical School, Nice, France

New York University, New York, NY, USA

University of Southern California, Los Angeles, CA, USA

Private Practice, Nice, France
e-mail: scortecci@wanadoo.fr

G. Odin
ENT and Maxillo-facial Surgery Department, Institut Universitaire de la Face et du Cou, University of Nice-Sophia Antipolis Medical School, Nice, France
e-mail: odin.g@chu-nice.fr

© Springer Nature Switzerland AG 2019

G. M. Scortecci (ed.), *Basal Implantology*, https://doi.org/10.1007/978-3-319-44873-2_4

Diskimplants® were developed thereafter, followed by improved implant emergence profiles (external hexagon, flat Monobloc emergence profile combining an external hexagon and a Morse cone, internal octagon).

The wide plate-form Diskimplants® that are used in combination with osteosynthesis screws were developed starting in January 2000 for the management of extremely atrophic jaws and fractured mandibles without recourse to prior bone grafting. The year 2005 saw the addition of bone matrix osseotensors for presurgery bone bed preparation to improve the blood supply and bone quality at the future implant site (Figs. 4.1, 4.2, 4.3, 4.4 and 4.5). In 2013, use of a temporary transpalatal bar for extremely atrophic, eggshell maxillae was generalized in order to guarantee absolute immediate stability of basal bone-anchored fixed full-arch restorations.

Today, basal implants are most often used to treat difficult anatomic situations where traditional root-form implants cannot be placed directly unless associated with other procedures such as bone grafting, nerve displacement, bone distraction, GBR, etc. This must be kept in mind when comparing statistics on success and failure rates. Excluding early implant failures, multicenter studies on the Diskimplant® system after, respectively, 9 and 30 years yielded success rates of 85–92%, which is comparable to the results reported for titanium root-form implants [71, 72]. For basal implants installed in atrophic jaws, the criterion for success is usually set at a minimum of 85% after 5 years of service and 80% after 10 years (Table 4.1).

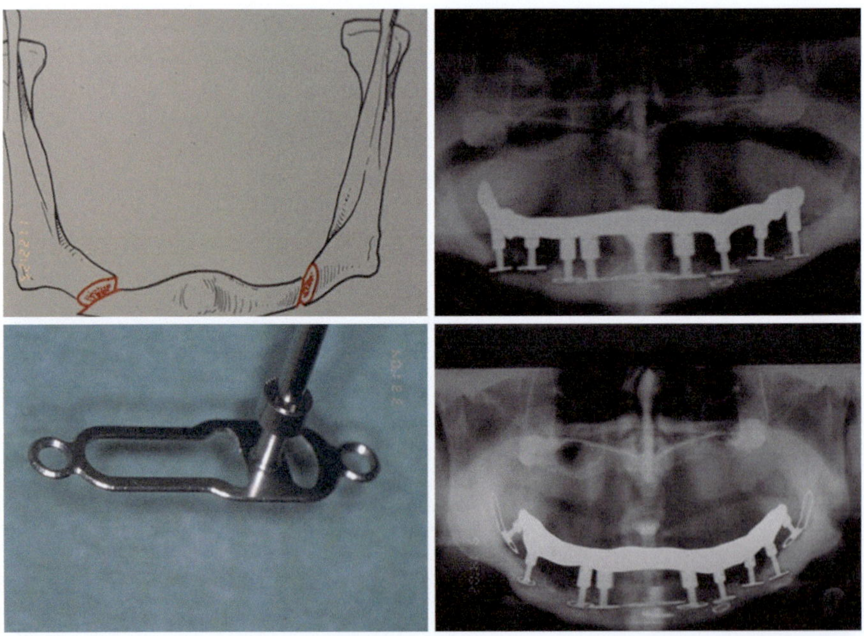

Fig. 4.1 Six years after Diskimplant® placement, this patient fell and fractured her posterior pencil mandible in December 1999. Two plate-form Diskimplants® were installed in January 2000. Panoramic aspect 4 years postop (Feb. 2004)

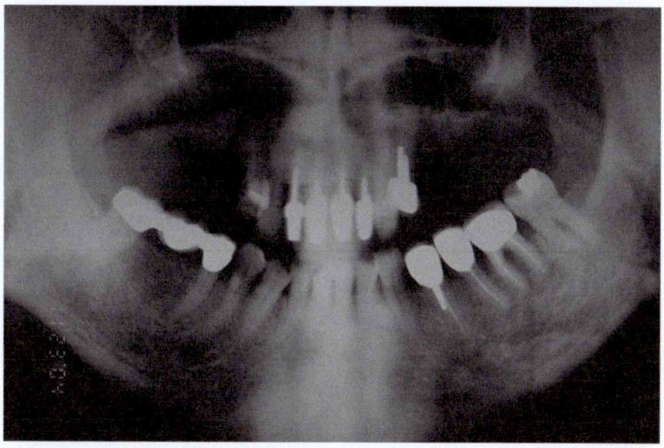

Fig. 4.2 Panoramic view of the initial status. First-generation, horizontal plate-form Diskimplants® were installed at a bone depth of 0.8–1.1 mm in the atrophic, upper right posterior maxilla of this 71-year-old woman (non-submerged approach)

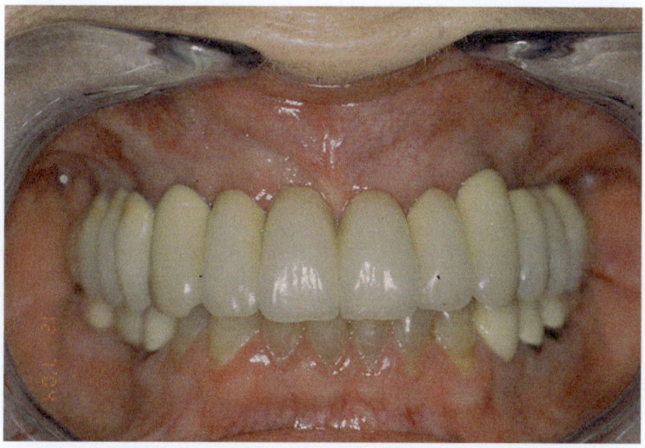

Fig. 4.3 Ceramic-baked-to-metal bridge screw-secured to basal implants placed after the patient used a screw-secured transitional fixed prosthesis with acrylic teeth for 1 year (same patient as Fig. 4.2)

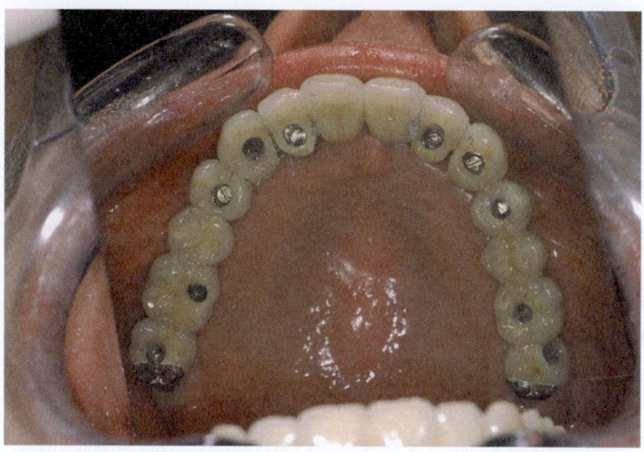

Fig. 4.4 Intraoral occlusal view of the screw-secured restoration. The screw access holes were closed with Teflon™ and composite

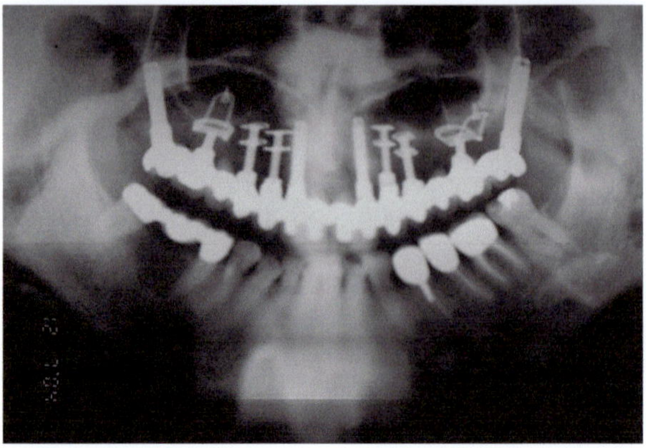

Fig. 4.5 Panoramic view 15 years postop (2000–2015). Two zygomatic plate-form Diskimplants® were placed in the infra-sinus, first molar region on both sides

Table 4.1 Proposed criteria for basal implant success

1. An individual basal implant is immobile in all directions when tested clinically
2. An individual basal implant with no complaints from the patient and no clinical symptoms (no pain, infection, or inflammation; soft tissues healthy) that is slightly mobile when tested manually does not need to be removed
3. A radiograph may demonstrate minor peri-implant radiolucency that is of no clinical significance (i.e., no pain or infection). Isolated radiologic findings of this nature are not the cause for removal of a Diskimplant®, especially if it has been in service for years without any complaint from the patient
4. Vertical bone loss around the implant is <0.2 mm annually following the first year of service
5. Individual implant performance is characterized by an absence of persistent and/or irreversible signs and symptoms, such as pain, mobility, infection, neuropathies, or paresthesia
6. The cosmetic outcome fulfills the patient's reasonable expectations in light of his or her initial status

4.2 Long-Term Clinical Studies of Basal Implants

Single-Center Study of Laterally Inserted T3D Basal Implants (Follow-Up 42 Years) (Fig. 4.6)

In 1974 and 1975, eight titanium T3D implants (the precursor of the Diskimplant®) with a machined surface finish were installed in seven patients (five women, two men) ranging in age from 28 to 42 years at the time of implant placement. All of the implants were immediately loaded (free-standing or connected with natural teeth). Two of these patients were available for follow-up in 2017. Their T3D implants were still functional, without any signs of peri-implantitis, and no bone loss had occurred. Due to the difficult freehand surgical protocol in which a carbide dental bur was used to laterally prepare the "T-shaped" osteotomy, T3D implants were abandoned in favor of easier-to-install Diskimplants®. Development of calibrated, one-piece titanium cutters greatly facilitated implant surgery and opened the way for widespread diffusion of the Diskimplant® technique.

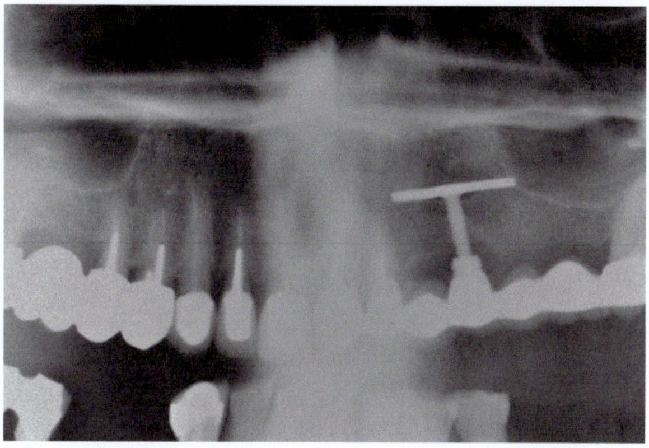

Fig. 4.6 T3D implant placed in 1974 and still in service in 2016 (42 years). Machined surface state, no sign of peri-implantitis

Table 4.2 Early multicenter study of 5848 Diskimplants® placed between 1979 and 1989

Year	Number of patients	Women	Men	Total implants/ year	Failed implants	Healthy implants
1979	11	7	4	31	0 (0)	31 (100%)
1980	92	62	30	246	40 (16%)	206 (84%)
1981	117	88	29	316	63 (20%)	253 (80%)
1982	128	97	31	381	58 (15%)	323 (85%)
1983	132	99	33	405	52 (13%)	353 (87%)
1984	146	116	30	438	46 (10.5%)	392 (89.5%)
1985	172	121	51	506	40 (8%)	466 (92%)
1986	189	122	67	612	38 (6.2%)	574 (93.8%)
1987	213	132	81	780	32 (4.1%)	748 (95.5%)
1988	272	185	87	960	46 (4.8%)	914 (95.2%)
1989	295	202	93	1203	85 (7%)	1118 (93%)
Total	1588	1061	527	5848	590 (10.9%)	5258 (89.1%)

NB: 1979–1984 corresponded to a period of limited clinical trials

Early Multicenter Analysis of the Outcome of 5848 Diskimplants® (1979–1989) (Table 4.2)

A total of 1588 patients (1061 women, 527 men) ranging in age from 14 to 84 years (average 58.2 years; 65% were older than 58 years) were equipped with Diskimplants® over a 9-year period, including early clinical trials (1979–1984). Two 14-year-old patients received implants during this period. Today, the consensus is to wait until patients reach 18–20 years and have completed their growth. An exception is young patients with total agenesis, as can occur in ectodermal dysplasia. These Diskimplants® were placed at 12 different centers (Germany, three; Italy, two; Switzerland, two; Belgium, two; and France, three centers). Only 482 patients were followed up regularly over 9 years; the 429 patients lost to follow-up were not included in the 1989 survey. As of June 2017, only four of the patients in this first treatment population were still being seen for their annual checkup (Figs. 4.7, 4.8, 4.9, 4.10, 4.11, 4.12, 4.13, 4.14, 4.15, 4.16, 4.17, 4.18 and 4.19).

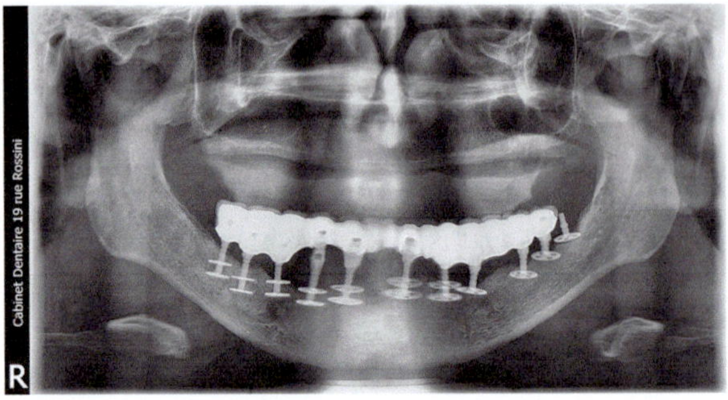

Fig. 4.7 This patient received 11 Diskimplants® in the lower jaw in 1984 (one of the implants is not prosthetically useful, but the patient refused to have it removed because there was no pain and the implant was completely stable, even though located in less than 1 mm of bone). The patient was lost to follow-up from 1985 to 2015 but returned in 2016 to request implants in the upper jaw, at which time this panoramic radiograph was taken

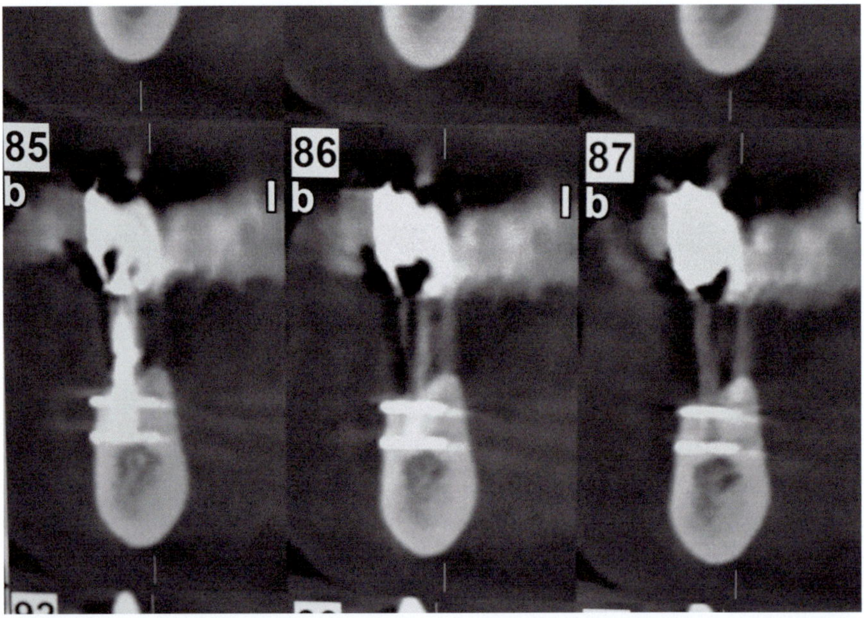

Fig. 4.8 Cone beam CT (same patient as Fig. 4.7). This double Diskimplant® (distance between two disks 3 mm) was placed 1.4 mm beneath the crest and is still in service after 32 years (non-modified titanium surface)

The criterion for determining success was survival of the implant and not the fixed prosthesis. Failure analysis was carried out by two radiologists and two experienced clinicians by means of a survey listing factors commonly observed with failed implants. Practitioners were requested to identify any factor or group of factors that may have contributed to failure and then make a subjective judgment as to

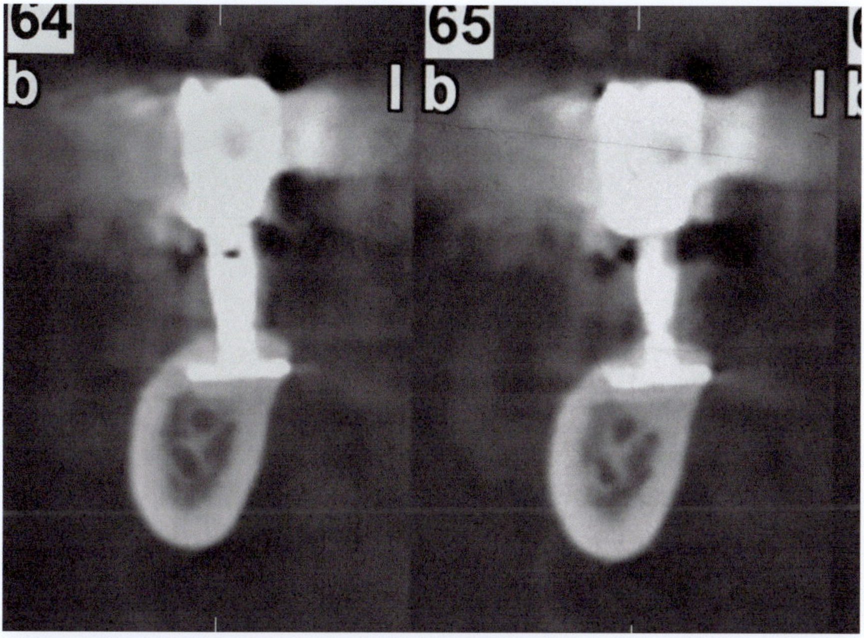

Fig. 4.9 Same patient as Fig. 4.7. Tomographic view after 32 years of service (1984–2016). This Diskimplant® (disk base diameter 7 mm) was installed 1.6 mm above the mandibular canal and 1.4 mm beneath the bone crest. No peri-implantitis or bone loss

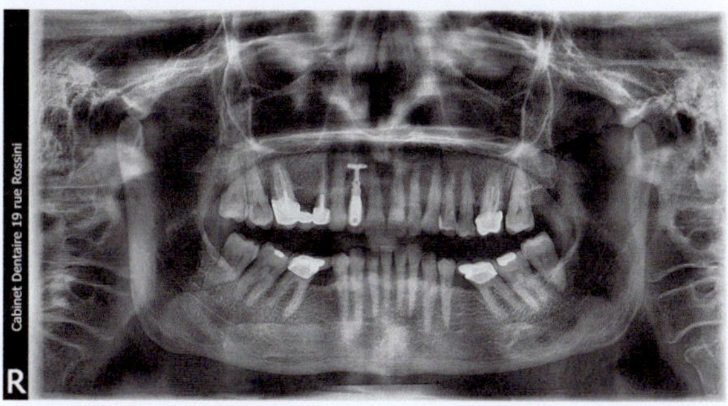

Fig. 4.10 Mono-disk Diskimplant® installed in 1984 for replacement of a single tooth (delayed loading protocol) (courtesy of Dr. Christian Bezzina). In 2016, after 32 years of service, a digital panoramic view showed the perfectly osseointegrated implant, without any bone loss

the primary cause (i.e., surgical wound healing failure, early peri-implantitis, late peri-implantitis, prosthodontic failure, unknown, etc.). Of the 590 failures identified in the database, 272 were included in completed surveys that were returned for analysis (89 were in the molar region, 82 were in the premolar region, and 101 were in the anterior area). Failed implants were generally not discovered until abutment connection was attempted, and the specific reasons for the lack of osseointegration were thus purely speculative.

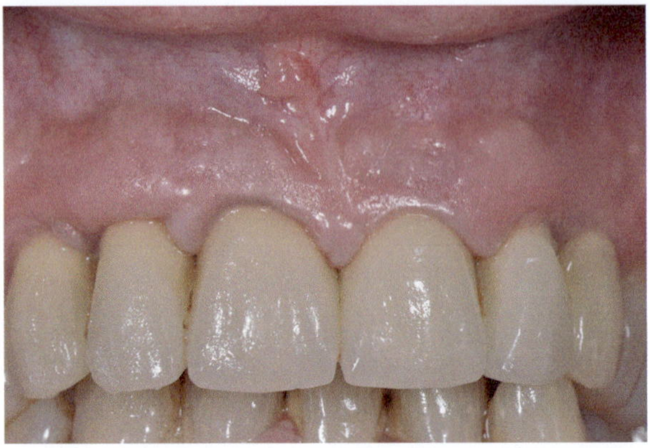

Fig. 4.11 Cosmetic aspect after 31 years of service: thick gingival biotype around the six Diskimplant®-supported front teeth (canine to canine)

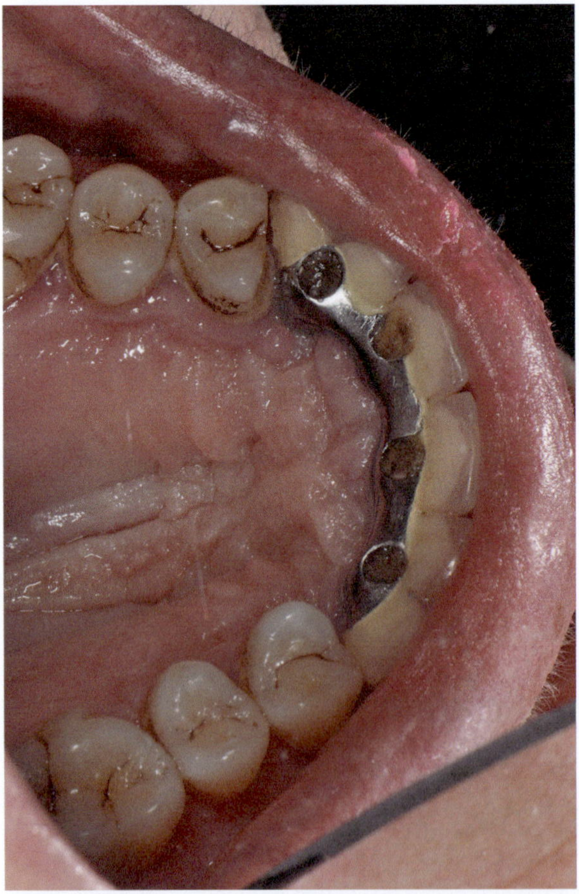

Fig. 4.12 Intraoral view of the screw-secured, 6-element ceramic-to-metal bridge supported by basal implants

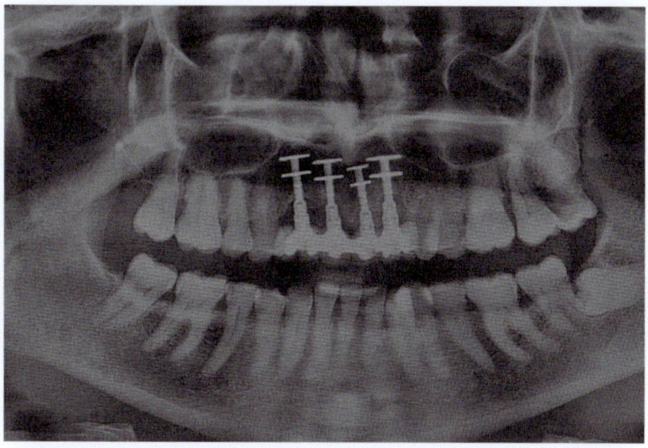

Fig. 4.13 Panoramic view after 31 years of service: the six front teeth were lost following facial trauma. Rehabilitation with four double Diskimplants® did not require bone grafting prior to implant installation

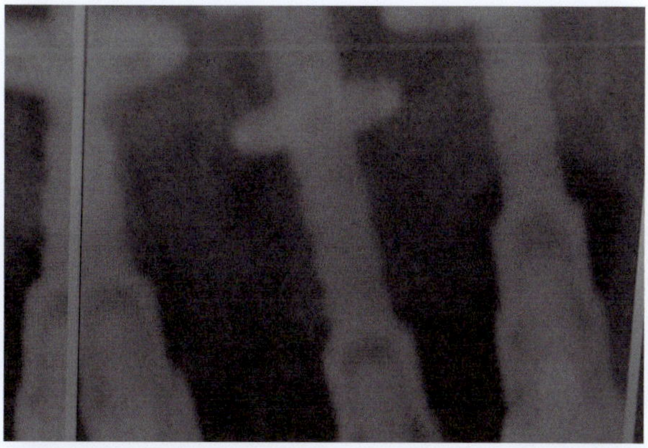

Fig. 4.14 Periapical radiograph at 31 years. No bone loss visible in this thin knife alveolar ridge

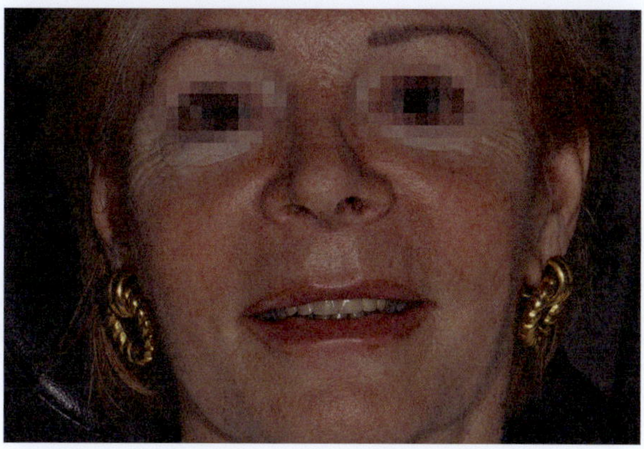

Fig. 4.15 This highly satisfied, 72-year-old patient (2016) had suffered severe trauma at the age of 41 years. No caries or periodontal disease

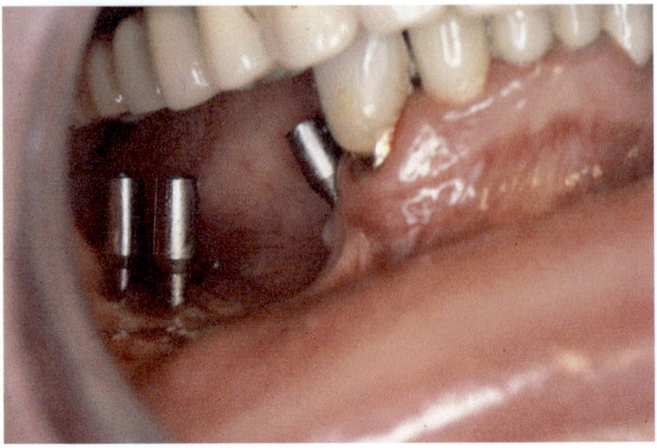

Fig. 4.16 Diskimplants® installed at a bone depth of 1.5–2 mm (lingual approach) immediately after removal of a failing subperiosteal implant in 1984 (patient aged 64 years)

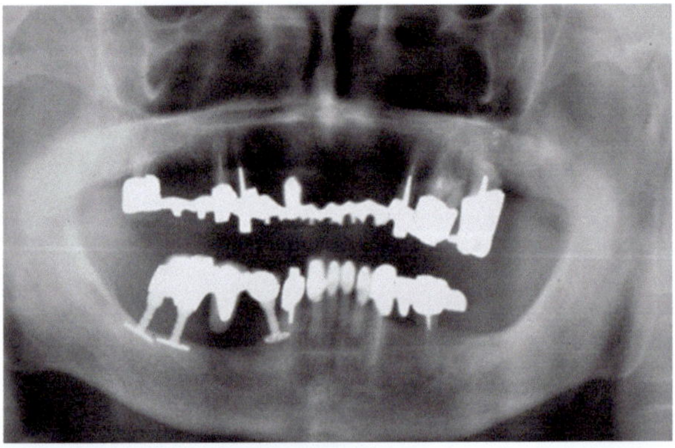

Fig. 4.17 The implant was left 6 months without functional prosthetic teeth. This technique works very well in calm patients. Today, basal implants placed in this area are left completely submerged to protect them from tongue thrusting

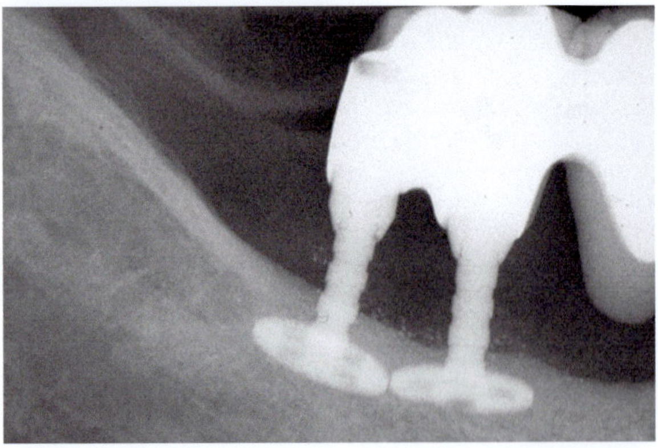

Fig. 4.18 Retroalveolar radiograph after 26 years of service. No bone loss (bone depth <1.5 mm) Disk diameter 7 mm. Occlusal conditions were favorable (no bruxism)

Significant medical compromise was present in patients in whom more than two implants were lost. Smoking was reported as a factor in 30% of the implant failures surveyed. Alcohol abuse was considered a factor in 3% of the implant losses. End-stage peri-implantitis was cited as a cause in only two Diskimplant® failures. This

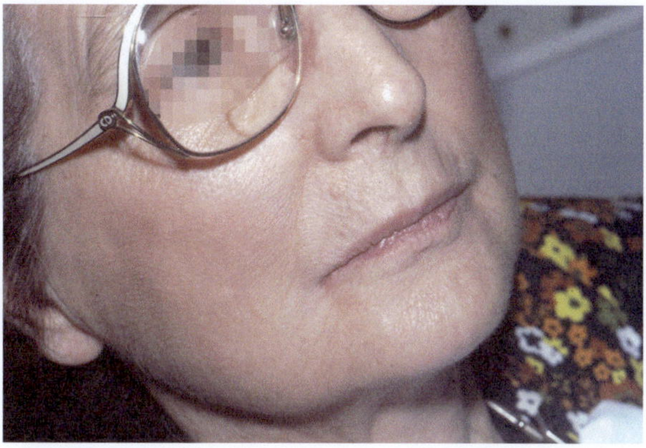

Fig. 4.19 Aspect of the patient in 2010 at age 90; this patient was highly compliant with recommendations concerning hygiene and maintenance, did not smoke, and paid particular attention to her diet

survey is merely a general descriptive tool since results were not analyzed statistically. However, average bone loss during the first year was <0.8 mm, and in certain cases, a bone gain was noted.

Long-Term Follow-Up (1984–2017) of Four Totally Edentulous Patients with an Extremely Atrophic Jaw Treated with Diskimplants®

In 1984 and 1985, a total of 37 titanium Diskimplants® with a machined *ad modum Brånemark* surface were installed in four patients (three women, one man). Initial available bone height for implant installation was less than 5 mm. A delayed (6 months) loading protocol was used for all patients. Two implants were lost in the first year due to non-osseointegration. Total vertical bone loss measured on perpendicular apical radiographs was $\leq$1 mm. In two patients, bone gain was $\geq$1 mm. Thirty-five implants were still in function in November 2017 (Figs. 4.20 and 4.21).

Immediately Loaded Basal Implants

Study results for 72 patients with completely edentulous maxillae treated from 1993 to 1997 are presented in Tables 4.3, 4.4, and 4.5.

The results obtained for 198 patients (112 women, 86 men) with severely atrophic, completely edentulous jaws aged 42–78 years at the time of treatment from 2000 to 2016 are presented in Table 4.6. The standard Diskimplants®, plate-form Diskimplants®, and root-form implants were all placed by the same team using an immediate functional loading protocol. A total of 18 implants were lost: 4 plate-form Diskimplants®, 3 Fractal® pterygoid implants, 4 Diskimplants®, and 7 root-form implants (Fratex®, Fractal®; Victory, France). Seventy percent of the patients (134) had been lost to follow-up by 2015.

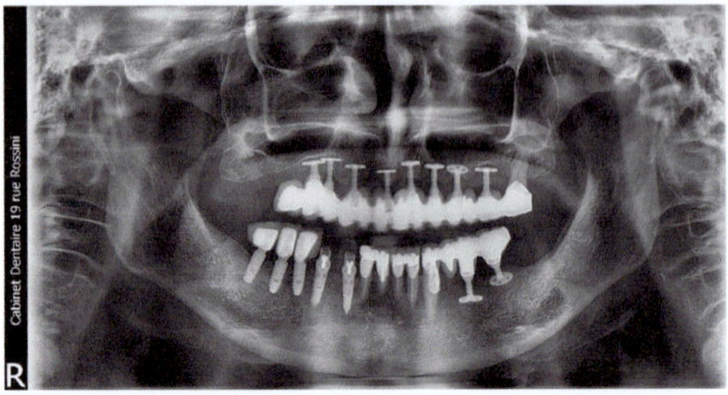

Fig. 4.20 Completely edentulous maxilla with first-generation Diskimplants® placed in 1984 after removal of a failing subperiosteal maxillary implant; implants still in service in November 2017 (33 years)

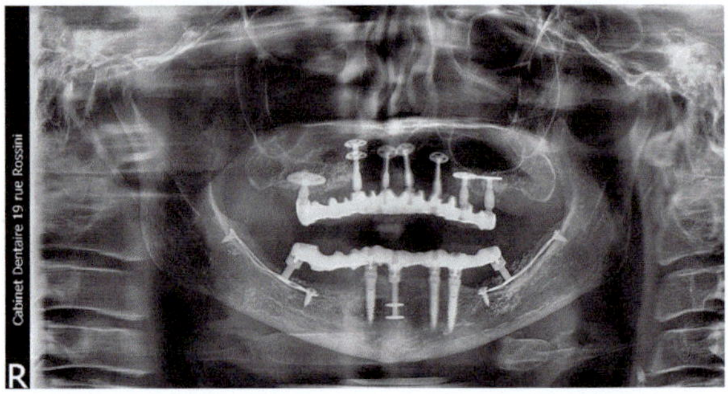

Fig. 4.21 Completely edentulous maxilla with first-generation Diskimplants® (1985) still in service after 32 years. The lower jaw was equipped in December 2017 (immediate functional loading procedure)

Table 4.3 Study population of 72 patients with completely edentulous maxillae treated with an immediate functional loading procedure (September 1993–February 1997)

Follow-up	Women	Men	Total
Fourth year	11	5	16
Third year	12	7	19
Second year	15	8	23
9 months	10	4	14
Total	48	24	72

Mean age at implant installation 62 years (range 42–85 years)

Table 4.4 Implant type and location by anatomic site (641 Diskimplants®, 142 Structure® root-form implants)

	Location in the upper jaw			
Implant type	Premaxilla[a]	Sinus area[b]	Tuberosity[c]	Total
Structure® root-form	24	0	118	142
Single disk	0	142	2	144
Double disk	105	35	8	148
Triple disk	309	24	16	349
Total by site	438	201	144	783

[a]First premolar, canine, incisors
[b]Second premolar, first molar, second molar
[c]Third molar

Table 4.5 Periotest® values in 72 patients (the lower the value, the higher the stability)

Location	Number of implants (72 patients: 48 women, 24 men)	Mean Periotest® value after 6 mo. of function (±SD)
Premaxilla[a]	438 (24 Structure® root-form implants, 504 Diskimplants®)	−2.2 (±2.05)
Sinus area[b]	201 Diskimplants®	0.8 (±1.9)
Tuberosity[c]	144 (118 Structure® root-form implants, 26 Diskimplants®)	−1.02 (±2.24)
Total	783 implants	−1.3 (±2.2)

[a]Incisors, canines, first premolar
[b]Second premolar, first molar, second molar
[c]Third molar

Table 4.6 Severely atrophic, completely edentulous jaws treated by the same team with standard Diskimplants®, plate-form Diskimplants® and root-form implants using an immediate functional loading protocol (2000–2016)

Year	Number of implants lost	Total implants placed	Number of patients	Maxilla	Mandible	Mandible: disks and plate-form disks	Maxilla: disks and plate-form disks	Fractal® pterygoid implants	Other root-form implants
2000	0	78	11	5	6	12	20	10	36
2001	0	90	13	7	6	12	29	13	36
2002	0	82	12	6	6	12	24	12	34
2003	1	67	9	5	4	8	20	10	29
2004	2	77	11	6	5	10	24	12	31
2005	2	90	13	7	6	12	28	14	36
2006	1	70	10	6	4	8	24	10	28
2007	3	83	12	7	5	10	28	14	31
2008	0	84	11	6	5	20	20	12	32
2009	0	95	14	8	6	12	22	15	36
2010	1	81	12	7	5	10	26	14	31
2011	1	84	12	7	5	10	28	14	32
2012	0	93	13	8	6	12	30	16	35
2013	2	93	14	9	5	10	33	18	32
2014	0	98	15	10	5	10	38	19	31
2015	3	101	16	9	7	14	31	17	39
2016	2	103	16	10	6	12	32	19	40
Total	18	1469	214	123	92	194	467	39	569

Conflict of interest statement Gérard M. Scortecci is the inventor of the Diskimplant and holder of several associated patents that are exploited by the Victory company. He is an unpaid consultant to this firm and a minority shareholder in the company. No money was received from any of the companies mentioned in the book or from any of the companies whose products are mentioned.

Recommended Reading

1. Scortecci GM. The diskimplant: a self-positioning pure titanium implant. Congress publication, 7th World Congres of Oral Implantology, Munich, West Germany; 1984.
2. English CE. Part III. An overview of the systems. CA Dent Assoc J. 1998;16:34–8.

3. Adell R, Eriksson B, Lekholm U, Brånemark PI, Jemt T. A long-term follow-up study of osseointegrated implants in the treatment of totally edentulous jaws. Int J Oral Maxillofac Surg. 1990;7:347–59.
4. Besch KJ. Consensus à propos des implants à intégration basale (BOI). Rev Mens Suisse Odontostomatol. 1999;109:996.
5. Bocklage R. Advanced alveolar crest atrophy: an alternative treatment technique for maxilla and mandible. Implant Dent. 2001;10(1):30–5.
6. Boyé G. Le double Diskimplant dans les régions parasinusiennes. Revue Française d'Implantologie Orale. 1989;1:27–46.
7. Brånemark PI. Introduction to osseointegration. In: Brånemark PI, Zarb GA, Albrektsson T, editors. Tissue-integrated prostheses: osseointegration in clinical dentistry. Chicago: Quintessence; 1985. p. 11–76.
8. Brånemark P, Hansson BO, Adell R, Breine U, Lindstrom J, Hallen O, et al. Osseointegration of implants in the treatment of the edentulous jaw. Experience from a 10-year period. Stockholm: Almqvist and Wiksell; 1977.
9. Cotten P. La implantologia basal. Una alternativa al injerto de hueso. Salud y Vida, suppl. de Lavanguardia; 2008, March.
10. Diederich H. Immediate loading of a maxillary full-arch rehabilitation by basal and crestal implants. Implant Dir. 2008;3(1):61.
11. Doglioli P, Scortecci G. Cytocompatibilité spécifique. Etude de l'activité enzymatique spécifique de la phosphatase alcaline. Projet de Norme: AFNOR Comité d'Etude 9 "Implants Dentaires"; 1990.
12. Doglioli P, Scortecci G. Characterization of endosteal osteoblasts isolated from human maxilla and mandible: an experimental system for biocompatibility tests. Cytotechnology. 1991;7:39–48.
13. Doms P. Biologie osseuse et recherches expérimentales en implantologie. Implantologie Orale. 1981;3:21–8.
14. Doms P. The tissue response to endosteal implants – microradiographic and tetracycline marking. In: Brånemark PI, Zarb G, Albrektsson T, editors. Tissue-integrated prostheses. Chicago: Quintessence; 1985. p. 143.
15. Doms P, Scortecci G. Nouvelles solutions thérapeutiques en prothèse: racines artificielles en titane pur. Implantologie Orale. 1985;18(2eme semestre):6–27.
16. Doms P. Expérience clinique en implantologie. Acta Stomatol Belg. 1986;83:87–97.
17. Donsimoni JM, Doms P, Besch KJ. Les progrès de l'implantologie basale: Diskimplants 1984-2001. Implantodontie. 1999;33:31–3.
18. Dubruille JH, Dubruille MT, Goudot P et al. Réhabilitation orale et implantologie. Encyclopédie Médico-Chirurgicale (Editions Scientifiques et médicales Elsevier SAS, Paris). Odontologie 23-330-A-10; 2000. 30 p.
19. Gapski R, Wang HL, Mascarenhas P, Lang NP. Critical review of immediate implant loading. Clin Oral Impl Res. 2003;14:515–27.
20. Goldring A, Harris G, et al. The synovial-like membrane at the bone-cement interface in loose total hip replacements and its proposed role in bone lysis. J Bone Joint Surg. 1983;65:158–9. (Abstract 5).
21. Gomez-Gonzalez M, Avila-Morales R. Réhabilitation du maxillaire avec une prothèse fixée implanto-portée suivant la technique classique du Diskimplant. Revue Française d'Implantologie Orale. 1990;3:5–7.
22. Haynes D, Hay S, Rogers S, Ohta S, Howie D, Graves S. Regulation of bone cells by particle-activated mononuclear phagocytes. J Bone Joint Surg (Br). 1997;79-B:988–94.
23. Ihde S. Restoration of the atrophied mandible using basal osseointegrated implants and fixed prosthetic superstructures. Implant Dent. 2001;10(1):41–5.
24. Ihde S. Adaptations fonctionnelles de la hauteur de l'os péri implantaire après implantation de BOI. Implantodontie – Implants et dentisterie esthétique. 2003;12(4):23–33.
25. Ihde S. Fixed prosthodontics in skeletal class III patients with partially edentulous jaws and age-related prognathism: the Basal Osseointegration Procedure. Implant Dent. 1999;8(3):241–6.

26. Ihde S. Comparison of basal and crestal implants and their modus of application. Smile Dent J. 2009;4(1):36–46.
27. Jaffin RA, Berman CL. The excessive loss of Brånemark fixtures in type IV bone: a 5-year analysis. J Periodontol. 1991;62:2–4.
28. Juillet JM. L'implant tridimensionnel T3D. Implantologie orale n° 2; 1981.
29. Kasemo B, Lausmaa J. Surface science aspect on inorganic biomaterials. CRC Crit Rev Clin Neurobiol. 1986;2:4.
30. Marcelat R. Contribution of CAD/CAM technology to implant-supported screw-retained restorations: use of a full-arch bridge in the maxillae: a case report. CAD/CAM. 2014;3:20–5.
31. Meningaud JP, Donsimoni JM. Facial allografts and oral rehabilitation. Rev Stomatol Chir Maxillofac Sept. 2012;113(4):350–2.
32. Meningaud JP, Donsimoni JM, Lantieri L. Facial allograft transplantation and basal implantology (cortically anchored disk-design implants). Rev Stomatol Chir Maxillofac. 2009;110(6):353–8.
33. Michel MC, Veyret D, Pantaloni J, Martin R. Analyse comparative par éléments finis d'implants odontologiques avec et sans appui cortical. Le Chirurgien-Dentiste France. 1990;510:83–9.
34. Mombelli A, van Oosten MAC, Schürch E, Lang NP. The microbiota associated with successful or failing osseointegrated titanium implants. Oral Microbiol Immunol. 1987;2(4):145–51.
35. Odin G, Balaguer T, Savoldelli C, Scortecci G. Immediate functional loading of an implant-supported fixed prosthesis at the time of ablative surgery and mandibular reconstruction for squamous cell carcinoma. J Oral Implantol. 2010;36(3):225–30.
36. Odin G, Misch CE, Binderman I, Scortecci G. Fixed rehabilitation of severely atrophic jaws using immediately loaded basal disk implants after in situ bone activation. J Oral Implantol. 2012;38(5):611–6.
37. Odin G, Petitbois R, Cotten P, Philip P. Distraction osteogenesis using bone matrix osteotensors in ectodermal dysplasia: a case report. Implant Dent. 2015;24(5):612–9.
38. Odin G, Petitbois R, Scortecci G. Soulevé de sinus et Ostéotenseur: le Fractal lift. La Lettre de la Stomatologie. 2009;44:4–11.
39. Odin G, Scortecci G. Améloblastome: Chirurgie subtotale et implantologie basale. A propos d'un cas (1986-2004). La Lettre de la Stomatologie; 2004:22.
40. Odin G, Scortecci G, Levratto F, Morin L. Techniques avancées en implantologie basale chirurgico-prothétique. Stratégie Prothétique. 2011;11(3):209–18.
41. Odin G, Sevalle M, Scortecci G. La "révolution ostéogénique". Le Chirurgien-Dentiste de France. 2009;1398:49–52.
42. Perel LM. Diskimplant system yields tricortical support to make the most of available bone. Dent Implantol Update. 1991;2(8):72–4.
43. Petitbois R. L'implant à plaque: une révolution en implantologie basale. Alpha Omega News. 2008;120:11–2.
44. Petitbois R, Manière R. La mise en charge immédiate en implantologie basale: protocoles. RFPD. 2008;3:36–41.
45. Petitbois R, Maniere R. A propos de la CAD-CAM en implantologie. Où en sommes-nous ? Le Chirurgien-Dentiste de France N° 1530, 31 mai 2012; 2012. p. 1–5.
46. Petitbois R, Scortecci G, Philip P. Dysplasie ectodermique et implantologie: gestion d'une situation extrême sans recours aux greffes osseuses. La Lettre de la Stomatologie. 2012;54:5–10.
47. Petitbois R, Scortecci G. La corticotomie alvéolaire: nouvelle approche chirurgicale grâce à l'ostéo-activation. Principe et protocole. Int Orthod. 2012;10(4):432–8.
48. Scortecci G. Le Diskimplant: racines artificielles en titane pur. Dent News. 1985;50:17-2.
49. Scortecci G. L'insertion latérale en implantologie (en italien) (translation by G. Huober). Il Dentista Moderno IV (N° 1); 1986.
50. Scortecci G. Impianto osteointegrato con appoggio tricorticale. Rapporto di 7 anni. Revue du XVIII Meeting Internationale Impianti e Trapianti Dentari del G.I.S.I. Bologne, Italie, mai 1988; 1988. p. 127–30.
51. Scortecci G. Patient treatment with dental implants. Proc. Joint ADA/FDI World Dental Congress, Washington, DC, USA; 8–14 October 1988.

52. Scortecci G. Osseointegrated dental implant with tricortical support. In: Proceedings of 37th Congress, Am Acad Implant Dentistry, Washington, DC; 1988.
53. Scortecci G. Thin maxillary ridges and fixed prosthodontics. Report on seven years' use in Europe. Pacific Coast Soc Prosthodontists Newsl. 1990;11(2):14.
54. Scortecci G. Prosthetic solutions with Diskimplants for the treatment of severe bone resorption. In: Abstract, 2nd international symposium on advanced application of osseointegration, Padova, Italy; 1991.
55. Scortecci G. A cosmetic solution for fixed implant prosthodontics. In: Abstract, Fortieth Annual Scientific Session, American Academy of Crown and Bridge Prosthodontics, Chicago, USA; 1991.
56. Scortecci G. Ostéointégration dans les faibles hauteurs de l'os. Abstract, Implantologie Endo-osseuse: cours pratique. Collège des Médecins Stomatologistes et Chirurgiens Maxillo-faciaux de France;1991. p. 171.
57. Scortecci G. Prothèse sur implant. In: Abstract, Journal of the Deutsche Gesellschaft für Zahnarztliche Implantologie, Wasserburg (RFA); 1992.
58. Scortecci G. Prosthodontic implant dentistry: How basal disk type implants combined with the patient's own stem cells can make the difference for functional fixed teeth in extremely atrophic jaws. In: Abstract. Annual Congress, The Academy of Prosthodontics, Chicago; 2009. p. 10–1.
59. Scortecci G. Pushing back the limits: repousser les limites du possible. DT Study Club Magazine, n° 3; 2015.
60. Scortecci G, Doglioli P. Behavior of human bone cells (maxilla and mandible) in contact with commercially pure titanium used for dental implants: in vitro study. Publication scientifique dans la Revue du Fourth World Biomaterials Congress, Berlin; 1992. p. 149.
61. Scortecci G, Doglioli P, Binderman I. Differentiation and characterization of human osteoblasts derived from maxillary and mandibular bone of healthy individuals. Abstract. Third Int. Workshop on Cells and Cytokines in Bone and Cartilage, 8–11 April 1990, Davis, Switzerland. Calcif Tissue Int. 1990;46(Suppl 2):A15–29.
62. Scortecci G, Doms P, Hoisington W. Osseointegrated system: tissue-integrated prosthesis for small bone volumes. In: Abstract, UCLA Symposium "Implants in the partially edentulous patient", Palm Springs, CA, n° 54; 1990.
63. Scortecci G, Donsimoni JM, Spahn FP, Binderman I. Ostéointégration et mise en fonction immédiate: sont-elles compatibles ? Alpha Oméga News. 1996:4–5.
64. Scortecci G, Hoisington W, Meyere P, Zattara H. Trans-sinusal technique: technical and Medico-legal aspects. In: Publication scientifique dans la Revue du 4th International Congress on Preprosthetic Surgery, Palm Springs, CA; 1991.
65. Scortecci G, Meyere P, Zattara H, Doms P. Intra-oral applications in small bone volumes. Patient selection and long-term results. In: Laney W, Tolman D, editors. Tissue integration in oral, orthopedic and maxillofacial reconstruction. Chicago: Quintessence; 1990. p. 350–5.
66. Scortecci G, Meyere P, Zattara H, Hoisington W. Type IV maxillary bone management with double Diskimplants in Europe. In: Abstract, 2nd UCLA Symposium "Implants in the partially edentulous patient", Palm Springs, CA; 1992.
67. Scortecci G, Meyere P, Zattara H. Technique infracanalaire avec les Diskimplants ostéointégrables. Rapport de 4 ans d'expérience. In: Abstract, Symposium Int. de la Société Belge de Chirurgie et d'Implantologie Orale, Bruxelles; 1992. p. 45.
68. Scortecci G, Misch CE, Odin G, Binderman I, Sers L. Implantologie basale: approche chirurgicale conforme aux données actuelles avérées. Dent Tribune. 2006;1:10–2.
69. Shen TC. The use of different implant modalities in the atrophied ridge. J Oral Implantol. 1999;25(2):109–13.
70. van Blitterswijk CA, Grote JJ, Kuypers W, Block-van Hoek CJ, Daems WT. Bioreactions at the tissue/hydroxyapatite interface. Biomaterials. 1985;6(4):243–51.
71. Scortecci G. Immediate function of cortically anchored disk-design implants without bone augmentation in moderately to severely resorbed completely edentulous maxillae. Journal of Oral Implantology. 1999;25(2):70–9.
72. Scortecci GM, Misch CE, Benner KU, editors. Implants and restorative dentistry. London: Martin Dunitz; 2001.

Books

Bert M, Leclercq P. L'occlusion en implantologie. Paris: Editions EDP Sciences; 2015. p. 311–4.

Bert M, Missika P, editors. Diskimplants. In: Les implants ostéo-intégrables. Paris: Editions CDP; 1991. p. 189–96; 361–9.

Cotten P. Implantologia basal y diskimplant. Una alternativa al injerto cuando hay déficit oseo moderado o severo. In: Matiz Cuervo J, editor. Odontogeriatria. Rehabilitacion oral del paciente adulto mayor. Bogota: Editorial Impresion Medica; 2013. p. 169–86.

Ihde S. Principles of BOI: clinical, scientific and practical guidelines to 4-D dental implantology. Berlin: Springer; 2005.

Laney R, William S, Tolman E. Tissue integration in oral, orthopedic and maxillofacial reconstruction. In: Second International Congress on oral, orthopedic and maxillofacial reconstruction. Mayo Medical Center, Rochester MN, Sept. 23–27, Quintessence Books; 1990.

Misch CE. Contemporary implant dentistry. St. Louis: Mosby Elsevier; 2008. p. 410–1030.

Missika P, et al. Gérer les difficultés et complications en implantologie. Paris: Espace ID; 2015. p. 78–80.

Scortecci G, Brenier P. Diskimplants: Technique de pose. In: Tarragano H, Missika P, Moyal F, Illouz B, Roche Y, editors. La chirurgie orale. Paris, France: JPIO, Editions CDP; 2010. p. 85–91.

Scortecci GM, Misch CE, Benner KU, editors. Implants and restorative dentistry. London: Martin Dunitz; 2000.

Scortecci G, Odin G, Morin L. Gestion per- et postopératoire de complications multiples. In: Missika P, et al., editors. Gérer les difficultés et complications en implantologie. Paris: Espace ID; 2015. p. 76–80.

Tarragano H, et al. La chirurgie orale: Editions CDP. Paris: Wolters Kluwer; 2010.

University Theses

Afota F. Stratégies chirurgicales pré-implantaires et implantaires des séquelles de fentes labio-maxillo-palatines: état de l'art et analyse de cas. Thesis N° 42-57-16-22, University of Nice-Sophia Antipolis, France; 2016.

Daher S. Utilisation des racines artificielles en titane pur en odonto-stomatologie. Thesis N° 42-57-85-38, University of Nice-Sophia Antipolis, France; 1985.

Gomez-Gonzalez MA. El implante endooséo: Diskimplant. Alternativa de tratamiento protesico en la odonto-estomatologia. Thesis, Universidad dei Pais Vasco, Spain; 1986.

Juillet JM. L'implant tridimensionnel. Thesis, University of Paris, France; 1972.

Odin G. Modélisation numérique de l'os mandibulaire appliquée à l'implantologie dentaire et maxillo-faciale. Paris, France: Ecole des Mines de Paris; 2008.

Scortecci G. L'implant dentaire tricortical: intégration biologique, recherche fondamentale et applications cliniques. Doctorat d'Etat en Odontologie (PhD thesis), Marseilles, France; 1988.

Initial Bone Bed Activation: Bone Matrix Osseotensors—Tissue Engineering

5

Itzhak Binderman, Gérard M. Scortecci, Patrick Philip, Joseph Choukroun, and Alexandre-Amir Aalam

5.1 Principles

Early techniques aimed at improving bone graft incorporation were performed using a variety of standard dental instruments (drills, burs, needles) to decorticalize the jaw bone surface after full-flap exposure and make it bleed. The results were painful and unpredictable, however, mainly because of heating, metal and bacterial pollution, non-calibrated trauma, and inappropriate instrument surface characteristics. In the early 1970s, Henry Goldman (Boston University, USA) described the

I. Binderman
Department of Oral Biology, University of Tel Aviv, Tel Aviv, Israel

G. M. Scortecci (✉)
University of Nice-Sophia Antipolis Medical School, Nice, France

New York University, New York, NY, USA

University of Southern California, Los Angeles, CA, USA

Private Practice, Nice, France
e-mail: scortecci@wanadoo.fr

P. Philip
Faculté de Médecine, Département d'Histologie, Unité d'Exploration Fonctionnelle Cellulaire et Tissulaire, Hôpital Pasteur, University of Nice-Sophia Antipolis, Nice, France
e-mail: pjmphilip@aol.com

J. Choukroun
SYFAC, Nice, France
e-mail: joseph@a-prf.com

A.-A. Aalam
Private Practice, Los Angeles, CA, USA
e-mail: DrAalam@ImplantPerioCenter.com

© Springer Nature Switzerland AG 2019

G. M. Scortecci (ed.), *Basal Implantology*, https://doi.org/10.1007/978-3-319-44873-2_5

use of an anesthesia needle to mechanically stimulate the periosteum in order to treat severe periodontal disease. Despite promising initial results, this manual needling procedure had a number of drawbacks (soft tissue contamination due to the hollow cylinder of the anesthesia needle, bacterial and metal contamination) and was thus progressively abandoned.

5.2 Stem Cell Activation, Distraction Osteogenesis, Neoangiogenesis

Complex interactions have been demonstrated between bone matrix tensions and signaling molecules (extracellular matrix/bone cells/cell nuclei). In addition to the existence of osteo-regulation processes based on mechano-transduction, osteotension triggers and regulates bone regeneration, thereby stimulating the human body's capacity for self-repair.

The philosophy behind minimally invasive mechanotherapy using an autologous, flapless approach is promotion of angiogenesis and osteogenesis by activation of local stem cells with minimal trauma. Recent work in mechanotherapy has revealed the "gene activation effect" of distraction osteogenesis. When the capacities of the human bioreactor (HBR) are ignited by osseotensors, the cascade of molecular events brings the mechanical signal into the nuclei and

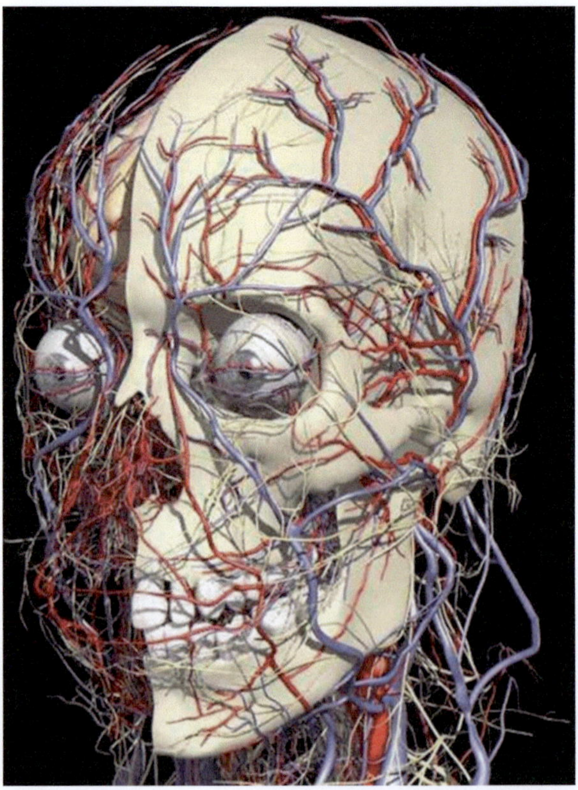

Fig. 5.1 The human bioreactor: the vascular route for BMP signaling molecules

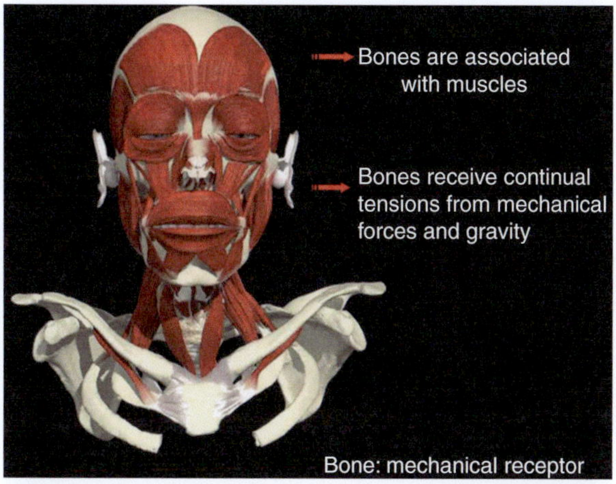

Fig. 5.2 Bone as a mechanical receptor is dependent on muscle activity

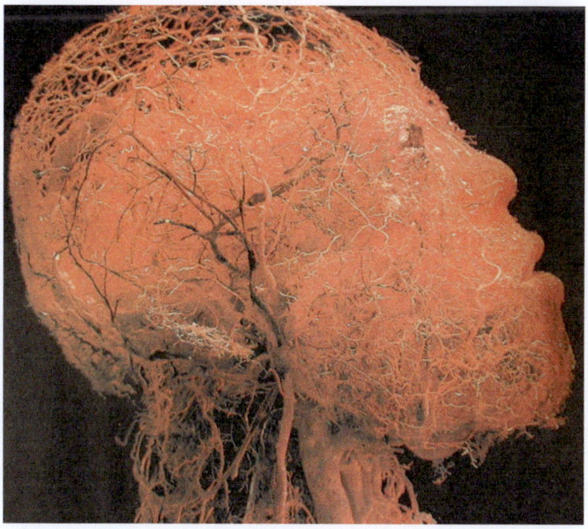

Fig. 5.3 Blood supply of the head, one of the most highly vascularized areas of the body

activates the appropriate gene for tissue regeneration (Figs. 5.1, 5.2, 5.3, and 5.4). Flapless application of mechanical stress to bone tissue (compression, distraction, trauma, microfracture, etc.) activates repair mechanisms via signaling molecules. Just as mechanical microtrauma of the periosteum induces subsequent repair, surgical trauma of the bone results in a burst of localized hard tissue remodeling via bone callus formation. The cascade of biological responses includes recruitment of stem cells, both locally and at a distance, that participate in bone remodeling. The localized micro-cracks caused by penetration of the osseotensor into the spongiosa induce the release of bone matrix growth factors (BMP, IGF-I and IGF-II, IGF-beta) that have a range of biologic properties. The trauma caused by the micro-cracks releases osteo-inductive proteins from the bone matrix; these proteins in turn recruit stem cells which participate in the bone remodeling process.

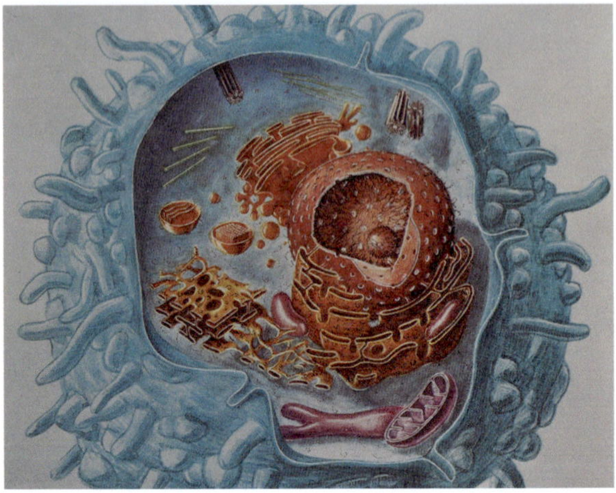

Fig. 5.4 After bone matrix osseotensor application, signaling molecules target specific receptors in the extracellular matrix, bone cells, and cell nuclei (DNA and gene activation)

These observations, along with research findings in such fields as mechanobiology, tensegrity, corticotomy, distraction osteogenesis, and angiogenesis, prompted the development of a specific instrument capable of producing calibrated microcracks without bacterial contamination, metal debris, or thermal damage to tissues. Bone matrix osseotensors were presented for the first time in 2005 at the Oral Implant Forum organized by the Medical School of the University of Nice-Sophia Antipolis, France. The ultimate goal of these purpose-designed calibrated instruments is (a) to minimize the inflammatory response and (b) to activate the patient's jaw stem cells in order to create new blood supply, stimulate progenitors, boost osteogenesis, and improve initial bone quality and quantity before installation of implants with or without guided bone regeneration (GBR). The autologous, flapless approach is particularly useful with basal implants which are primarily placed in small bone volumes. Osseotensors are also indicated when sinus lift procedures (Fractal® lift) and bone grafting are planned. In this last case, both the donor and recipient sites are activated.

Since 2005, these instruments have become an integral component of presurgery management to improve the bone quality several days or weeks (depending on initial bone density) before installation of Diskimplants® or root-form implants.

Diphasic Effect of Bone Matrix Osseotensors (Figs. 5.5, 5.6, 5.7, 5.8, 5.9, 5.10, and 5.11)

Transparietal penetration of the DLC-coated (diamond-like carbon) tip of the instrument through the osteogenic compartments (periosteum, bone matrix, endosteum, vascular walls, bone marrow) instantly modifies the bone matrix tensions implicated in bone homeostasis. The resultant distraction osteogenesis induces two time-related antagonist effects.

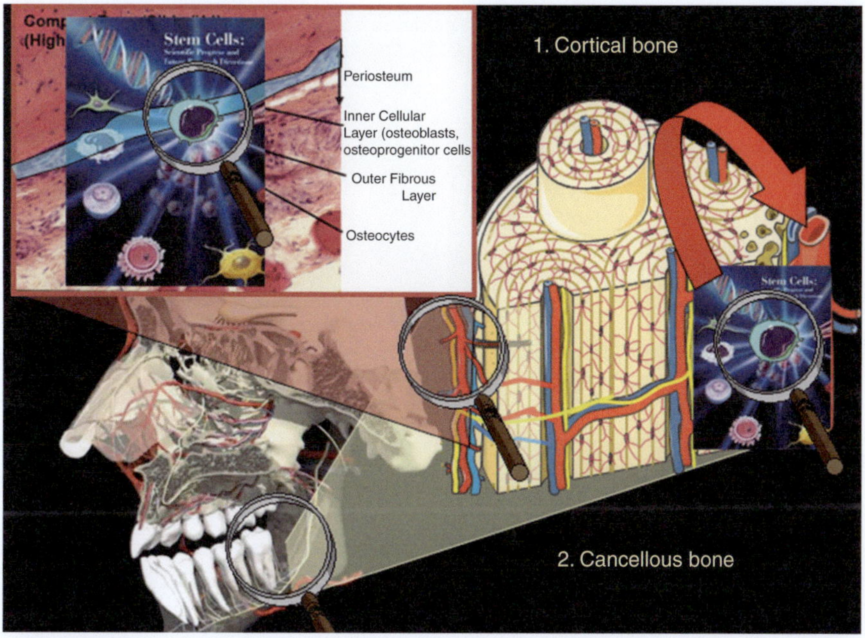

Fig. 5.5 Stem cell sites in human jaws (inner periosteal layer, endosteum, perivascular sheath, bone marrow). The intrabony blood supply in extremely atrophic bone is limited. When a jaw fracture occurs, the majority of the cells involved in the repair process come from the inner layer of the periosteum. This explains why bone grafting procedures performed before implant installation are often unsuccessful. Basal implants are an alternative to bone grafts because they are placed directly in the remaining living native bone

(a) ***Catabolic Phase from t = 0 to t = 21 Days***
The bone is softened due to macrophage type 1 phagocytosis and osteoclast activity. During this initial catabolic phase, which begins 3 minutes after trauma with an inflammatory response, the bone "softens" as the result of primary macrophage activity the first 3 days. Macrophage 1 activity then ceases progressively. Macrophage type 2 activity, which promotes neoangeogenesis, begins after 3 days. This ongoing process of stem cell differentiation for tissue repair develops over 3 weeks.

(b) ***Anabolic Phase from t = 21 to t = 45 Days***
The anabolic phase that follows the catabolic response is characterized by osteoblastic activity with reconstruction and strengthening of the bone due to formation of a callus. The suitable waiting period for implant installation and/or bone grafts in type IV or III bone is 45 to 90 days, depending on the initial bone condition and the patient's age.

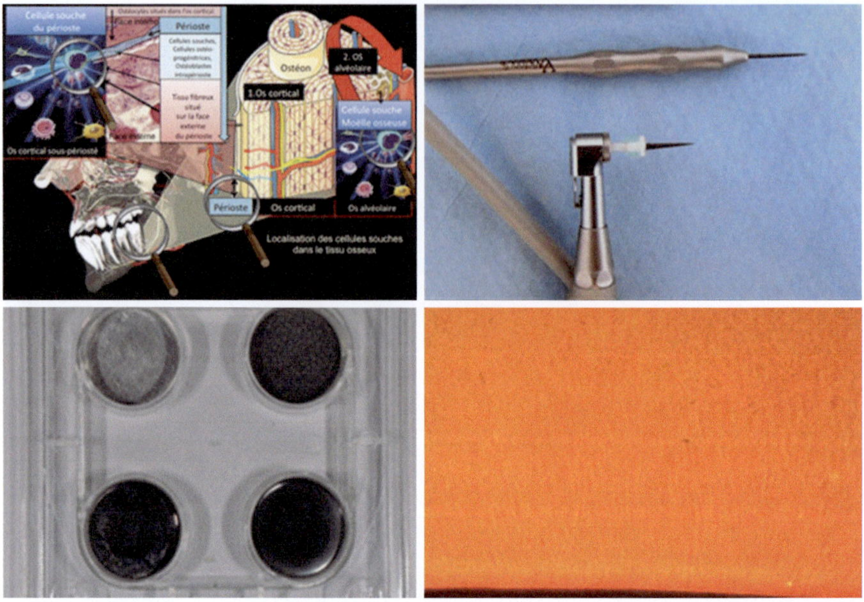

Fig. 5.6 Manual and rotary bone matrix osseotensors. Different materials and surface states were tested in cultures of cells from human jaws. Mirror-smooth, diamond-like carbon (DLC) gave the best results. Human osteoblasts from the maxilla attached perpendicularly to the DLC surface via their pseudopods

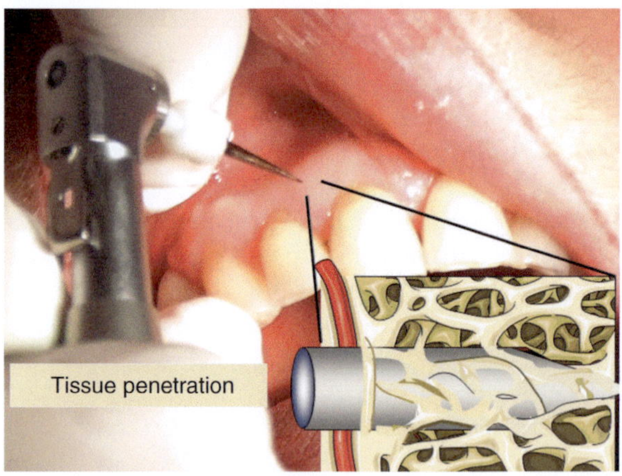

Fig. 5.7 Transparietal tissue penetration under local anesthesia: the bone matrix osseotensor must pass through the sinus membrane

5.3 Practical Use of Bone Matrix Osseotensors (Figs. 5.12, 5.13, 5.14, 5.15, 5.16, and 5.17)

Manual Osseotensors for D3 and D4 Bone Densities

The purpose-designed Osseotensor® for spongy bone is a manual, size-calibrated surgical steel instrument with a diamond-like carbon-coated (DLC) tip specially

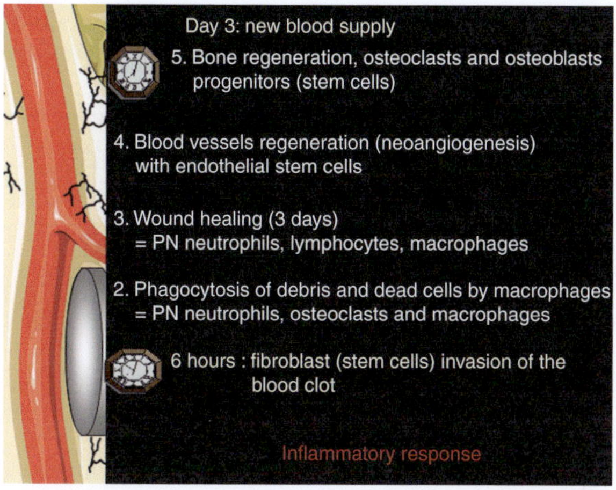

Fig. 5.8 The cascade of biological events that occur after tissue penetration

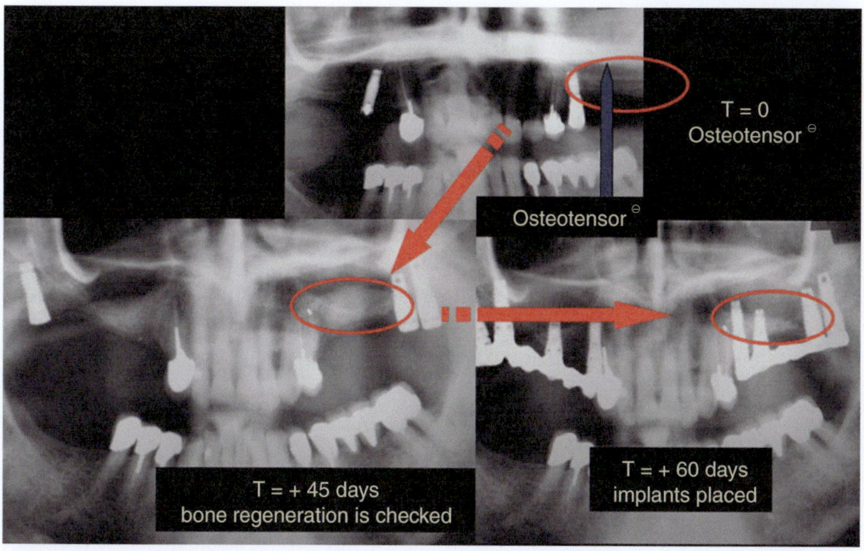

Fig. 5.9 Clinical application of osseotensors in the sinus area. Implants were placed using a flapless procedure 60 days later; they were left submerged 4 to 6 months as a function of bone thickness and quality. No bone substitute material was used. The dense area in the left maxillary sinus is the result of callus formation caused by bleeding under the Schneiderian membrane following osseotensor penetration

designed to condense and expand type III and type IV soft bone without any drilling effect. After topical and local anesthesia of the gingiva, a manual osseotensor is "press fit" through the gum and the periosteum into the spongiosa; this flapless procedure is performed with slight manual rotation. The operator must first check the bone surface mm by mm with a manual osseotensor and select the weakest area of bone that is easy to penetrate manually. A manual osseotensor should never be

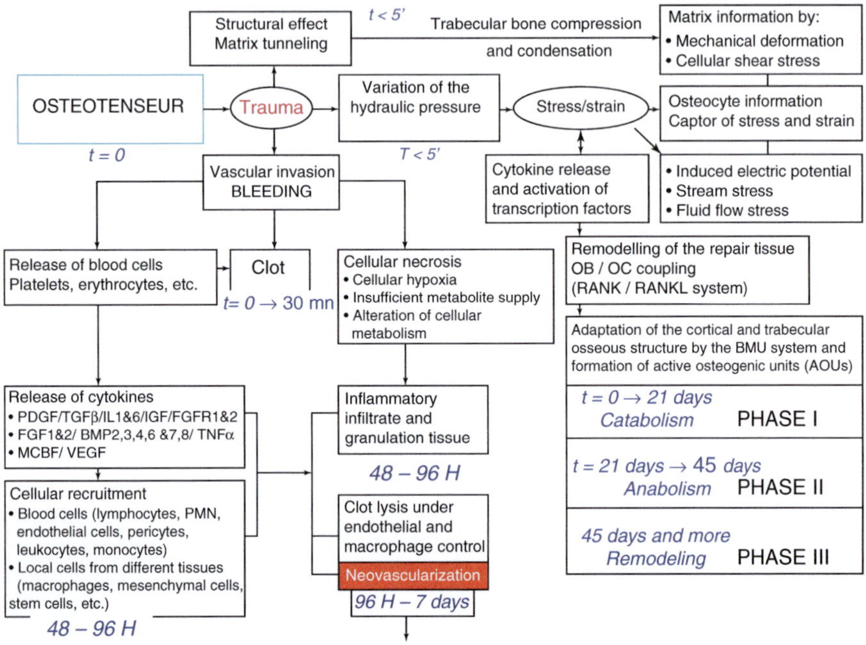

Fig. 5.10 Timetable of the biological events that occur following the use of bone matrix osseotensors

forced into areas of already-dense cortical bone as this could damage the tip. The number of manual impacts in very soft and/or eggshell-thin D4 or D5 bone is not limited, but a minimum distance of 2 mm should always be respected between two impact sites. In contrast, in dense D1 or D2 bone, a single impact with a rotary osseotensor suffices.

The size of each manual impact is smaller than the tip of a transfusion needle. The solid design of the diamond-like carbon-coated instrument avoids transportation of metal debris, bacteria, and soft tissue into the sterile bony environment. When used in the sinus regions, it can easily traverse the eggshell-thin bony sinus wall and pass through the Schneiderian membrane. Blood from the well-irrigated connective tissue extravasates under the respiratory epithelial lining of the sinus cavities and acts as a balloon that atraumatically elevates the Schneiderian membrane. Penetration of the sinus membrane is comparable to the use of a needle for local anesthesia, but without the risk of foreign body transportation since the osseotensor tip is closed. Consequently, the manual osseotensor tip can completely pass through the sinus floor and the healthy sinus membrane without provoking hemorrhagic bleeding inside the sinus cavity. When the operator pulls outs the manual osseotensor, the Schneiderian membrane closes up immediately, just like when a transfusion needle is removed. The immediate closure of the membrane is due to gravity, atmospheric pressure, and cell-to-cell adhesion of the respiratory sinus epithelium. Any blood is maintained under the respiratory epithelium in the connective

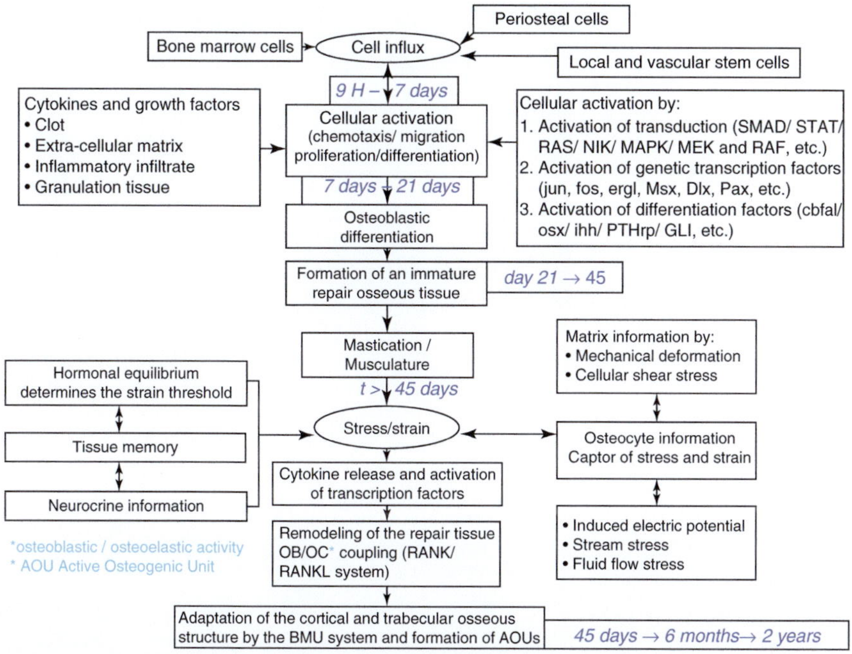

Fig. 5.11 Timetable (continued)

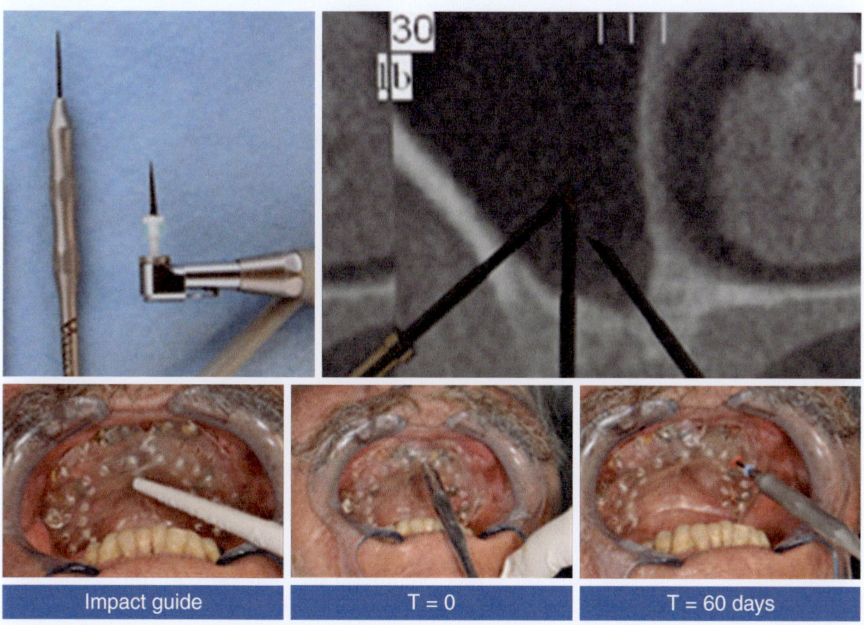

Fig. 5.12 Clinical and radiological views of the use of bone matrix osseotensors in the sinus area

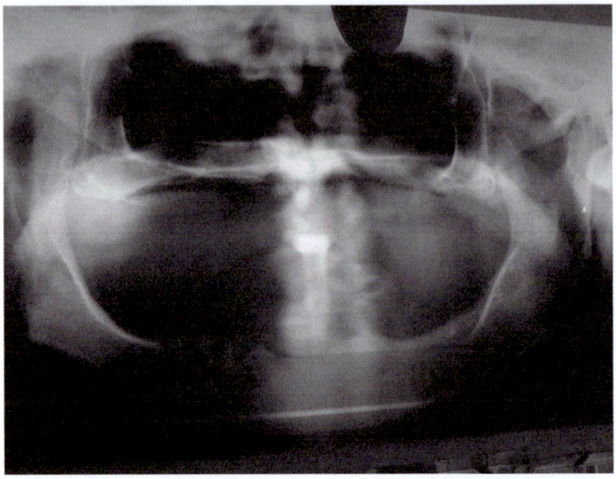

Fig. 5.13 Panoramic view of an atrophic maxilla before application of bone matrix osseotensors (same patient in Figs. 5.14, 5.15, 5.16, 5.17, 5.18, 5.19, 5.20, 5.21, 5.22, 5.23, and 5.24)

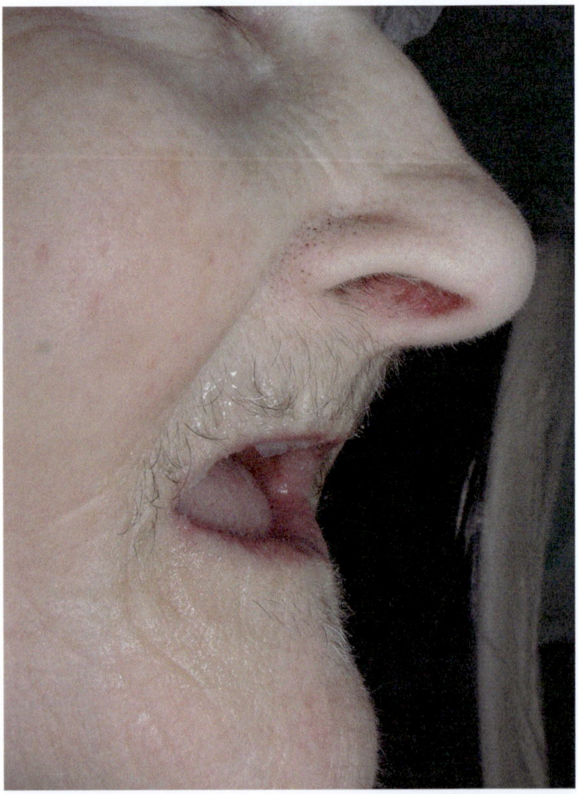

Fig. 5.14 77-year-old, female oral invalid

tissue compartment. The balloon effect of the slow blood flow in the connective tissues that gently raises up the Schneiderian membrane creates a space for formation of a callus on the sinus floor. The bone gain measured by 3D cone beam CT imaging generally ranges in height from 1.3 to 6 mm (Figs. 5.18, 5.19, 5.20, 5.21, 5.22, 5.23, 5.24, 5.25, 5.26, 5.27, 5.28, 5.29, 5.30, 5.31, and 5.32).

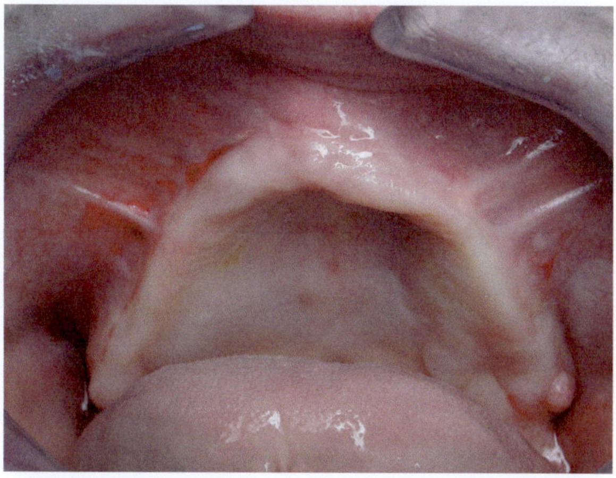

Fig. 5.15 Intraoral view

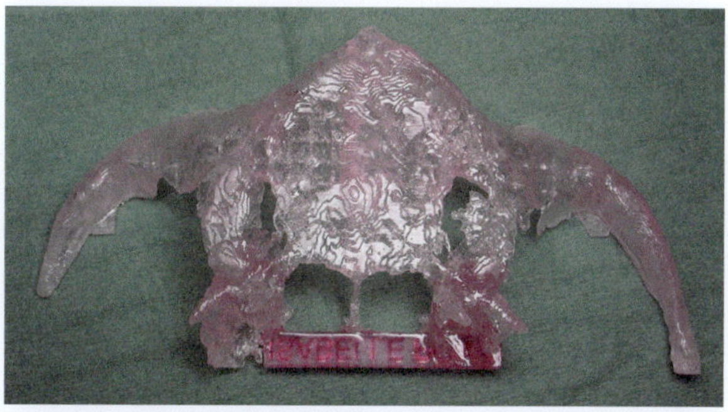

Fig. 5.16 The 3D stereolithographic reconstruction helps the surgeon to identify the weakest areas of the bone for application of a manual osseotensor in order to induce callus formation

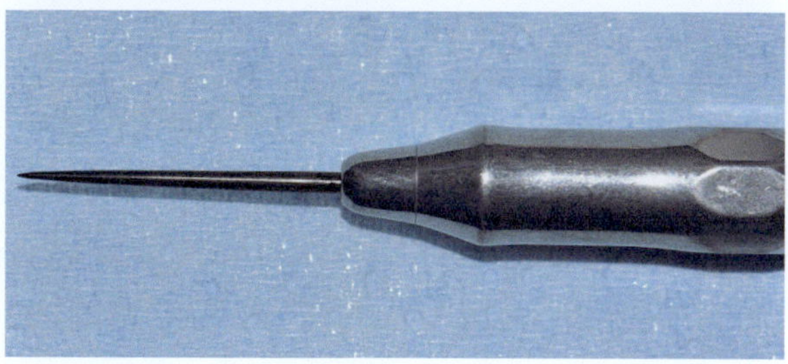

Fig. 5.17 Manual bone matrix osseotensor: the instrument of choice for bone stimulation in patients with atrophic maxillae

Regional Accelerated Phenomenon (RAP)

Each osseotensor impact site is the point of departure of accelerated reparative osteogenesis. Mineralization of the subperiosteal blood clot leads to formation of a bone callus after 45 to 90 days; this corresponds to the bone consolidation constantly observed for closed fractures without displacement. For type III and type IV soft bone, the micro-cracks (similar to distraction osteogenesis) created in the spongy bone 45 to 90 days prior to implant surgery and/or bone grafting procedures

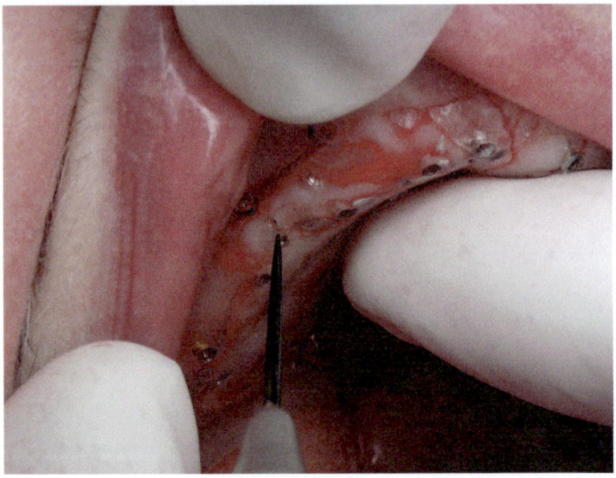

Fig. 5.18 The osseotensor procedure is performed using a flapless approach under local anesthesia. A transparent acrylic osseotensor guide allows evaluation of the improvement in bone density at the exact same bone sites 45 to 60 days later

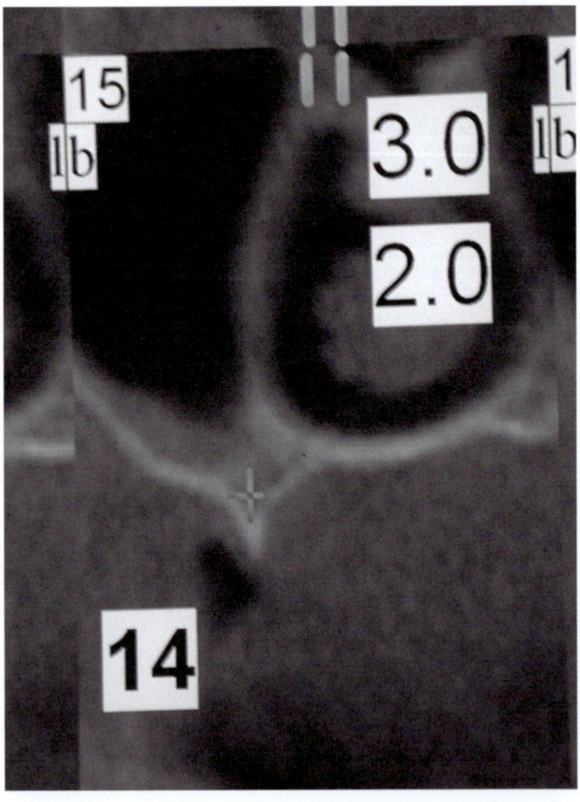

Fig. 5.19 Cone beam CT 60 days after application of bone matrix osseotensors in the right maxillary sinus area (bone gain 2–3 mm)

induce local bony condensation and expansion without destroying the outer architecture of the area, which remains intact.

Type III and type IV bone can thus be "hardened" into active type II bone. Depending on the severity of bone atrophy and the age of the patient, the procedure must be repeated at intervals of 45 to 90 days until the surgeon can manually feel a

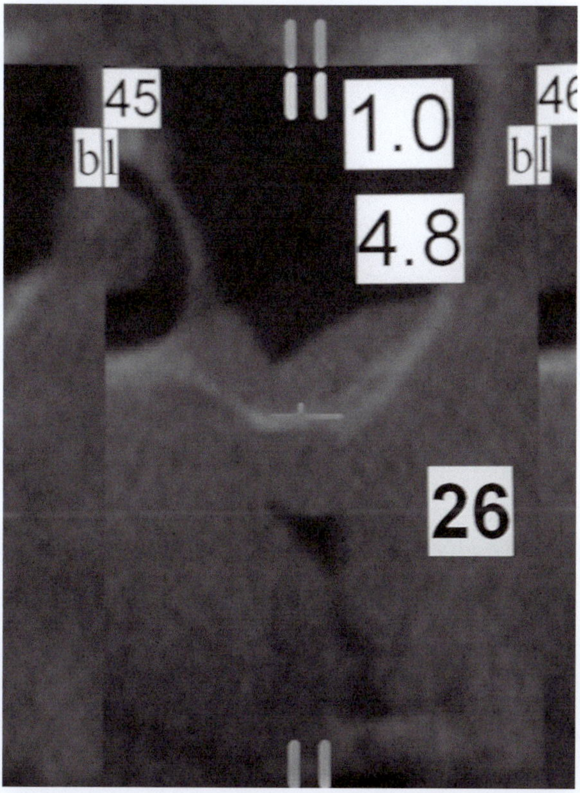

Fig. 5.20 Left maxillary sinus area 60 days after bone matrix osseotensor application (bone gain 4.8 mm)

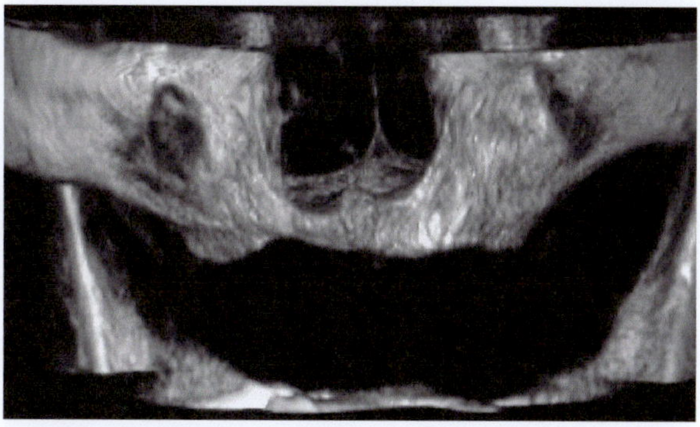

Fig. 5.21 3D reconstruction before implant installation

marked improvement in bone quality in the area. However, a single session suffices in the great majority of cases. For extremely atrophic maxillae, several months of treatment may be required before basal implants can be installed safely. Such waiting periods are usually well-accepted by oral invalids who have previously experienced implant failure or an unsuccessful bone graft. Cone beam CT alone cannot always visualize the improvement of the initial bone density. This change must be confirmed by tactile perception, by probing the area with a manual osseotensor.

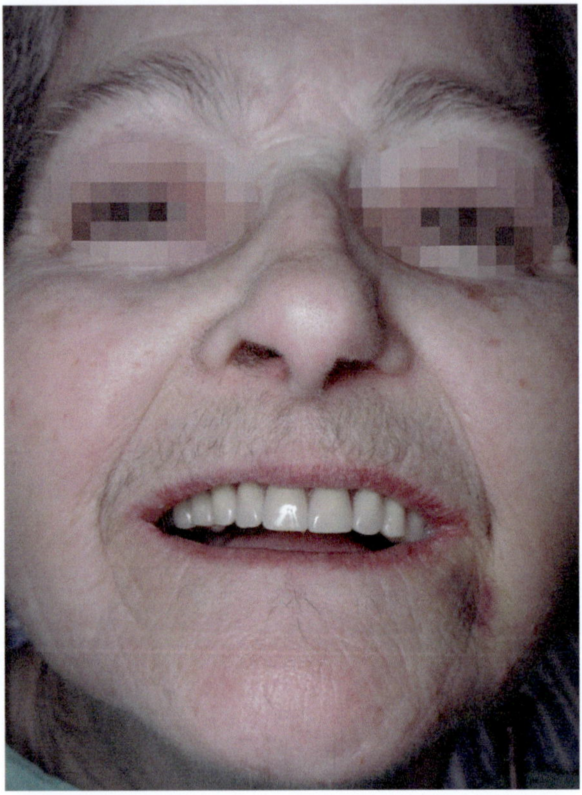

Fig. 5.22 Prosthesis secured to basal implants 72 h after surgery (immediate functional loading). Cosmetic outcome

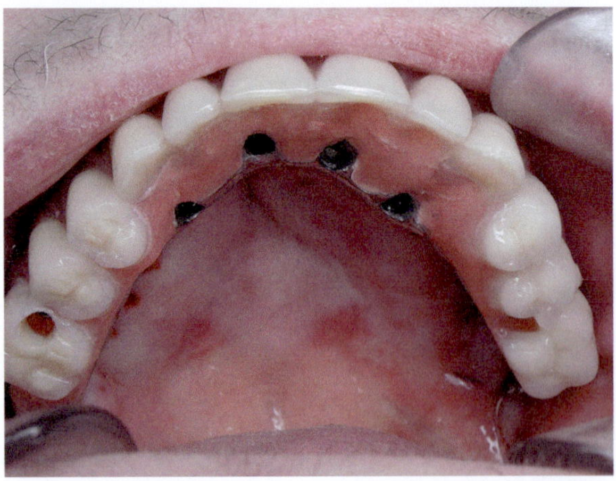

Fig. 5.23 Intraoral view

Rotary Osseotensors for D1 and D2 Bone Densities

Mounted on handpieces (20,000 rpm) and used under copious irrigation, rotary osseotensors are reserved for D1 and D2 dense cortical bone, which is encountered almost exclusively in the mental area of the mandible. Limited areas of D2 bone occur in the maxilla (pterygoid process, zygomatic process, nasal floor, vertical nasal wall). A single axial impact into the bone per future implant site suffices using a flapless approach (impact depth from 3 to 11 mm). At the same time, outside of the cortex, periosteal stem cells can be activated with a manual osseotensor by tunneling the surrounding periosteum; the bleeding that occurs under its inner layer of bone cell progenitors will promote new blood supply. Performed under local anesthesia, the procedure is painless and remains sterile because no flap is elevated. Subperiosteal bleeding is contained and the original bony architecture and peripheral blood supply are maintained.

Rotary osseotensors are the opposite of a conventional drill since they essentially condense the bone rather than remove it. They work by perforating the outer cortex and pushing the endosteal trabeculae against the remaining buccal, lingual, or palatal bone wall. The drilling effect is minimal because only the tip has a cutting function; the remainder of the DLC-coated surface is smooth. D1 bone shows little, if any, bleeding and is unsuitable for direct implant placement. Root-form implants, in particular, are likely to fail in such an environment because D1 bone contains less than 1% living cells and almost no intrabony blood supply capable of promoting osseointegration. In such cases, even with absolute initial stability, an implant may fail because the new bone regeneration cascade requires a new blood supply. This is why a rotary osseotensor should be used for D1 bone sites 8 days prior to implant installation in order to promote neoangiogenesis (a single 10-mm deep impact suffices for each implant site).

Hyperdense, D1 sclerotic bone and D2 bone are "softened" into active D2 bone (i.e., bone with osteoclastic activity) in 6 to 8 days (8 days marks the end of the post-trauma catabolic macrophage-1 phase). This is the best moment for implant placement, distraction, or bone grafting on dense bone; there is no need to wait more than 8 days for an increase in bone density since the bone is already hyperdense. When bone grafting is scheduled, the donor and recipient sites are both activated 8 days before surgery. The effects of bone softening do not last indefinitely, however. Bone splitting, for example, should be performed 8 days post-application, during the initial catabolic phase, before the bone begins to consolidate. This procedure is very helpful for removal of a fractured osseointegrated implant or an impacted canine or wisdom tooth 1 week after use of a rotary osseotensor. In these situations, four impacts down to the level of the apex of the tooth or the implant to be removed are recommended, taking advantage of the initial catabolic phase.

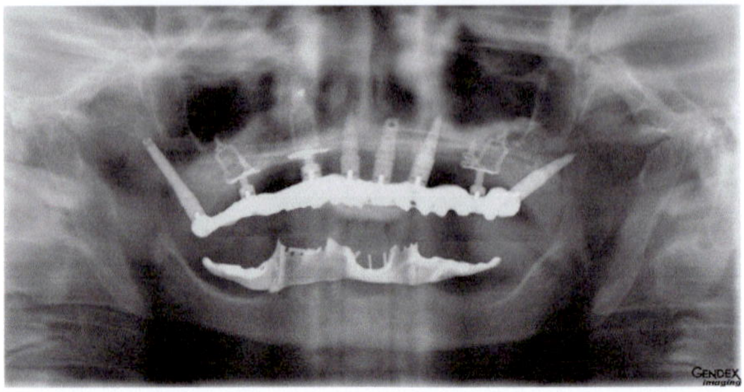

Fig. 5.24 Panorex at 12 years post-op

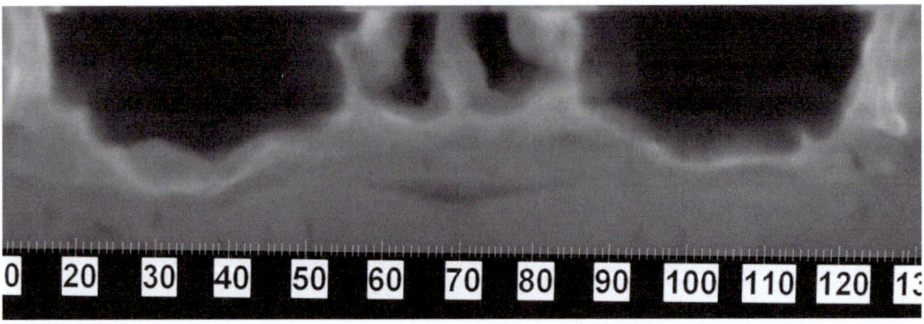

Fig. 5.25 Cone beam CT before osseotensor application (69-year-old patient); initial condition of the atrophic maxilla

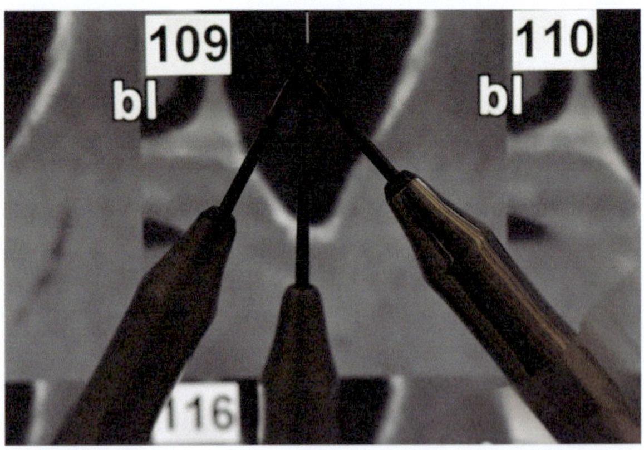

Fig. 5.26 Manual osseotensor applied 60 days before basal implant installation

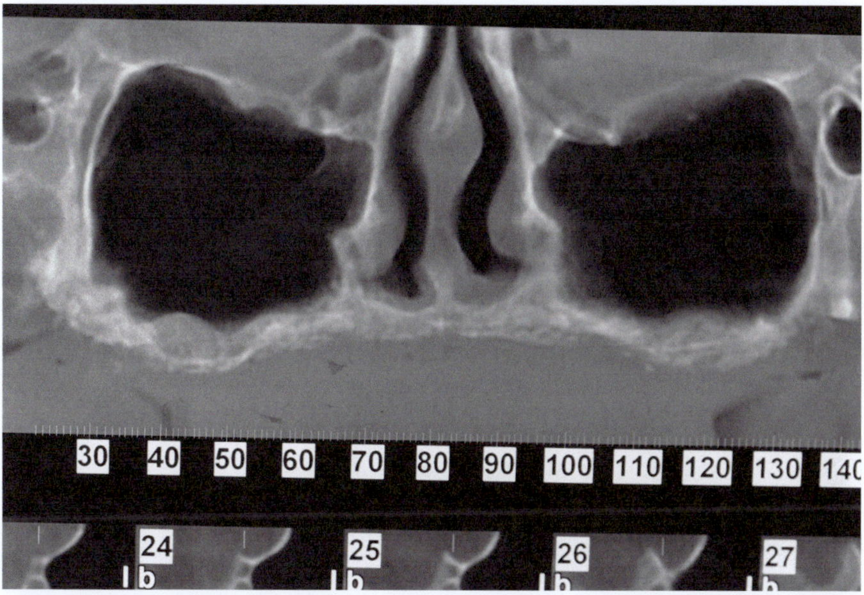

Fig. 5.27 Cone beam CT 90 days after osseotensor application; both the bone volume and density have increased

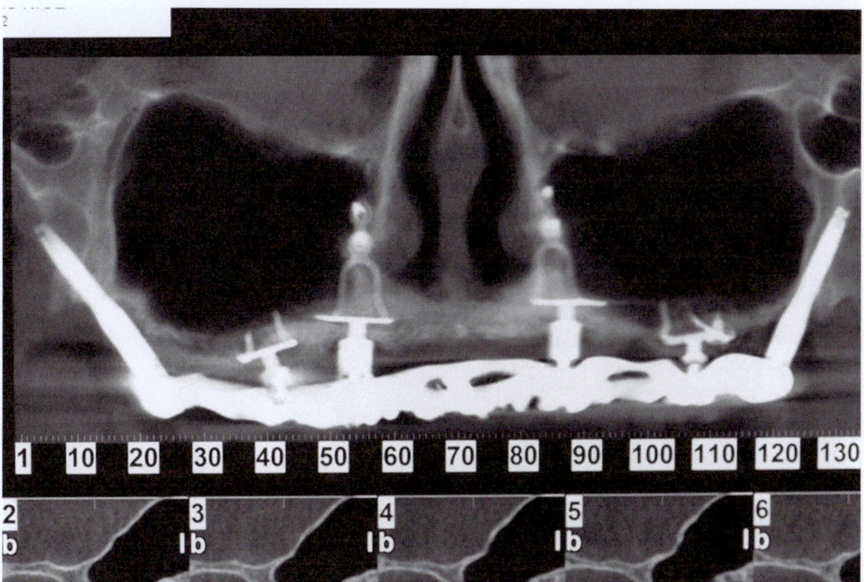

Fig. 5.28 Cone beam panoramic view after basal implant installation in the major maxillary buttresses

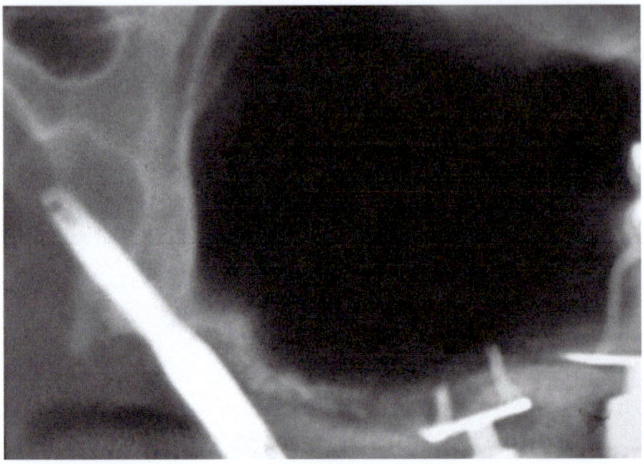

Fig. 5.29 Pterygoid and zygomatic anchorage of basal implants

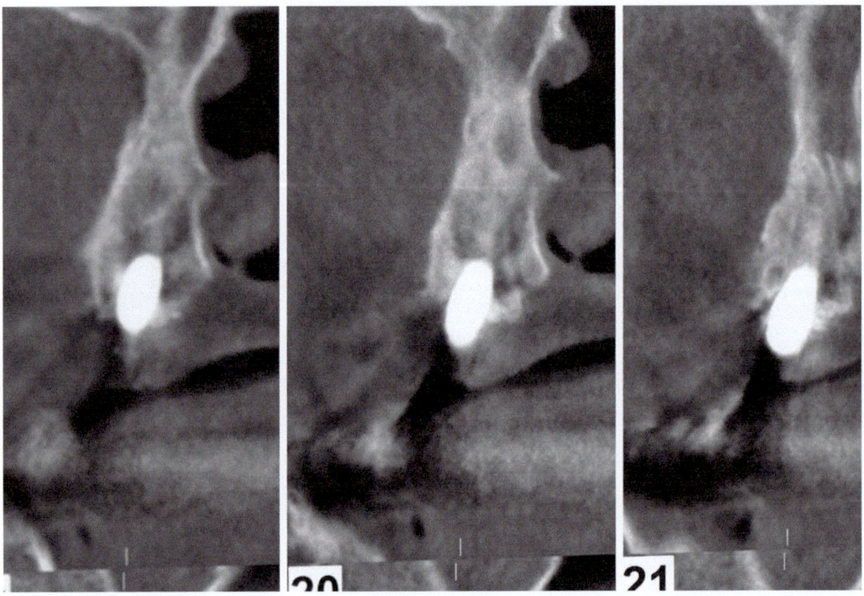

Fig. 5.30 Anchorage of a 20-mm-long root-form implant (Fractal®, Victory) in the dense bony pterygoid process

5.4 Indications and Contraindications for Osseotensors

Successful clinical use of osseotensors for over a decade has led to the establishment of safe, reliable protocols and identification of potential complications (bending of the instrument, fracture of the tip, bone necrosis due to excessive impacts with a rotary osseotensor, infection due to application through an infected sinus, etc.).

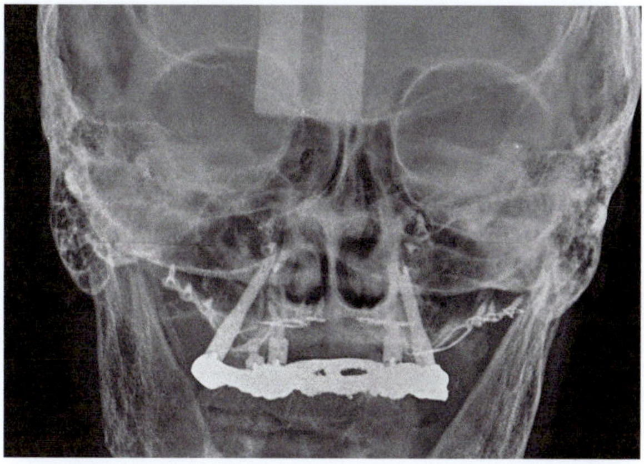

Fig. 5.31 Front view of basal implants firmly anchored on the zygomatic processes (major bony buttresses of the maxilla) using 5–6-mm-long orthopedic screws

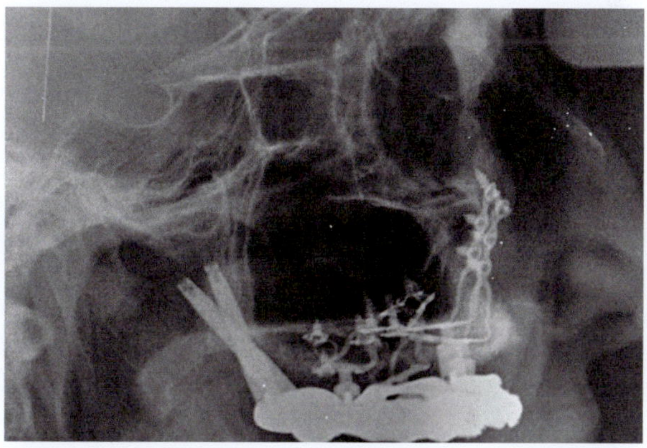

Fig. 5.32 Sagittal view of an angulated root-form implant in the pterygoid process, a zygomatic plate-form Diskimplant®, and basal implants secured with orthopedic screws on the canine buttresses (same patient as Fig. 5.31)

Indications for Manual Osseotensors (Used Mainly in the Maxilla)

Manual osseotensors can be used in three different ways: transparietal penetration of the bone site, tunneling of the periosteum, and as a manual probe to check bone quality.

- Flapless application 45–60 days before implant installation and/or sinus elevation. Only insert the osseotensor through "weak," easy-to-penetrate areas of cancellous bone identified by tactile perception. The number of manual impacts depends on the anatomic situation. When a sinus elevation procedure is planned, the manual osseotensor must pass through the lateral eggshell-thin sinus plate and the sinus membrane. Wait 45 days, and then manually recheck the site. If the density is satisfactory, an immediate loading protocol can be used for management of total edentulism. A submerged protocol is required for partial edentulism (allow a 6- to 9-month waiting period before loading implants placed in initially weak bone).

- Flapless tunneling of the periosteum in order to increase the initial blood supply and activate periosteal stem cells:
  (a) One week before GBR and afterward as a manual probe for verification of bone density
  (b) One week before autologous free and/or pedicle bone grafts

Caution: Never attempt to penetrate dense cortical bone with a manual osseotensor as there is a risk the instrument tip will bend or break. Always try to locate and manually penetrate areas of soft, cancellous, and/or eggshell-thin bone that will harden following formation of a callus.

Indications for Rotary Osseotensors (Used Mainly in the Mandible)

The rotary osseotensor must penetrate to a bone depth of 10 mm under copious irrigation. Indications include:

- Flapless application 1 week before implant placement (a single intrabony impact suffices).
- Flapless application 1 week before extraction of an impacted tooth or mobilization of an impacted canine (four or five impacts around the tooth to be extracted).
- Flapless application 1 week before retrieval of a fractured, osseointegrated implant (three or four impacts around the implant to be removed).
- Flapless application 1 week before distraction and/or crestal expansion (combined with use of a manual osseotensor for the periosteum). A single impact with a rotary osseotensor is sufficient to reduce the density of high knife-ridge cortical bone and allow ulterior distraction/expansion.

Use of Osseotensors for Diskimplants® and Plate-Form Diskimplants®

- Rotary osseotensor 1 week before implant placement in type I or type II bone (anterior mandible) (a single impact at each recipient site). For atrophic mandibles, a single impact in the mental area and an impact in each of the posterior areas above the nerve suffice.
- Manual osseotensor 45–90 days before surgery for type III or type IV bone (mainly encountered in the maxilla). The number of manual impacts is not limited in soft or eggshell-thin bone, but already-dense bone areas should be avoided.
- Manual osseotensor for periosteal stimulation of the posterior mandible 1 week before placement of a ramus plate-form Diskimplant®.

Use of Osseotensors for Root-Form Dental Implants

- Rotary osseotensor 1 week before implant installation in type I or type II bone (anterior mandible); one impact per intended implant site.
- Manual osseotensor 45–90 days before implant placement in type III or type IV bone (maxilla); the number of manual impacts is not limited (usually one impact every 2 mm in eggshell-thin or "butter-like" bony areas).

Verification of Bone Density with a Manual Osseotensor After Sinus Lift Procedures and GBR

Manual osseotensors allow easy tactile evaluation of the results of sinus lift procedures and GBR. After mild local anesthesia (articaine 1:200 000) plus a flash of 2 g amoxicillin, the instrument is inserted using a flapless approach through the mucosa and into the bony area in order to evaluate the density of the grafted material. Once the density of the grafted bone site is judged acceptable, i.e., when the osseotensor no longer easily penetrates the bony area using manual pressure, basal and/or root-form implants can be installed and left submerged for 4 to 6 months (delayed loading protocol).

Contraindications

Since oral implantology and regenerative medicine are elective procedures, bone matrix osseotensors should only be used for physically and mentally healthy individuals. In particular, patients on intravenous, high-dose bisphosphonates are not candidates for osseotensors. Patients with sinusitis, oral infections, inadequate oral hygiene, or poor dental conditions must first be treated and educated before osseotensors can be considered. Finally, patients with mental disorders should be evaluated by a psychiatrist before they can be considered candidates for the procedure.

5.5 Minimally Invasive Sinus Lift: Fractal® Lift

Forty-five to sixty days after osseotensor application, specially designed Fractal® root-form implants (Victory, Nice, France) can be installed in the posterior maxilla, where 2 to 4 mm of residual bone generally remains beneath the sinuses. Installation requires just a single osteotomy with a step drill (Fractal® final drill or pilot drill). Thanks to their reverse micro-thread design, these implants act as stem cell elevators (Fig. 5.9) that prevent perforation of the sinus membrane during implant installation. The apex raises up the Schneiderian membrane without tearing it. Lateral openings and channels permit evacuation of hydraulic pressure at the crestal level. The Fractal® lift procedure does not require placement of any biomaterial.

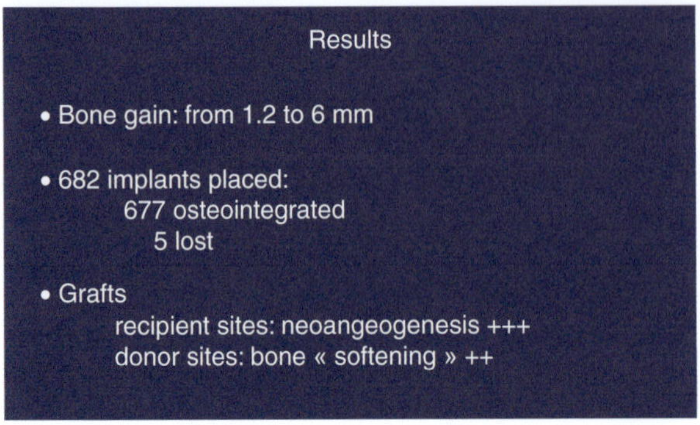

Fig. 5.33 Root-form implant: bone gain after osseotensor application in the sinus area (flapless crestal approach). No bone substitute material was used

When 2–4 mm of bone height are available beneath the sinus floor, an 8 mm Fractal® implant can be placed 60 days after bone matrix activation with a manual osseotensor. If there are at least 4 mm of available bone, an 11-mm Fractal® implant can be installed. When only 2–3 mm of bone are available, only one implant should be placed at a time, at intervals of 45 days, to avoid interrupting the blood supply. A lateral window or a basal implant is appropriate when there are less than 2 mm of initial bone height available under the sinus.

Delayed loading is mandatory for single-tooth replacement and cases of partial edentulism. A waiting period of 6 months or more is necessary for reduced bone heights. Bone density should always be verified manually with an osseotensor before proceeding with osteotomy. If bone density is inadequate, an additional osseotensor session should be performed, with a waiting period of 60 days rather than 45 days before surgery.

Results (Fig. 5.33)

Cone beam CT scans (Planmeca) were used by Vermeulen in 2012 to analyze a series of 682 implants placed 45 to 60 days after application of bone matrix osseotensors; a bone gain of 1.2 to 6 mm was noted in the sinus area (677 of the implants were osseointegrated; 5 had been lost). Results for use of osseotensors in combination with bone grafting revealed that bone graft incorporation and new bone formation were significantly increased at the recipient sites thanks to the initial improvement of the blood supply.

5.6 Tissue Engineering and PRF

Biomaterials (BioOss®, CoreBone®, autologous dentin prepared with a Dentin Grinder®, Ivory® Dentin, etc.) and PRF are often used in GBR tissue engineering and regenerative medicine as scaffolding for the new blood supply, new bone formation, and tissue augmentation. Application of osseotensors is thus essential for initial preparation of target sites for applied tissue engineering protocols. These instruments are also helpful as probes for verification of the result of GBR before implant placement. To increase the initial blood supply and stimulate recruitment of bone progenitor stem cells, manual osseotensors and rotary osseotensors should be used, respectively, 45 days (in D4/D3 bone) to 1 week (in D1/D2 bone) before surgery.

5.7 Platelet-Rich Fibrin (PRF): A Natural and Biological Blood Concentrate

Joseph Choukroun and Alexandre-Amir Aalam

Wound healing is a complex biologic process that includes active participation of cells, connective tissue, extracellular matrix (ECM), and soluble factors and their continuous interaction. Numerous studies have demonstrated that local delivery of multiple growth factors can enhance soft and hard tissue formation. However, since angiogenesis is closely linked with osteogenesis, the ideal scenario is to deliver a cascade of multiple growth factors to induce bone formation.

During the normal wound healing process, a fibrin clot forms immediately after trauma and contains platelets, fibrin, and ECM proteins. In the field of platelet concentrates, the concept of platelet-rich fibrin (PRF) is to obtain a fibrin clot by a centrifugal spin. The PRF clot with integrated growth factors and cytokines provides a favorable environment for cell migration and rapid vascularization.

Platelet-Rich Fibrin (PRF): A Natural Fibrin Matrix Concept

PRF was first developed in France by Choukroun et al. in 2001 [1]. The concept of PRF is to collect an autologous growth factor-concentrated fibrin clot. This technology requires a centrifuge and a blood collection system (PRF Duo, Process for PRF, France). The PRF protocol is very simple: the absence of anticoagulant and a specific tube design allow for quick activation of the blood sample platelets that are in contact with the tube walls and the release of the physiologic coagulation cascade. Fibrinogen is initially concentrated in the top layer of the tube before the circulating thrombin transforms it into fibrin. A fibrin clot is then obtained in the middle layer, just between the red corpuscles at the bottom and acellular plasma (PPP) at the top.

What Is Fibrin?

Fibrin is an activated form of fibrinogen, which is a soluble fibrillar glycoprotein abundantly present in both plasma and platelet alpha-granules. It plays a determinant role in platelet aggregation during hemostasis. It is transformed into a biologic glue which aids in establishing the initial platelet clumping and results in a protective wall for the ruptured endothelial vessel lining. Fibrinogen is transformed into an insoluble fibrin by thrombin, while the polymerized fibrin gel constitutes the first healing matrix for the injured site [2].

Platelets and Cytokines

Platelets are trapped in large numbers in the fibrin mesh. They are formed in bone marrow from pinched off cytoplasmic fragments of megakaryocytes and are released into the circulation. They are discoidal and anuclear structures with an 8- to 10-day life span. Platelets contain alpha-granules, dense granules, and other granules that are secreted at the time of activation. Alpha-granules contain platelet-specific proteins (β-thromboglobulin), non-platelet-specific proteins (fibronectin, thrombospondin, fibrinogen) and other coagulation factors, growth promoters, fibrinolysis inhibitors, and immunoglobulins. Dense granules contain adenosine diphosphate (ADP), adenosine triphosphate (ATP), ionized calcium, histamine, and serotonin. The platelet phospholipid double layer membrane contains glycoproteins that function as receptors for collagen and other molecules. Activation is fundamental to initiate hemostasis due to platelet aggregation at the injured site and in the interaction with coagulation mechanisms [3, 4].

Cytokines

Cytokines and growth factors are small proteins released from platelet alpha-granules after clotting whose function is mediated through specific cell receptors. The release of cytokines during degranulation stimulates cell migration and proliferation within the fibrin matrix, launching the first stages of healing [2]. There are numerous cytokines in PRF:

- Transforming growth factor ß1 (TGF-ß1) is the most powerful fibrosis agent of all the cytokines.
- PDGF (platelet-derived growth factor). Mesenchymal cell mitogen is an essential regulator for migration, proliferation, and survival of mesenchymal cells, according to its specific receptor distribution.
- The IGF axis: protective cell agent (insulin-like growth factors—IGFs).
- EGF.
- FGF.

Slow release of growth factors by the PRF membrane: Several studies clearly demonstrate that the PRF membrane sustains a substantial slow release of key growth factors for at least 1 week [5, 6].

Leukocytes: A Key Parameter

The literature dealing with platelet concentrates often ignores the impact of leukocytes, which are key participants: they produce large amounts of VEGF and PDGF which are crucial for promotion of angiogenesis [4, 7].

Evolution of PRF

1. Advanced Platelet-Rich Fibrin (A-PRF)
   Since 2012, considerable evidence has been accumulated about the role of white cells in vascularization and bone formation [8]. Granulocytes play a major role in vascularization and improve the function of monocytes which are now named "supercells for bone regeneration" [9]. Monocytes and macrophages produce BMP-2 [10]. The synergy of fibrin and monocytes is evident. Understanding the g-force role on white cell loss during the spin leads to a reduction of the centrifugal force (in rpm). Thus, the matrix function is improved [11].
2. Injectable Platelet-Rich Fibrin (i-PRF)
   With the same concept of a non-additive system, the i-PRF was designed in 2014. Blood is drawn into a specially designed tube that is centrifuged at very low speed for a short time (3 min). The objective was double:
   - To enhance the amount of physiological inflammatory cells and mesenchymal stem cells (detected by flow cytometry analysis according to the characteristics published by the International Society for Cell Therapy): we found 20 times more white cells in the supernatant than in the PRP, and 1–2% of the cells in this supernatant are MSCs.
   - To obtain a liquid form of PRF at the end of the spin that clots after several minutes. This technique allows liquid injection into the site (gingiva or PDL) or into the bone graft. When the i-PRF is injected into the bone graft (already mixed with the A-PRF fragments), it clots very quickly (1 min) and permits a more cohesive and malleable bone graft.

This technique is specifically interesting for sinus lift procedures where a more solid bone graft reduces bone graft particle migration into the maxillary sinus. The stability of the bone graft particles embedded in a fibrin clot allows much easier adaptation and more rapid vascularization.

Clinical Use and Indications (Figs. 5.34, 5.35, 5.36, 5.37, 5.38, 5.39, 5.40, and 5.41)

Clinically, PRF is used as a tissue matrix and as a recipient bed for growth factors. Clots are prepared in a metal PRF container (PRF Box), which permits their slight compression into membrane or plug form. This form permits the easiest clinical application. All clinical situations in oral surgery may be improved by the use of A-PRF or i-PRF: socket preservation, bone grafts, and soft tissue management [12].

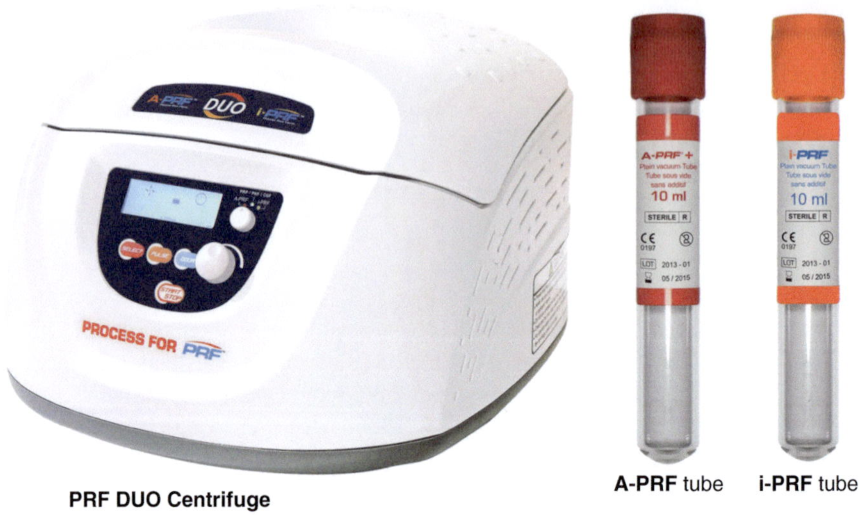

Fig. 5.34 PRF Duo centrifuge and A-PRF and i-PRF tubes

Fig. 5.35 Blood tube after centrifugation

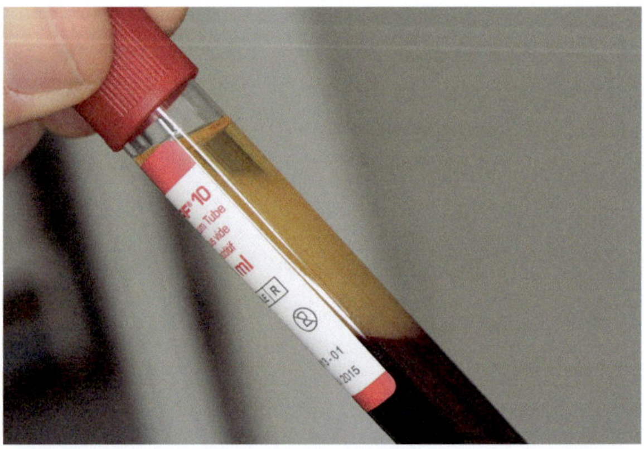

Fig. 5.36 PRF membranes

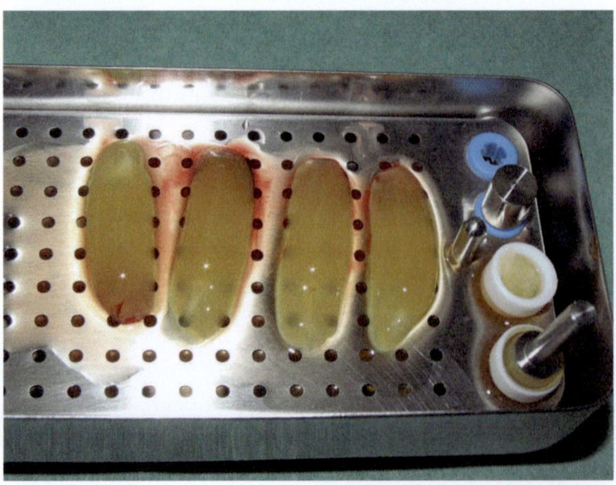

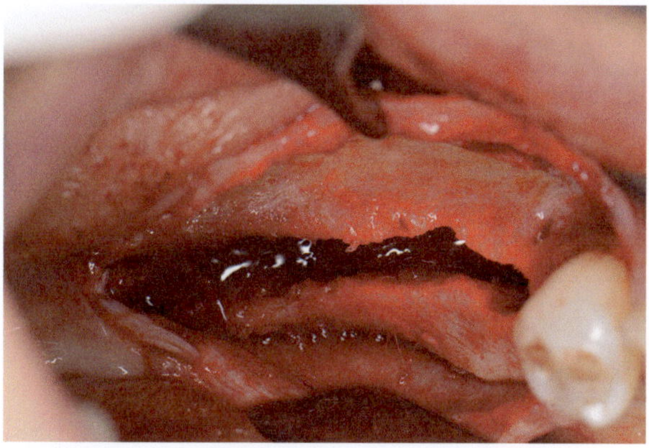

Fig. 5.37 Sockets after extraction

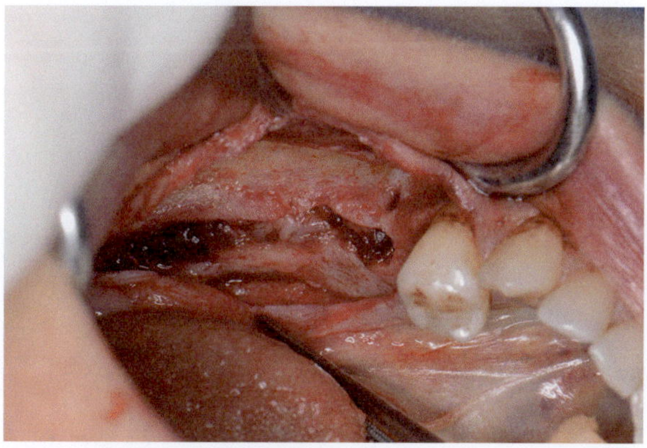

Fig. 5.38 Filling with A-PRF

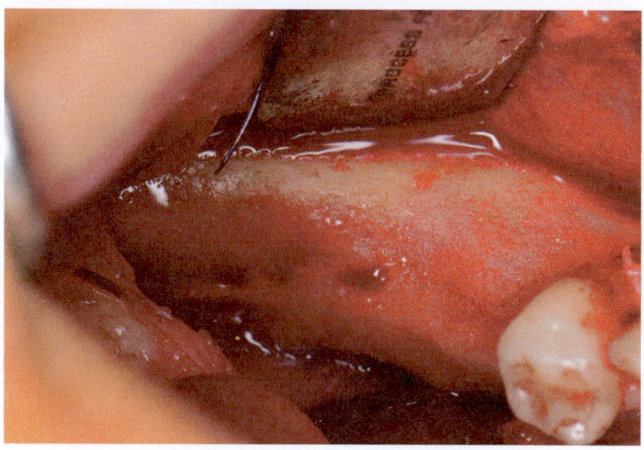

Fig. 5.39 Follow-up at 4 months

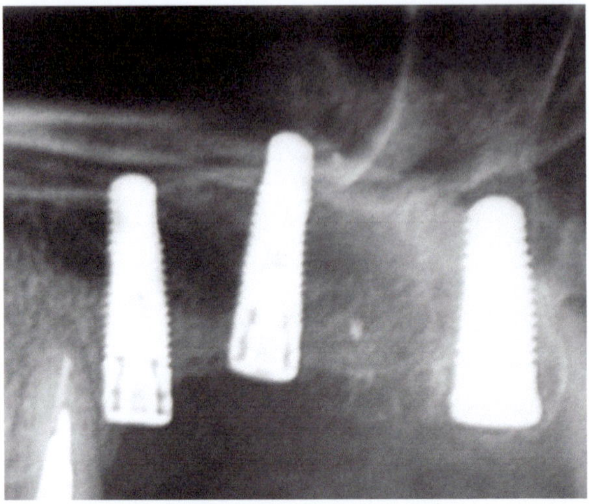

Fig. 5.40 Follow-up at 4 months; sinus lift with only PRF

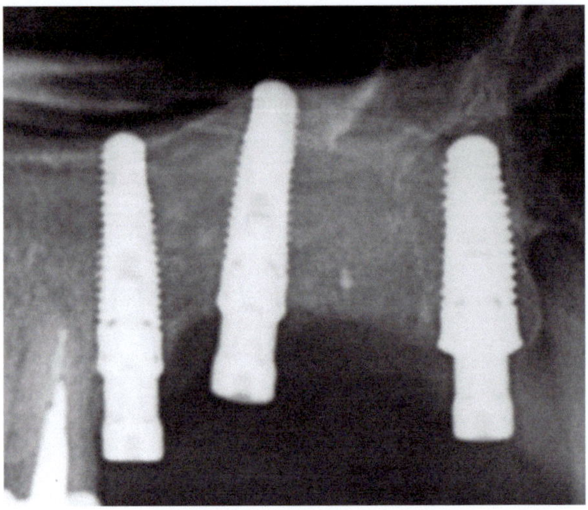

Fig. 5.41 Follow-up at 6 months

5.8 Conclusion

The very simple and inexpensive PRF technique provides an autologous fibrin matrix with slow release of growth factors. With over 15 years of experience in the use of PRF, more than 500 articles on the subject are available in Medline, confirming the validity of the approach. However, it remains a technique in progress, and future enhancements will be made with the evolution of tissue engineering.

Conflict of interest statement Gérard M. Scortecci is the inventor of the Diskimplant and holder of several associated patents that are exploited by the Victory company. He is an unpaid consultant to this firm and a minority shareholder in the company. No money was received from any of the companies mentioned in the book or from any of the companies whose products are mentioned.

Recommended Reading

1. Choukroun J, Adda F, Schoeffler C, Vervelle A. Une opportunité en paro-implantologie: le PRF. Implantodontie. 2001;1(42):55–62.
2. Mosesson MW, Siebenlist KR, Meh DA. The structure and biological features of fibrinogen and fibrin. Ann N Y Acad Sci. 2001;936:11–30.
3. Weibrich G, Kleis WK, Kunz-Kostomanolakis M, Loos AH, Wagner W. Correlation of platelet concentration in platelet-rich plasma to the extraction method, age, sex, and platelet count of the donor. Int J Oral Maxillofac Implants. 2001;16:693–9.
4. Weibrich G, Kleis WK, Hafner G, Hitzler WE, Wagner W. Comparison of platelet, leukocyte, and growth factor levels in point-of-care platelet-enriched plasma, prepared using a modified Curasan kit, with preparations received from a local blood bank. Clin Oral Implants Res. 2003;14:357–62.
5. Fujioka-Kobayashi M, Miron RJ, Hernandez M, Kandalam U, Zhang Y, Choukroun J. Optimized platelet rich fibrin with the low speed concept: growth factor release, biocompatibility and cellular response. J Periodontol. 2016;2:1–17.
6. Shamloo A, Xu H, Heilshorn S. Mechanisms of vascular endothelial growth factor-induced pathfinding by endothelial sprouts in biomaterials. Tissue Eng Part A. 2012;18(3–4):320–30.
7. Maciel J, Oliveira MI, Colton E, McNally AK, Oliveira C, Anderson JM, Barbosa MA. Adsorbed fibrinogen enhances production of bone- and angiogenic-related factors by monocytes/macrophages. Tissue Eng Part A. 2014;20(1–2):250–63.
8. Kawazoe T, Kim HH. Tissue augmentation by white blood cell-containing platelet-rich plasma. Cell Transplant. 2012;21(2–3):601–7.
9. Soltan M, Rohrer MD, Prasad HS. Monocytes: super cells for bone regeneration. Implant Dent. 2012;21(1):13–20.
10. Pirraco RP, Reis RL, Marques AP. Effect of monocytes/macrophages on the early osteogenic differentiation of hBMSCs. J Tissue Eng Regen Med. 2013;7(5):392–400.
11. Ghanaati S, Booms P, Orlowska A, Kubesch A, Lorenz J, Rutkowski J, Landes C, Sader R, Kirkpatrick C, Choukroun J. Advanced platelet-rich fibrin: a new concept for cell-based tissue engineering by means of inflammatory cells. J Oral Implantol. 2014;40(6):679–89.
12. Miron RJ, Fujioka-Kobayashi M, Bishara M, Zhang Y, Hernandez M, Choukroun J. Platelet-rich fibrin and soft tissue wound healing: a systematic review. Tissue Eng Part B Rev. 2016;23(1):83–99.
13. Alikhani M. Accelerated orthodontics. Integrating a new concept in your daily practice. Presented at: XXXI World ICOI Congress; the Future of Implant Dentistry; October 3–5, 2014, Tokyo, Japan; 2014.
14. Barone A, Nannmark U. Bone biomaterials & beyond. Milano: Edra Milano; 2014.
15. Binderman I, Zor U, Kaye AM, et al. The transduction of mechanical force into biochemical events in bone cells may involve activation of phospholipidase A2. Calcif Tissue Int. 1988;42:261–6.
16. Bonewald F. The amazing osteocyte. J Bone Miner Res. 2011;26(2):229–38.
17. Bouletreau PJ, Warren SM, Spector JA, Peled ZM, Gerrets RP, Greenwald JA, Longaker MT. Hypoxia and VEGF up-regulate BMP2 mRNA and protein expression in microvascular endothelial cells: implications for fracture healing. Plast Reconstr Surg. 2002;109:2384–97.
18. Chappard D. Les cellules osseuses, le modelage et le remodelage osseux. In: Guillaume B, Audran M, Chappard D, editors. Tissue osseux et biomatériaux en chirurgie dentaire, vol. 2. Paris: Quintesssence International; 2014. p. 21–41.
19. Chenyu H, Ogawa R. Mechanotransduction in bone repair and regeneration. FASEB J. 2010;24(10):3625–32.
20. Dolan EB, Vaughan TJ, Nieburg GL, Casey C, Tallon D, McNamara LM. How bone tissue and cells experience elevated temperatures during orthopaedic cutting: an experimental and computational investigation. J Biomech Eng. 2014;136:021019.
21. Dolan EB, Haugh MG, Voisin MC, Tallon D, McNamara LM. Thermally induced osteocyte damage initiates a remodelling signalling cascade. PLoS One. 2015;10:e0119652.

22. Eghbali-Fatourechi GZ, Lamsam J, Fraser D, Nagel D, Riggs BL, Sundeep K, Khosla S. Circulating osteoblast-lineage cells in humans. N Engl J Med. 2005;352:1959–66.
23. Ekström K, Omar O, Granéli C, Wang X, Vazirisani F, Thomsen P. Monocyte exosomes stimulate the osteogenic gene expression of mesenchymal stem cells. PLoS One. 2013;8(9):e75227. https://doi.org/10.1371/journal.pone.0075227.
24. Frost MH. The biology of fracture healing. An overview for clinicians. Part II. Clin Orthop Relat Res. 1989;248:294–309.
25. Huang C, Ogaxa R. Mechanotransduction in bone repair and regeneration. FASEB J. 2010;24:3625–32.
26. Ilizarov GA. The principles of the Ilizarov method. Bull Hosp Joint Dis Orthop Inst. 1988;48:1–11.
27. Ilizarov GA. The tension stress effect on the genesis and growth of tissues. Part I. The influence of stability of fixation and soft-tissue preservation. Clin Orthop Relat Res. 1989a;238:249–81.
28. Ilizarov GA. The tension stress effect on the genesis and growth of tissues. Part II. The influence of the rate and frequency of distraction. Clin Orthop Relat Res. 1989b;239:263–85.
29. Ilizarov GA. Clinical application of the tension stress effect for limb lengthening. Clin Orthop Relat Res. 1990;250:8–26.
30. Ingber DE. Tensegrity: the architectural basis of cellular mechanotransduction. Annu Rev Physiol. 1997;59:575–99.
31. Ingber DE. Mechanobiology and diseases of mechanotransduction. Ann Med. 2003;35:564–77.
32. Kazanjian VH. The interrelation of dentistry and surgery in the treatment of deformities of the face and jaws. Am J Orthod Oral Surg. 1941;27:10–30.
33. Kuroda R, Matsumoto T, Kawakami Y, Fukui T, Mifune Y, M Kurosaka M. Clinical impact of circulating CD34-positive cells on bone regeneration and healing. Tissue Eng Part B Rev. 2014;20(3):190–9. https://doi.org/10.1089/ten.TEB.2013.0511.
34. Marx JL. Angiogenesis research comes of age. Science. 1987;237:23–4.
35. Matsumoto T, Kawamoto A, Kuroda R, Ishikawa M, Mifune Y, Iwasaki H, Miwa M, Horii M, Hayashi S, Oyamada A, Nishimura H, Murasawa S, Doita M, Kurosaka M, Asahara T. Therapeutic potential of vasculogenesis and osteogenesis promoted by peripheral blood CD34-positive cells for functional bone healing. Am J Pathol. 2006;169(4):1440–57.
36. McNulty MA, Virdi AS, Christopherson KW, Sena K, Frank RR, Sumner DR. Adult stem cell mobilization enhances intramembranous bone regeneration: a pilot study. Clin Orthop Relat Res. 2012;470(9):2503–12.
37. Misch CE. Contemporary implant dentistry. St Louis, MO: Mosby Elsevier; 2008. p. 1034–5.
38. Misch CE, Qu Z, Bidez MW. Mechanical properties of trabecular bone in the human mandible. Implications of dental implant planning and surgical placement. J Oral Maxillofac Surg. 1999;57:700–6.
39. Morgan EF, Gleason RE, Hayward LNM, Leong PL, Palomares KTS. Mechanotransduction and fracture repair. J Bone Joint Surg Am. 2008;90(Suppl 1):25–30.
40. Mukherjee S, Raje N, Schoonmaker JA, Liu JC, Hideshima T, Wein MN, Jones DC, et al. Pharmacologic targeting of a stem/progenitor population in vivo is associated with enhanced bone regeneration in mice. J Clin Invest. 2008;118(2):491–504.
41. Odin G, Misch CE, Binderman I, et al. Fixed rehabilitation of severely atrophic jaws using immediately loaded basal disk implants after in situ bone activation. J Oral Implantol. 2012;38:611–6.
42. Odin G, Petitbois R, Cotten P, Philip P. Distraction osteogenesis using bone matrix osteotensors in ectodermal dysplasia: a case report. Implant Dent. 2015;24(5):612–9.
43. Scortecci G. Activation of osteogenesis via bone matrix osteotensors prior to implant placement and/or bone grafting procedures. Nine years of clinical follow-up and research. Presented at XXXI ICOI World Congress; The Future of Implant Dentistry; October 3–5, 2014, Tokyo, Japan; 2014.
44. Scortecci G, Misch CE, Benner KU. Implants and restorative dentistry. London: Martin Dunitz; 2000. p. 79–85.

45. Sundelacruz S, Levin M, Kaplan DL. Membrane potential controls adipogenic and osteogenic differentiation of mesenchymal stem cells. PLoS One. 2008;3(11):e3737. https://doi.org/10.1371/journal.pone.0003737.
46. Sundelacruz S, Levin M, Kaplan DL. Comparison of the depolarization response of human mesenchymal stem cells from different donors. Sci Rep. 2015;5:18279. https://doi.org/10.1038/srep18279.
47. Suya H. Corticotomy in orthodontics. In: Hosl E, Baldauf A, editors. Mechanical and biological basics in orthodontic therapy. Heidelberg: Hütlig Buch; 1991. p. 207–26.
48. Urist MR. Bone formation by auto-induction. Science. 1965;150:893–9.
49. Vermeulen J. Euro Implanto lecture. France: Nice; 2012.
50. Zaidi N, Nixon AJ. Stem cell therapy in bone repair and regeneration. Ann N Y Acad Sci. 2007;1117:62–72.
51. Zhang W, Zhu C, Wu Y, Ye D, Wang S, Zou D, Zhang X, Kaplan DL, Jiang X. VEGF and BMP-2 promote bone regeneration by facilitating bone marrow stem cell homing and differentiation. Eur Cell Mater. 2014;27:1–11.

Part II

Step-by-Step Basal Implantology

Indications and Contraindications

6

Gérard M. Scortecci

6.1 Medical and Dental Risk Assessment in Basal Implantology

Basal implant therapy requires respect of the same principles and diagnostic methodology as for root-form implants. The medical and dental history, vital signs, comprehensive clinical examination of the head and neck, and laboratory studies indicate whether the patient is in good health. They may reveal significant pathological conditions and serve as the basis for risk assessment. They also document the need to obtain a medical consultation to diagnose a suspected systemic disease and, if necessary, obtain treatment by a specialist. The family physician or medical specialist also provides his expertise and experience to fully evaluate physical or mental status and the special risks of general anesthesia or the use of intravenous sedation together with local anesthesia in medically compromised patients. Medications that are prescribed pre- and postoperatively may interact with the patient's existing drug regimen.

The following guidelines are means to avoid unforeseen complications.

- *Primum non nocere* (Hippocrates, fifth century BC): the physician's mission is to safeguard the health of the people and not aggravate it. The normal course of any therapy is to improve the patient's health. This is especially the case for dental implant installation, which is not an emergency procedure.
- Examination, diagnosis, and prevention of problems: many potential complications can be avoided by simple preventive measures, the best of which is an

G. M. Scortecci (✉)
University of Nice-Sophia Antipolis Medical School, Nice, France

New York University, New York, NY, USA

University of Southern California, Los Angeles, CA, USA

Private Practice, Nice, France
e-mail: scortecci@wanadoo.fr

© Springer Nature Switzerland AG 2019

G. M. Scortecci (ed.), *Basal Implantology*, https://doi.org/10.1007/978-3-319-44873-2_6

adequate patient history and examination, including vital signs and the psychological status of the patient. All pertinent information obtained during initial and subsequent preoperative visits should be conserved.

- Long-term objectives for implant treatment: poor oral hygiene, drug and tobacco abuse, and difficult mechanical and occlusal conditions can all compromise long-term success and patient compliance. Risk/benefit analysis is required before a decision is made.
- Reliable treatment planning: overly risky basal implant treatment options must be avoided. Alternative conventional denture treatment should be considered first and discussed with the implant candidate. This includes the possible use of bone grafting prior to placement of root-form or basal implants. Three-dimensional implant planning using appropriate planning software with a basal implant library and stereolithographic models allows determination the optimum number of basal implants and their positions.
- Informed consent and cost: the patient must be clearly informed of the risks and benefits of basal implant treatment. Psychologically unstable patients are not good implant candidates. The procedure must be fully explained to the patient prior to the start of therapy, including prosthetic considerations and maintenance and timing. The total duration of the basal implant treatment must be explained. Patients must be informed of potential risks and the fact that the occurrence of unforeseeable events may require modification and/or corrections with possible return to a conventional appliance.

  The total cost must be also indicated as soon as possible.

- Strategy for management of potential failures: preference should be given to easy-to-retrieve or easy-to-manage basal implant systems permitting rapid return to the pre-implant surgery situation without compromising the use of conventional removable prosthetic devices.
- Osteogenic activation with bone matrix osseotensors before implant surgery to improve the bone density of the future recipient bone bed.

6.2 Contraindications to Implant Therapy

Relative Contraindications

As for axial implants, there are a number of relative contraindications for basal implant treatment that require particular attention before a decision is made to proceed with implant placement. Successful implant therapy will obviously be compromised in heavy smokers and individuals with poor oral hygiene unless lifestyle changes are made. A history of substance abuse or chronic ethylism should also prompt thorough assessment of the patient's capacity for compliance. Finally, implant installation is generally not advisable during pregnancy.

Implant candidates with inadequately controlled diabetes, erythropoietic or phosphocalcic metabolic disorders, or immunodeficiency syndrome can receive

Table 6.1 Oral manifestations of aging

Manifestation	Cause/consequence
Loss of teeth	Primarily caused by degeneration of periodontal and/or dental (caries) structures Atrophy of the posterior mandibular and maxillary sectors due to tooth loss and subsequent wear of a removable denture
Alveolar bone loss	Periodontal disease, bone atrophy, iatrogenic effect of denture(s)
Basal bone loss	The bone remaining after alveolar bone loss is mainly basal bone, which has a poor blood supply and algodystrophic areas. This bone can continuously disappear if stress is applied by a removable denture.
Attrition	Rate is influenced by diet and masticatory habits (bruxism)
Oral mucosa	Loss of elasticity with dryness and atrophy; tendency to hyperkeratosis
Gingivae	Loss of stippling, edematous appearance; keratinized layer thin or absent; tissue friable and easily injured. Bleeding due to medication Highly sensitive mobile mucosa with very little attached gingiva
Saliva	Diminished function of salivary glands with relative or absolute xerostomia owing to atrophy of cells lining the intermediate ducts; xerostomia also results in abnormal taste sensations and stomatodynia
Tongue	Atrophic glossitis, probably caused by concurrent vitamin B complex deficiency
Lips	Angular cheilosis is very common and probably is related to concurrent vitamin B deficiency and close bite; cheilitis and "purse-string" mouth caused by dehydration
Masticatory muscles	Myoatrophy caused by hypofunction
Maxillary sinus pneumatization	Descent of the bone structure and upper molars following sinus expansion
Oral invalidity	Patient is unable to wear a full or partial denture for physical (including gag reflex) and/or psychological reasons; remains without teeth and eats only soft meals directly on the gums; is incapable of adapting to any type of removable appliance
Oral manifestations of neurodegenerative diseases/ Parkinson's disease	The constant rotational movement of the tongue seen in patients with Parkinson's disease makes it difficult to wear a removable denture
Alzheimer's disease	Patient unable to cope with a removable denture. Possible loss of the removable appliance

implants in certain cases, but expert medical advice should be sought first (Table 6.1). This is also the case for patients undergoing radiotherapy, individuals with a history of prolonged use of corticosteroids, and those taking anticoagulants or at risk for cardiac disease. Likewise, IV administration of bisphosphonates has been linked to osteonecrosis of the jaw.

Absolute Contraindications

The so-called "absolute" contraindications comprise systemic diseases that are life-endangering or may seriously jeopardize the patient's health, as well as compromise the long-term success of implants [1]. At-risk patients should always be referred to their general physician or a specialist before a final decision is made to proceed with implant therapy. The following is a non-exhaustive list of common absolute contraindications:

- Heavy bruxism, clenching, uncontrolled malocclusion, and/or a history of fractured teeth, especially when associated with psychological problems
- High-dose IV bisphosphonates for treatment of severe osteoporosis or cancer (risk of osteonecrosis of the jaw)
- Facial and trigeminal neuropathies associated with a depressive state, epilepsy
- Severe heart disease, recent stroke, or heart attack (risk of infectious endocarditis)
- Severe or uncontrolled diabetes
- Untreated renal insufficiency
- Ongoing radiotherapy for cancer (risk of osteoradionecrosis of the jaw, especially after radiation of the head and neck region)

Basal Implants in Childhood and Adolescence

Basal implants represent an interesting therapeutic approach with very specific indications in young patients. The limitations and contraindications to their use are related primarily to their long-term impact. One of the main problems is the fatigue resistance of the implanted material: fracture of the implant body may require either repeat surgery or abandon of the fractured implant in situ and return to a conventional approach. Basal implants should not be installed in adolescents who have not yet completed their growth. The current consensus is that implants should not be installed before 18–20 years of age, except for patients with complete agenesis, as can occur in certain cases of ectodermal dysplasia. In Europe, the USA, and Japan, the life expectancy of teenage implant patients is approximately 60 years. The outcome of basal implants subjected to the stress of mastication for such long periods is still not known. To date, the longest observation period for a continuously functioning freestanding central incisor Diskimplant® is 33 years (1984–2018).

Cosmetics remains a difficult problem because osseointegrated implants do not follow the same pattern of continuous eruption as natural teeth. The implant margin remains fixed, whereas the natural tooth margin tends to descend in the upper incisor area of young patients, which is the most critical site for esthetics.

Psychological Contraindications

The following conditions are generally regarded as psychiatric contraindications to implant treatment:

- Psychotic syndromes, i.e., schizophrenia or paranoia
- Alcohol or drug abuse, if not diagnosed with great certainty as secondary to the oral problem

- Severe character disorders and neurotic syndromes, i.e., hysteroid and borderline personality
- Body dysmorphic disorder (BDD) and patients with extreme and unrealistic expectations and demands regarding the cosmetic outcome of the operation rather than functional results
- Syndromes associated with cerebral lesions and presenile dementia

Patients presenting with the above disorders must be identified as early as possible. However, it is equally important to offer treatment to those patients whose edentulism is a causal factor of their psychiatric or social problems. Owing to the importance of correct patient selection, a psychiatrist should be consulted when necessary. In general, dysmorphophobic and bipolar patients are not suitable candidates for extensive basal implant treatments, but they can be accepted after psychiatric evaluation and treatment for limited implant protocols, such as single-tooth replacement, if oral conditions are not extreme.

There are also patients who consider a complete, fixed implant-supported restoration the ultimate solution to all of their problems. They may believe that the elimination of any remaining teeth will forever eliminate all of the discomfort and pain they have endured in the past, thus obviating the need for any future dental care. These patients may therefore demand the removal of teeth that perhaps can be restored successfully. For other individuals, however, the loss of remaining teeth is a tremendous psychological blow, and it may take some time for them to accept the diagnosis. Basal implantology offers an alternative to conventional removable dentures in many cases and makes it possible to help patients who, for anatomical or psychological reasons, have been unable to cope with conventional prosthetic treatment.

6.3 Indications for Basal Implant Treatment [2–26]

1. Bone volume incompatible with direct placement of axial (crestal) root-form implants (Figs. 6.1 and 6.2).
2. Bone volume suitable for root-form implants but bone quality is poor (D4). Basal implants can be considered in such cases thanks to their wide base providing multicortical anchorage. Osseotensors should be used to improve bone density 45 days prior to implant placement.
3. Reduced buccal opening preventing axial drilling (premolar/molar mandibular sectors).
4. Bone grafting and/or sinus floor elevation refused by the patient or contraindicated (Figs. 6.2, 6.3, 6.4, 6.5, 6.6, 6.7, 6.8, 6.9, 6.10, 6.11 and 6.12).
5. Salvage surgery after failure of root-form implants and/or bone grafting (Figs. 6.2, 6.3 and 6.4); an immediate loading protocol can be used for completely edentulous patients (Figs. 6.13, 6.14 and 6.15).
6. Extraction-immediate Diskimplant® implantation with simultaneous GBR when the entire buccal plate has been destroyed (Figs. 6.16 and 6.17).
7. High, thin knife ridge (buccal-lingual width <3 mm) with simultaneous GBR at Diskimplant® installation.

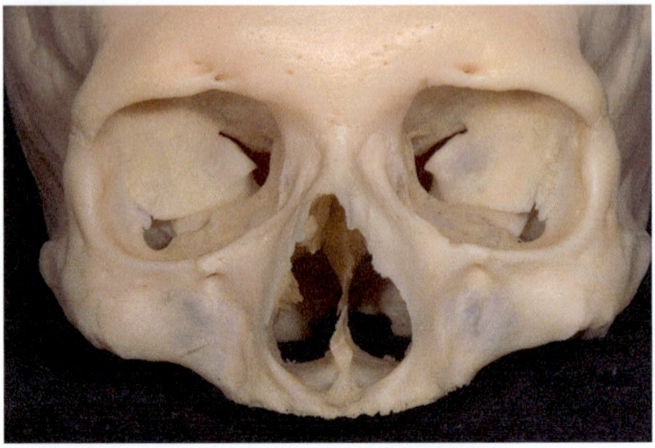

Fig. 6.1 The bone quality and volume of this extremely atrophic dry maxilla are incompatible with installation of root-form implants unless bone grafting is performed first. This is a typical indication for plate-form Diskimplants®

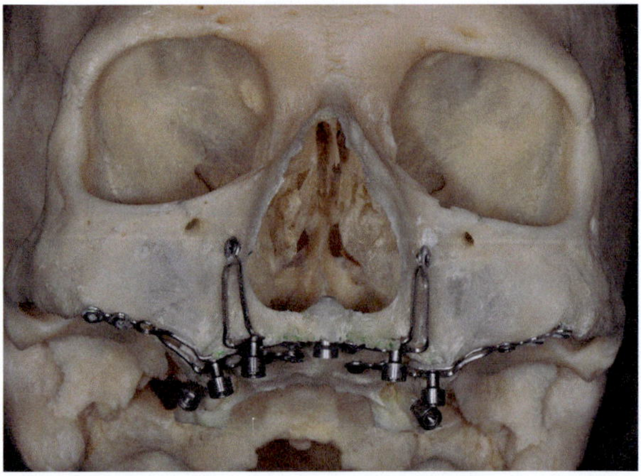

Fig. 6.2 Extremely atrophic dry maxilla: this is not an indication for prior bone grafting. Plate-form Diskimplants® are indicated in the canine pillar and zygomatic areas. An immediate loading protocol is mandatory with a highly rigid, screw-secured fixed prosthesis acting as an external orthopedic fixation appliance. Use of a removable denture would irrevocably compromise the basal implant rehabilitation

8. Severe maxillary and/or mandibular atrophy: ultrashort monodisk Diskimplants® (bone height <4 mm) (Fig. 6.8) or plate-form Diskimplants® (Fig. 6.9) can be installed without prior bone grafting.
9. Totally edentulous patients: 45–60 days after local stem cell activation with a manual osseotensor, a rapid return to fixed teeth is possible for eggshell-thin maxillae using an immediate functional loading procedure with simultaneous placement of bone substitute material and/or GBR (Figs. 6.10, 6.11, 6.12, 6.13, 6.14, 6.15, 6.16, 6.17, 6.18, 6.19 and 6.20).
10. Partially edentulous patients: immediate functional loading for the posterior maxilla and mandible may be an option if clinical parameters are favorable and at least three or four implants are connected together. Delayed loading remains safer for single-tooth replacements and two implants.
11. Connection with strong, healthy natural teeth is possible in selected cases.

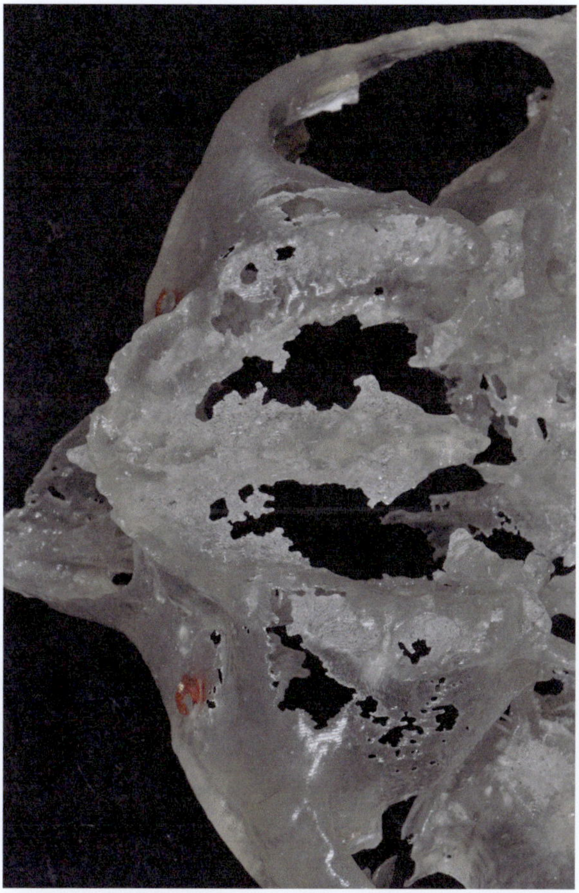

Fig. 6.3 Stereolithographic model of an eggshell-thin maxilla (64-year-old woman)

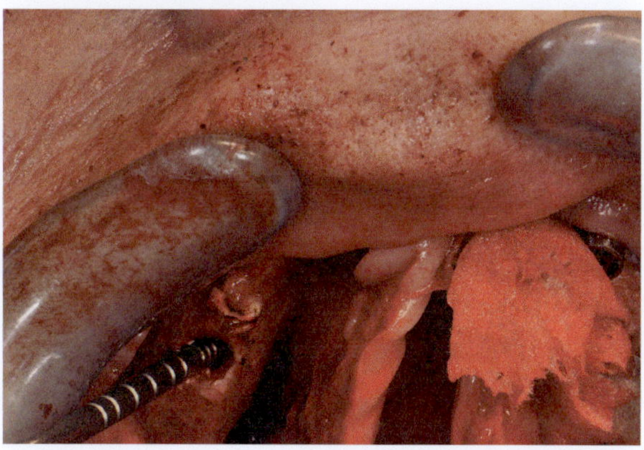

Fig. 6.4 Fenestration of the sinus: the Schneiderian membrane is delicately pushed up with a specific round-tipped instrument

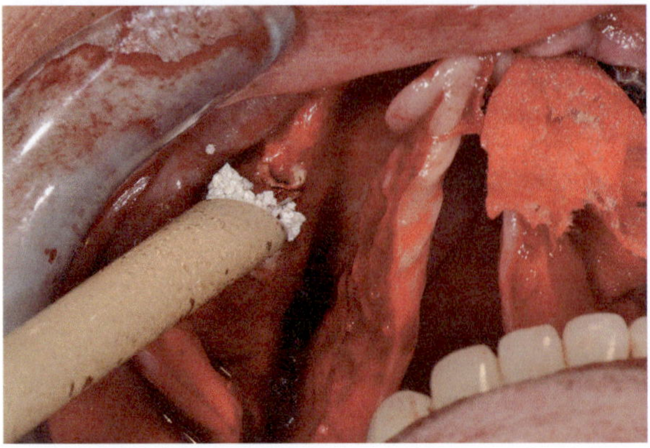

Fig. 6.5 Sinus membrane elevation with bone substitute material

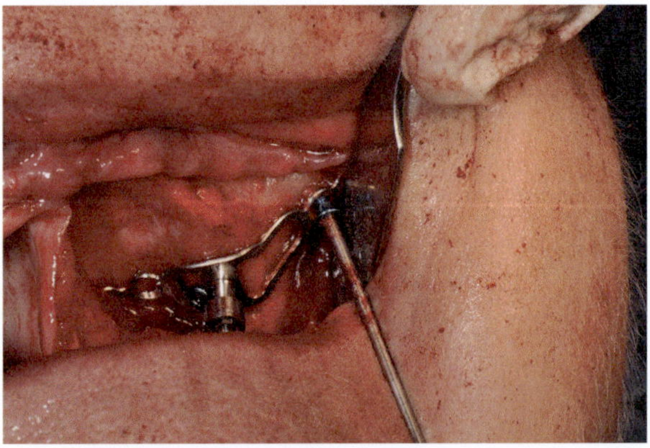

Fig. 6.6 Basal implant screw-secured onto the dense zygomatic bone

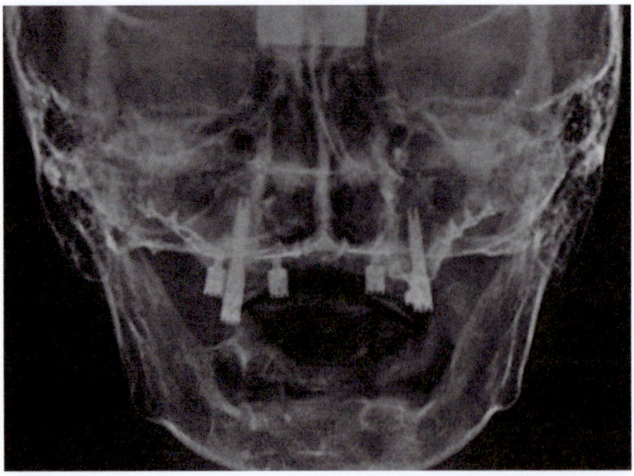

Fig. 6.7 Teleradiograph at 6 months (fixed prosthesis removed) (same patient as Figs. 6.3, 6.4, 6.5, and 6.6)

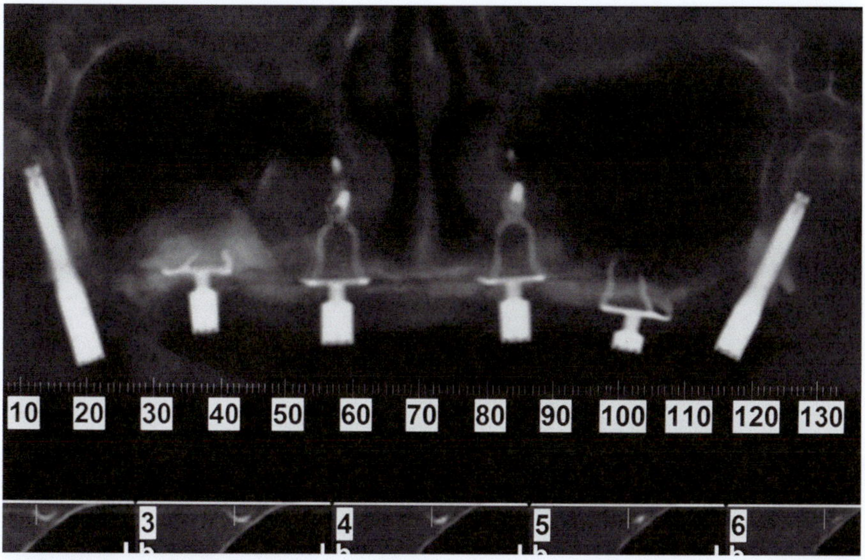

Fig. 6.8 Cone beam CT at 6 months. The maxillary sinuses are clear and healthy (same patient as Figs. 6.3, 6.4, 6.5, 6.6 and 6.7)

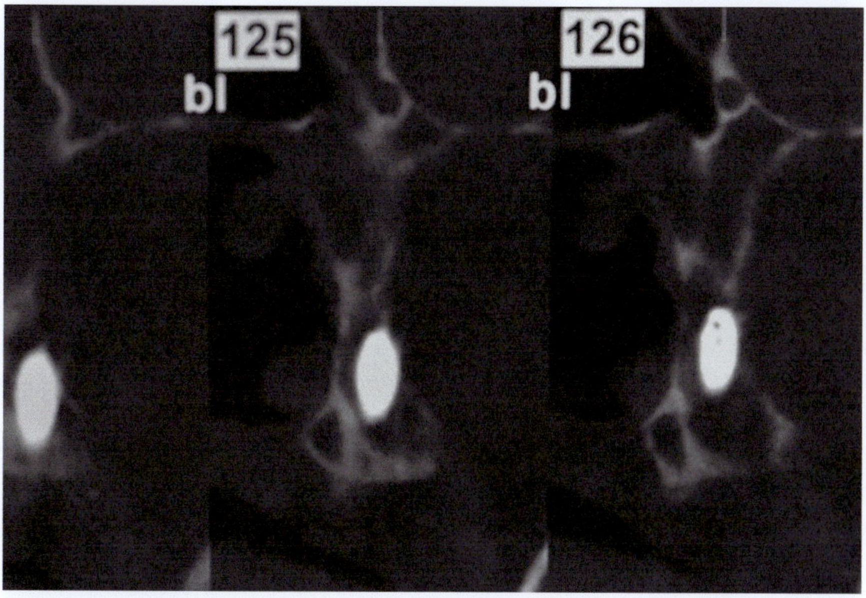

Fig. 6.9 Cone beam CT of the pterygoid implant placed between the two pterygoid processes (same patient as Fig. 6.8)

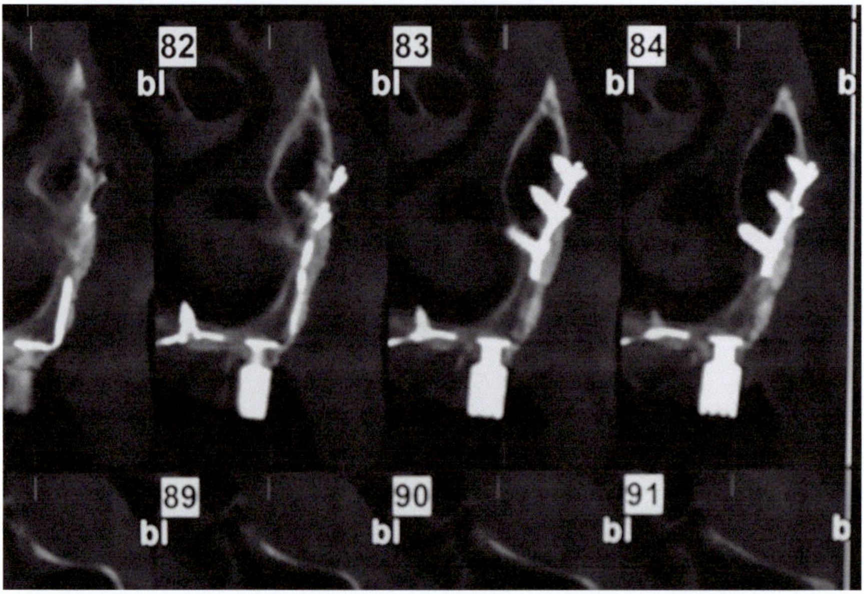

Fig. 6.10 Cone beam CT showing a basal implant installed on the canine pillar

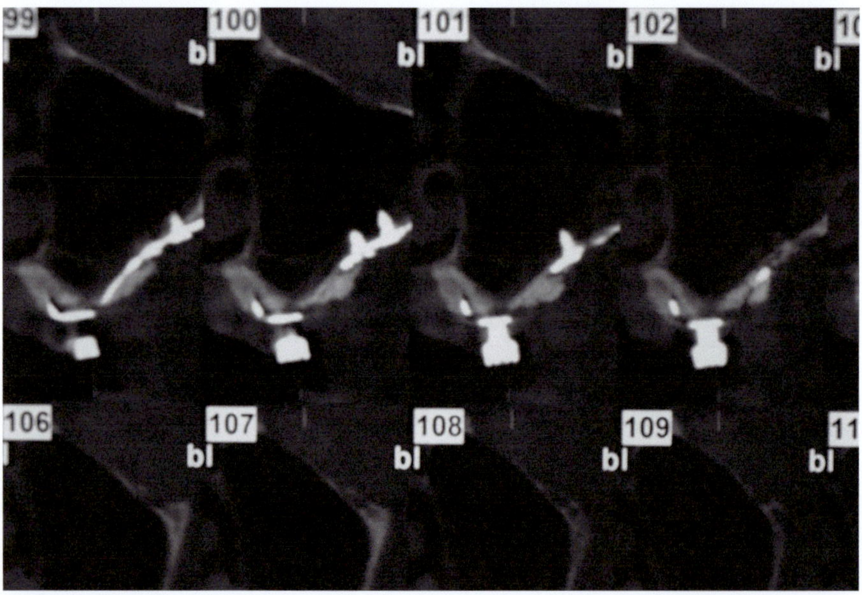

Fig. 6.11 Cone beam CT showing a plate-form Diskimplant® screw-secured onto the right zygomatic process. Note the bone substitute material 6 months after sinus membrane elevation. The sinuses appear clear and healthy

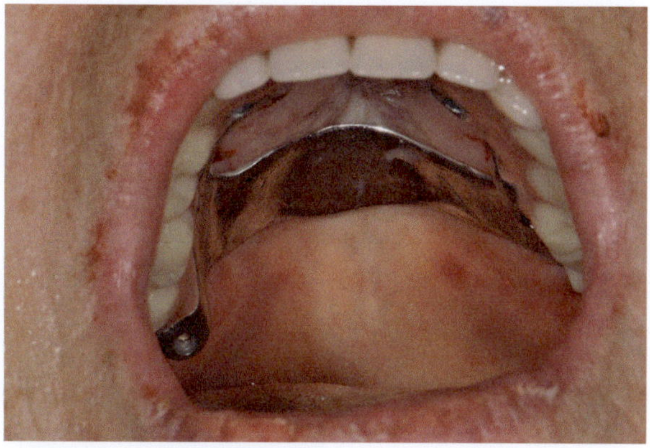

Fig. 6.12 Intraoral view of the fixed, screw-retained, immediately functional prosthesis with a wide transpalatal bar (to be removed after 6 months) (same patient as Fig. 6.3)

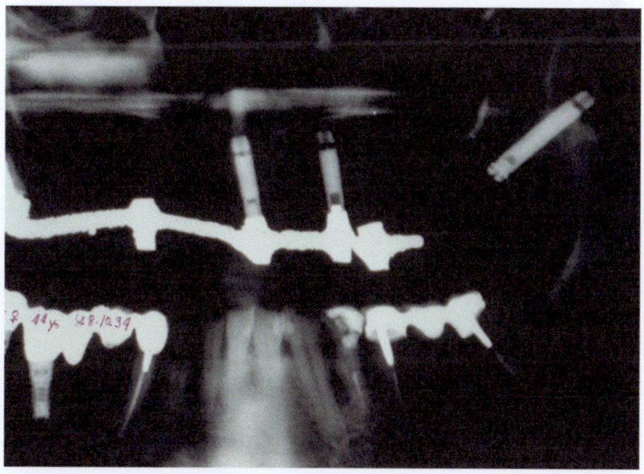

Fig. 6.13 Failing root-form implant 4 years post-op. Although a panoramic radiograph alone is not sufficient for accurate implant treatment planning, it provides a good overview of the patient's oral status before more invasive investigations are conducted

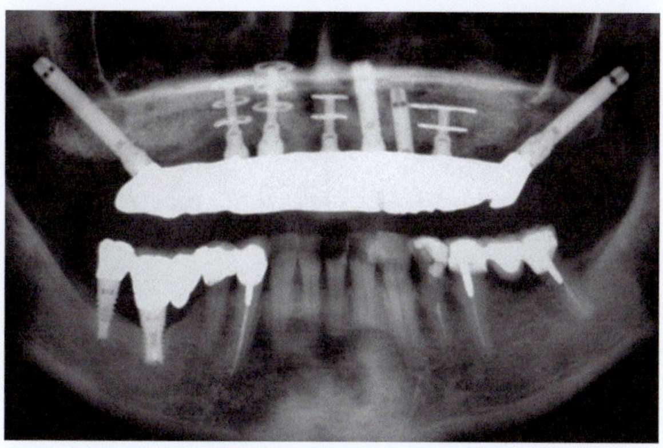

Fig. 6.14 Same patient as Fig. 6.13: the situation was corrected using basal Diskimplants® (single, double, triple disk models) and root-form implants (immediate functional loading protocol). Panorex after 16 years of service (2001–2017)

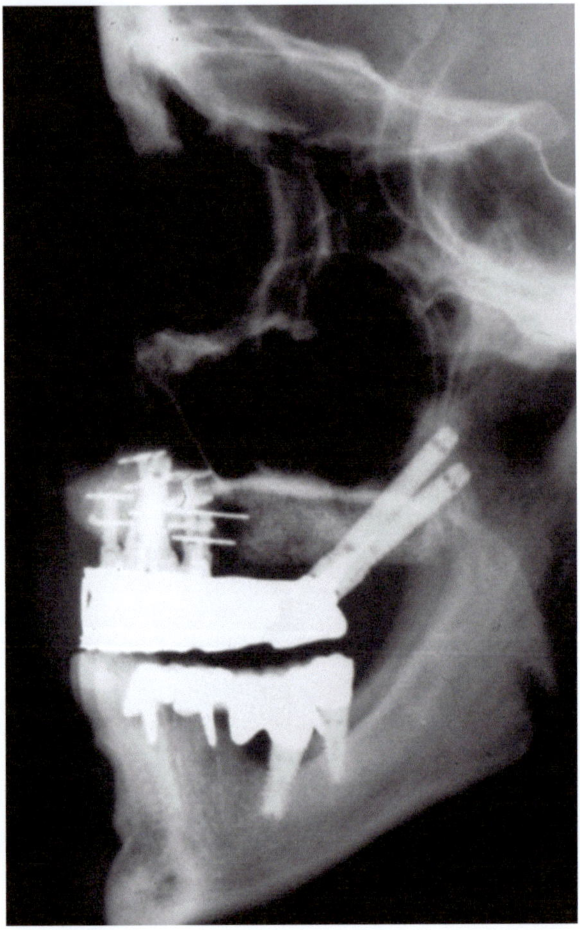

Fig. 6.15 Same patient as Figs. 6.13 and 6.14: Sagittal view of the final rehabilitation after 16 years. The sinus is healthy. Note the strong distal anchorage obtained with bilateral pterygoid implants

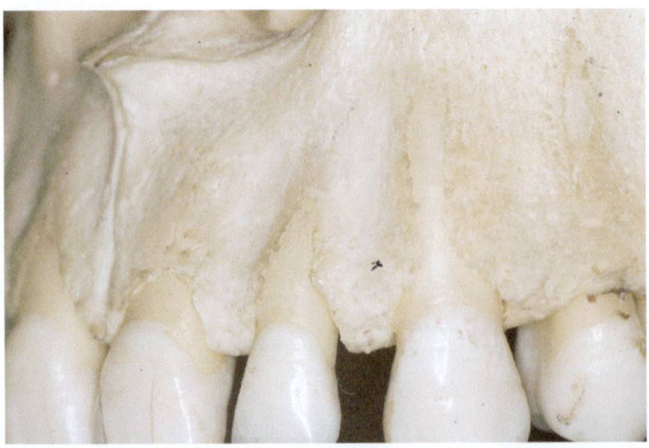

Fig. 6.16 The maxillary front teeth have no buccal plate. This is a good indication for immediate extraction of the hypermobile teeth and installation of a double Diskimplant® and GBR to fill in the buccal defect

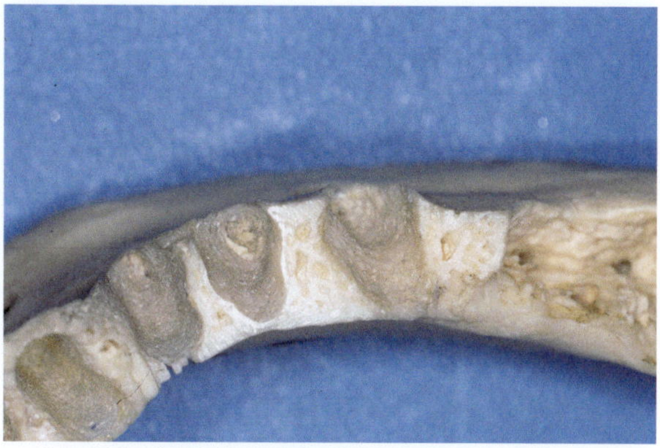

Fig. 6.17 Mandibular teeth without any buccal plate following tooth loss. This is another indication for double Diskimplants® and GBR. In both situations (Figs. 6.5 and 6.6), delayed loading is safest (6 months) unless the clinical conditions are highly favorable

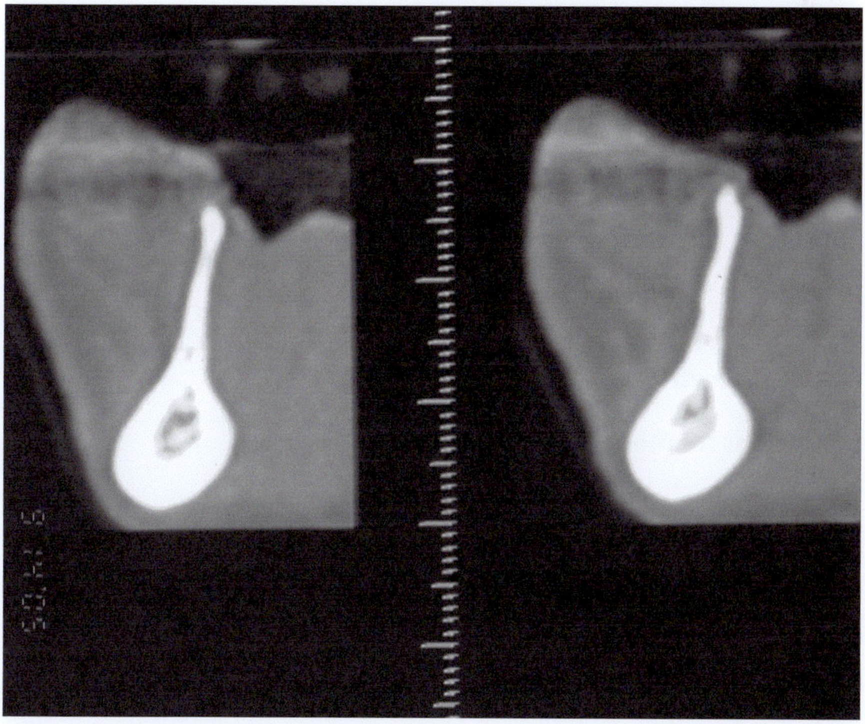

Fig. 6.18 This mandibular high knife ridge (D1 bone) can be directly managed with a double or triple Diskimplant® plus GBR and PRF. Because the bone is <3 mm thick at the crest level, placement of root-form implants would necessitate a bone graft or extensive reduction of the bone height in order to dispose of an acceptable bone width

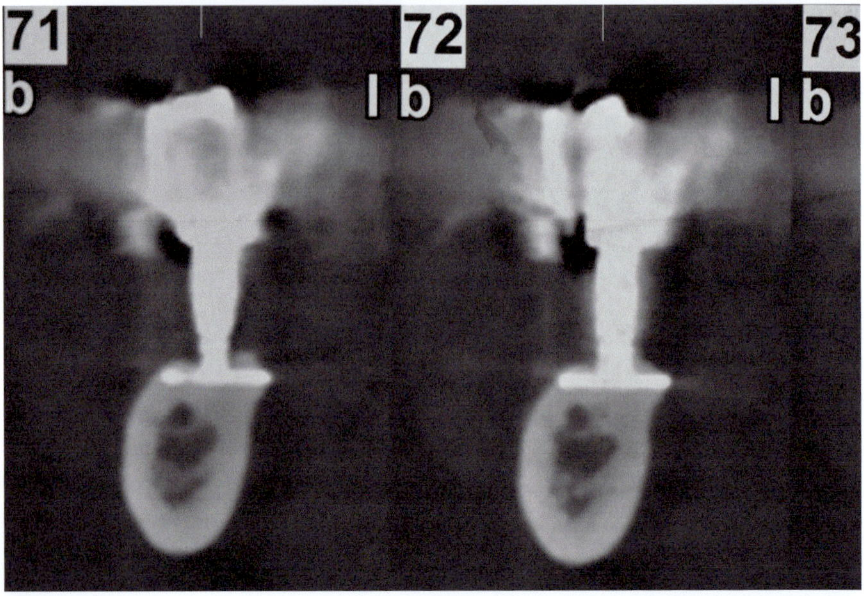

Fig. 6.19 A flat posterior mandible is an indication for monodisk Diskimplants® or a plate-form Diskimplant® (2 mm of available bone above the mandibular canal). Cone beam CT after 28 years of service (1989–2017)

6.4 Indications by Type of Diskimplant®

Indications for Monodisk Implants

- Wide round atrophic crest (height <5 mm, apical width >7 mm)
- Available bone height ≥2 mm
- Posterior maxilla/resorbed anterior maxilla
- Posterior mandible/resorbed anterior mandible

Indications for Multidisk Implants (Two or Three Disks, Inter-disk Distance 3 mm)

- High, thin maxillary or mandibular knife ridges (crest width ≤3 mm; bone height ≥6 mm)
- Single-tooth replacement when the vestibular bone wall has been completely lost at the time of extraction or after failure of a bone graft or GBR

Indications for Screw-Secured, Plate-Form Diskimplants®

Plate-form Diskimplants® (33 or 43 mm in length, 7 or 9 mm in width) can be installed even where there is <1 mm of bone height; they can also be installed directly on the bone crest. These implants can also be used to span a bone opening in the sinus area. When sufficient bone height is available, the wide basal disk is inserted laterally 2–5 mm under the top of the ridge. Crestal bone loss is minimal, and clinical results are better than with wide-diameter, screw-type implants installed in similar clinical situations. Plate-form Diskimplants® are maintained in place by preparing an endosseous notch with a 7 or 9 mm cutter. After positioning the implant in the notch, mini osteosynthesis screws (4, 5, or 6 mm in length) are placed through specially designed eyelets to hold the implant down tightly against the dense bone. Partial juxta-osseous support and sectorial endosseous anchorage, reinforced by the mini orthopedic screws, are essential to prevent plate mobility deleterious to osseointegration. Using GBR, these basal implants must always be completely covered by autologous bone chips, a bone substitute material, and/or a membrane such as PRF, in order to obtain osseointegration of the subperiosteal portion.

In the maxilla, these implants are installed on the canine pillar and in the infra-sinus/zygomatic zone. In the mandible, they are installed in the posterior sector.

Specific indications include:

- Severe to extreme bone atrophy
- Flat, shallow bone areas above the mandibular canal (idem for the maxilla)
- Bone height $\leq$2 mm
- Bone width 7–9 mm
- Minimum mesiodistal length of available bone 25 mm

Contraindication: Plate-form Diskimplants® are never indicated for single-tooth replacements. They must always be used in conjunction with other implants or connected to healthy natural teeth by means of a fixed bridge.

6.5 Indications by Implant Site

Maxilla: Upper Canine Pillar

When neither root-form implants nor standard Diskimplants® are indicated, a plate-form Diskimplant can often be screw-secured onto the canine pillar. The plate must be placed as close as possible to the vertical border of the nasal canine wall. The surgeon must bend the plate at a 90° angle and introduce it through a crestal bone cut prepared with a 9 mm diameter cutter. Alternately, the crest can merely be flattened and the implant placed on top of the crest and then screw-secured to the palatal bone and the canine pillar.

Severely Atrophic Maxillae (Available Bone Height <2 mm): Zygomatic Diskimplants®

Anchorage in the dense zygomatic bone is possible using 43 × 9 mm or 33 × 9 mm plate-form Diskimplants® screw-secured by two to five mini orthopedic screws. The malar bone is always very dense, but the palatal bone is weak. This eggshell-thin residual buccal and palatal basal bone must be densified using osseotensors 45 days or more before implant installment in order to allow formation of dense new bone in the form of a callus.

Zygomatic Plate-Form Diskimplants® and Simultaneous Sinus Floor Elevation

If there is an opening in the wall or floor of the sinus, a sinus lift procedure with placement of PRF and bone substitute material is necessary before a plate-form Diskimplant® can be installed (the implant must never be in direct contact with the sinus membrane).

Pterygoid Process: Tubero-Pterygoid Implants

Cylindroconical Fractal® root-form implants (Victory, Nice, France) with a monobloc crestal emergence diameter of 4.5 mm require at least 6 mm of bone width at the crest level of the tuberosity. With their atraumatic, 2.5 mm diameter rounded apex and micro-threads that render them entirely self-tapping over their total length (20 and 23 mm), these pterygoid implants are compatible for use in any bone density. In type I, II, and III bone, the implant can be screwed into place. In type IV bone, the implant can be impacted (press fit), thanks to the external micro-threads interrupted by four parallel guide channels, and then locked in place by slight rotation (the "press and turn" technique). When there is not enough available bone, single, double, or triple Diskimplants® can be installed in this sector. Since the residual basal bone in the tuberosity is very weak (type IV), the use of osseotensors 45–60 days prior to implant installation is mandatory.

Mandible

Wide, Round Shallow Ridges: Wide-Diameter, Ultrashort Root-Form Implants Versus Diskimplants® and Horizontal Plate-Form Diskimplants® for the Posterior Mandible (Bone Height ≤5 mm)

Routine use of wide diameter (4.75 mm or more) and short (7 or 8 mm) or ultrashort (≤6 mm) root-form implants remains controversial. Osteotomy for wide-diameter screw-type implants (ø 5 mm or more) entails considerable bone destruction, especially at the crest level. Threads are more likely to be exposed with time during mastication due to the powerful pull of the masseter muscles, opening the way for rapid onset of peri-implantitis. As a consequence, crestal bone may continue to resorb after initial osseointegration of the implant body during function. Laterally inserted Diskimplants® can be placed in bone heights of 5 mm or less; available base diameters range from 7 to 11 mm. The shaft diameter at the crestal alveolar bone level is 2.35 mm.

Wide, Flat Shallow Ridges with Less than 3 mm Above the Mandibular Nerve

In highly atrophic mandibles, installation of screw-secured plate-form Diskimplants® (43 × 9 mm or 33 × 9 mm) is indicated in the posterior area. Full arch restorations including these plate-form implants necessitate an immediate loading protocol. In contrast, plate-form Diskimplants® installed to treat partial edentulism are compatible with both submerged and non-submerged protocols. As mentioned earlier, plate-form Diskimplants® must be fully covered by autologous bone chips and/or a bone substitute material (Bio-Oss®, CoreBone®, InterPore®, etc.) and PRF.

Maxilla and Mandible

High Knife-Edge Ridges: Double Diskimplants® and Triple Diskimplants® Versus Small-Diameter Root-Form Implants (Figs. 6.18, 6.19)

Conventional screw-type implants often necessitate technical reduction of the crest that must be flattened before axial osteotomy can be performed. In contrast, because lateral osteotomy is initiated at the base of the jaw rather than on the crest, Diskimplant® installation eliminates the need for surgical reduction of thin maxillary or mandibular knife ridges. Subsequent crestal bone loss and gingival retraction, if any, are less severe. A better esthetic outcome is thus possible without prior systematic bone grafting although bone substitute materials are often placed at the moment of basal implant installation in order to promote GBR.

Basal Implant Treatment for Ectodermal Dysplasia (Figs. 6.20, 6.21, 6.22, 6.23, 6.24, 6.25, 6.26 and 6.27)

The conventional approach to treatment of these challenging situations involves bone grafting followed by installation of root-form implants after a waiting period. Basal implant placement can obviate the need for grafting and makes it possible to equip the jaws using an immediate loading protocol.

When a crestal bone width of at least 3 mm is available, small-diameter (3.3 mm) root-form Fratex® (Victory, Nice, France) implants can be safely installed after bone preparation with an osseotensor 2 weeks beforehand. Fratex® implants can expand a 3 mm thick alveolar crest up to 6.6 mm. If less bone is available, bone splitting and horizontal bone distraction are not technically possible. Preimplantation bone grafting is sometimes an option but involves a waiting time of at least 3 months before implants can be installed. A more attractive, less time-consuming solution offering

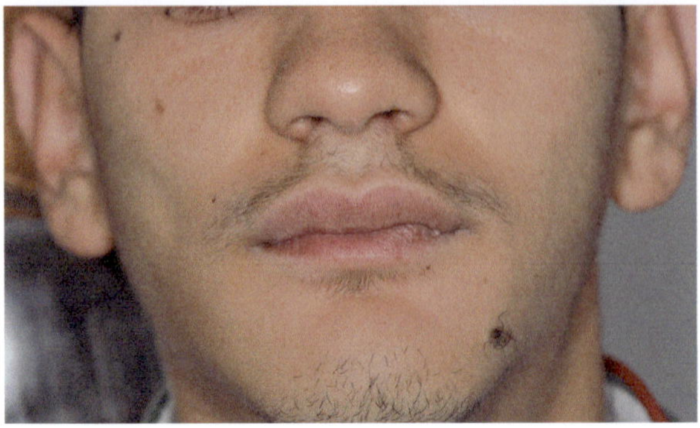

Fig. 6.20 A 22-year-old patient with ectodermal dysplasia

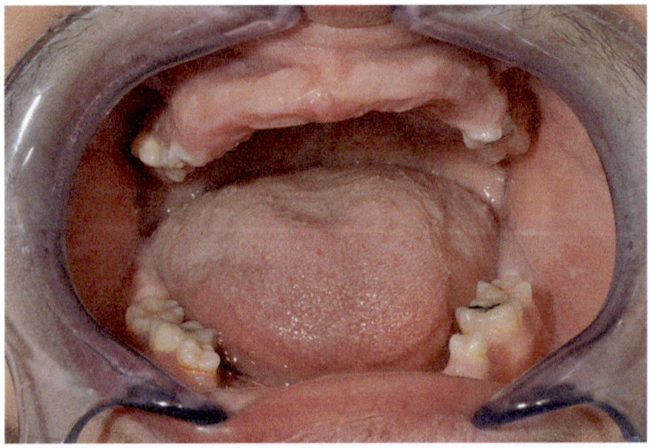

Fig. 6.21 Intraoral view of the patient with his baby teeth

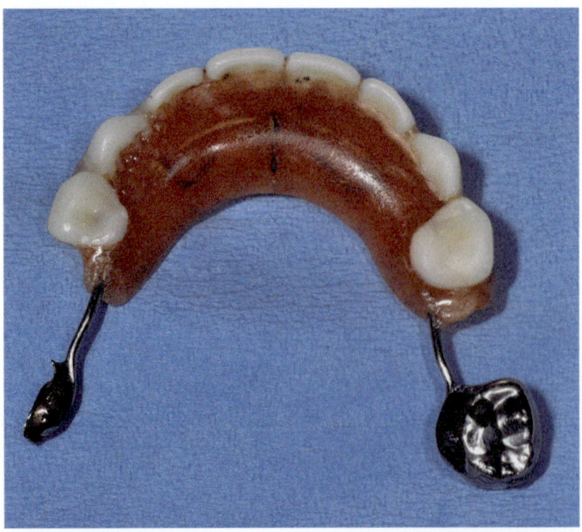

Fig. 6.22 Removable appliance worn since the age of 12 years

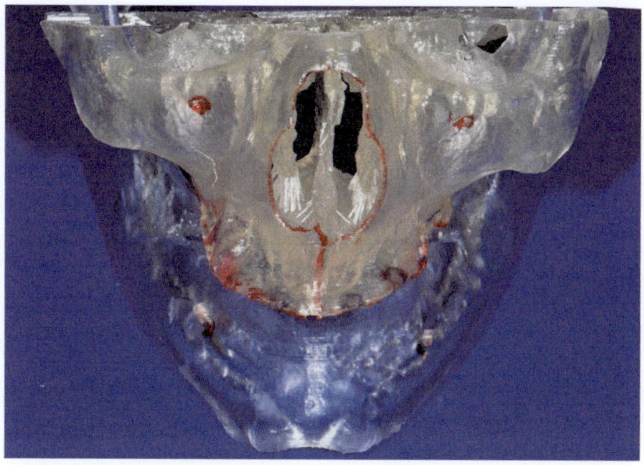

Fig. 6.23 Preoperative stereolithographic model

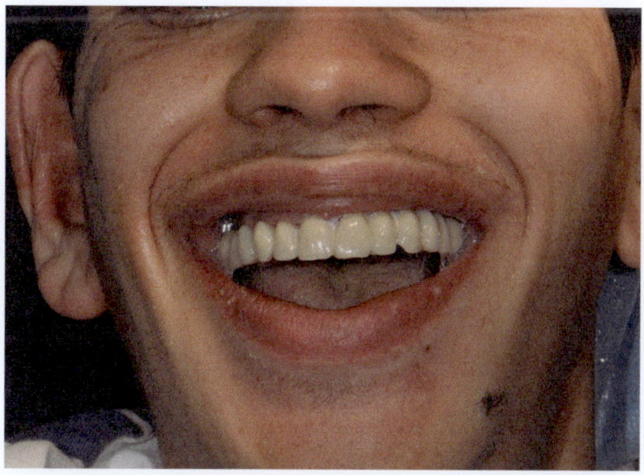

Fig. 6.24 Cosmetic result 1 year post-op

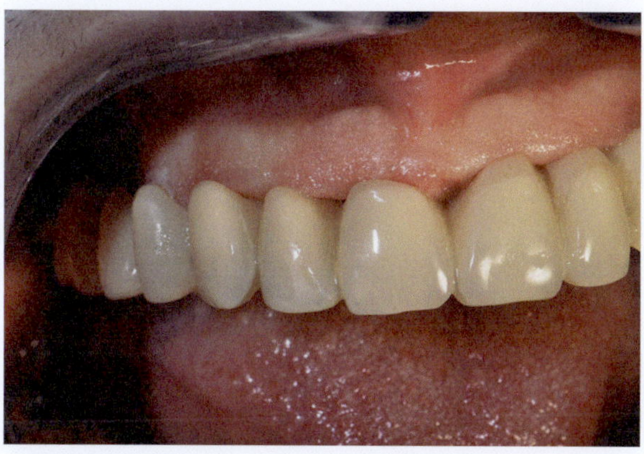

Fig. 6.25 Close-up view of the upper rehabilitation

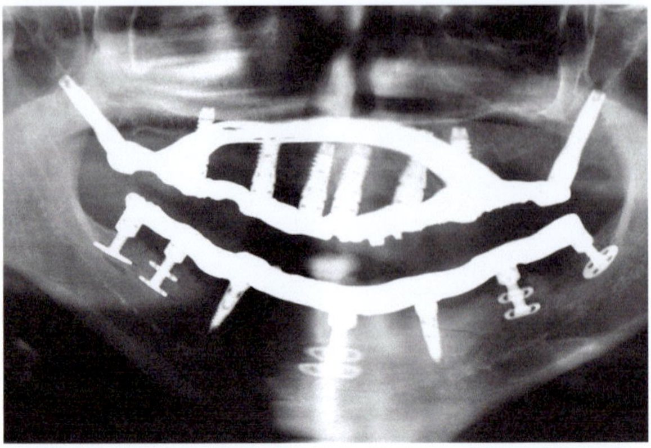

Fig. 6.26 Panoramic view of the total rehabilitation after 1 year

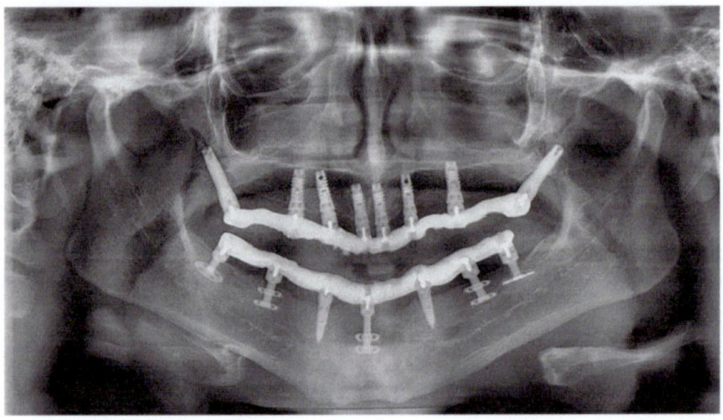

Fig. 6.27 The transpalatal bar was removed 6 months later. Panoramic view after 6 years (January 2018)

predictable long-term results is lateral insertion of a double Diskimplant®. The protruding double disks are covered over by bone substitute material and serve as scaffolding for GBR. As always, absolute primary Diskimplant® stability is essential. Insertion of a 5 or 6 mm long mini orthopedic screw against the apical base of the double Diskimplant® can help prevent micromovement.

Conflict of interest statement Gérard M. Scortecci is the inventor of the Diskimplant and holder of several associated patents that are exploited by the Victory company. He is an unpaid consultant to this firm and a minority shareholder in the company. No money was received from any of the companies mentioned in the book or from any of the companies whose products are mentioned.

Recommended Reading

1. Baden E. Diagnostic methodology. In: Scortecci G, Misch CE, Benner KU, editors. Implants and restorative dentistry. London: Martin Dunitz; 2001.
2. Bain CA, Moy PK. The association between the failure of dental implants and cigarette smoking. Int J Oral Maxillofac Impl. 1993;8:609–15.
3. Barnes R, Veith RC, Raskind MA. Depression in older persons: diagnosis and management. West J Med. 1981;135:463–8.

4. Chanavaz M. Patient screening and medical evaluation for implant and preprosthetic surgery. J Oral Implantol. 1998;24(4):222–9.
5. Dufour C. Chronic liver disease and cirrhosis. In: Everhart J, editor. Digestive diseases in the United States: epidemiology and impact. Washington, DC: US Department of Health and Human Services, Public Health Service, National Institutes of Health; 1994.
6. Feldman RS, Bravacos JS, Rose CL. Association between smoking different tobacco products and periodontal disease indexes. J Periodontol. 1983;54:841–7.
7. Fleg JL. Alterations in vascular structure and function with advancing age. Am J Cardiol. 1986;57:3344.
8. Fleming KC, Adams AC, Peterson RC. Dementia: diagnosis and evaluation. Mayo Clin Proc. 1995;70:1093–107.
9. Folkow B, Svanborg A. Physiology of cardiovascular aging. Physiol Rev. 1993;73:725–64.
10. Gardner ID. The effect of aging on susceptibility to infection. Rev Infect Dis. 1980;2:801–10.
11. Gerstenblith G, Lakatta EG, Weisfeldt ML. Age changes in myocardial function and exercise response. Prog Cardiovasc Dis. 1976;19:1–21.
12. Gorman LM, Lambert PM, Morris JF, et al. The effect of smoking on implant survival at second-stage surgery: DICRG Interim Report No. 5. Dental Implant Clinical Research Group. Implant Dent. 1994;3:165–8.
13. Henry RG, Wekstein DR. Providing dental care for patients diagnosed with Alzheimer's disease. Dental Clin North Am. 1997;41:915–42.
14. Hurwitz M. Predisposing factors in adverse reactions to drugs. Br Med J. 1969;1:536–9.
15. Hypertension and Follow-up Program Cooperative Group. Five-year finding of the hypertension detection and follow-up program. II. Mortality by race, sex and age. J Am Med Assoc. 1979;242:2572–7.
16. Ismail A, Burt BA, Eklund SA. Epidemiologic patterns of smoking and periodontal disease in the United States. J Am Dent Assoc. 1983;106:617–21.
17. Joint National Committee (JNC) on Detection, Evaluation and Treatment of High Blood Pressure. The fifth report of the Joint National Committee on the Detection, Evaluation and Treatment of High Blood Pressure (JNC-V). Arch Intern Med. 1993;153:154–83.
18. Jones JK, Triplette RG. The relationship of cigarette smoking to impaired intra-oral wound healing. J Oral Maxillofac Surg. 1992;50:237–9; discussion 239–40.
19. Kannel WB, Gordon T. Evaluation of cardiovascular risk in the elderly: the Framingham study. Bull NY Acad Med. 1978;54:573–91.
20. Khachaturian ZS. Diagnosis of Alzheimer's disease. Arch Neurol. 1985;42:1097–105.
21. Krall EA, Dawson RB. Smoking and bone loss among postmenopausal women. J Bone Miner Res. 1991;6:331–8.
22. Lewis WH Jr, Alving AS. Changes with age in the renal function in adult men. I. Clearance of urea nitrogen in the blood. III. Concentrating ability of the kidneys. Am J Physiol. 1938;123:500–15.
23. Resnik R, Misch CE. Misch's avoiding complications in oral implantology. St. Louis, MO: Elsevier; 2017.
24. Stoelting RK, Miller RD. Basics of anesthesia. 2nd ed. New York: Churchill Livingstone; 1989. p. 114.
25. Thoman M. Role of interleukin-2 in the age-related impairment of immune function. J Am Geriatr Soc. 1985;33:781–7.
26. US Bureau of the Census, Day JC. Population projections of the United States by age, sex, race, and Hispanic Origin: 1995–2050. Current population reports. Washington, DC: US Government Printing Office; 1996. p. 25–1130.

Treatment Planning

7

Gérard M. Scortecci and Guillaume Odin

7.1 Reliable Basal Implant Treatment Options

The treatment plan must take into account both clinical and economic factors. If the patient and/or his or her insurance company cannot or will not accept the treatment plan that will reasonably guarantee the long-term (10 years) success of the restorative implant therapy, a conventional alternative solution is advisable.

Creation of acceptable function and esthetics requires determination of the optimum number, type, position, and orientation of the planned basal implants. With study models mounted on an articulator, the clinician or technician can produce a self-cured acrylic template depicting the teeth in the area where the implants are to be located. CT imaging is then performed with the diagnostic template seated intraorally. Treatment planning software (Materialise, Dentsply) containing the Diskimplant® library allows the clinician to accurately plan the location of basal implants, taking into account the optimal prosthetic locations marked on the diagnostic template, including implant dimensions and angulation.

A wax-up and mock-up can then be fabricated to simulate the suggested treatment result and to show the patient the anticipated outcome. Based on the wax-up, a surgical stent is fabricated. After obtaining the consent of the patient, initial bone

G. M. Scortecci (✉)
University of Nice-Sophia Antipolis Medical School, Nice, France

New York University, New York, NY, USA

University of Southern California, Los Angeles, CA, USA

Private Practice, Nice, France
e-mail: scortecci@wanadoo.fr

G. Odin
ENT and Maxillo-facial Surgery Department, Institut Universitaire de la Face et du Cou, University of Nice-Sophia Antipolis Medical School, Nice, France
e-mail: odin.g@chu-nice.fr

© Springer Nature Switzerland AG 2019

G. M. Scortecci (ed.), *Basal Implantology*, https://doi.org/10.1007/978-3-319-44873-2_7

bed preparation with manual osseotensors is followed 45–60 days later by basal implant surgery in type III or IV bone. For type I and type II bone, surgery is possible 8–15 days after application of a rotary osseotensor (a single impact per implant site). The prerequisites for diagnosis and treatment planning in basal oral implantology are discussed hereafter.

7.2 Delayed Versus Immediate Loading

The decision to use a submerged technique, an immediate loading protocol, or a removable appliance has a direct impact on the success and reproducible osseointegration of basal implants.

Total Edentulism

- Removable dentures on basal implants are not recommended for extremely atrophic jaws as such appliances promote micro movements and continuous bone resorption.
- Immediate loading with a functional, screw-secured bridge acting as an external orthopedic fixator is recommended for totally edentulous, extremely atrophic jaws. Delayed loading is not an option in these situations because use of a full denture during the 6-month waiting period can damage and/or mobilize the basal implants.
- Immediate fabrication of a transitional screw-secured CrCo/titanium prosthesis is advisable as this appliance allows evaluation of esthetics, proper fit, occlusion, hygiene, phonetics, etc.

Partial Edentulism

- Except for a very few favorable clinical situations, immediate loading is not recommended for partial edentulism. Temporization must be well planned from the outset to avoid damage to basal implants during the healing phase (6 months). In the esthetic zone, an Invisalign®-like appliance with a commercial tooth or teeth is recommended. When implants are installed in the posterior sectors, the patient is advised not to wear this removable denture during meals.

7.3 Recommended Number of Basal Implants (Figs. 7.1, 7.2, 7.3, 7.4, 7.5, 7.6, 7.7, 7.8, and 7.9)

The rule of one implant per tooth is generally the safest solution for partial edentulism. For the completely edentulous maxilla, 6–10 basal implants usually suffice for 12–14 teeth. For the mandible, 5–9 implants may be sufficient for 12–14 teeth using an immediate loading procedure.

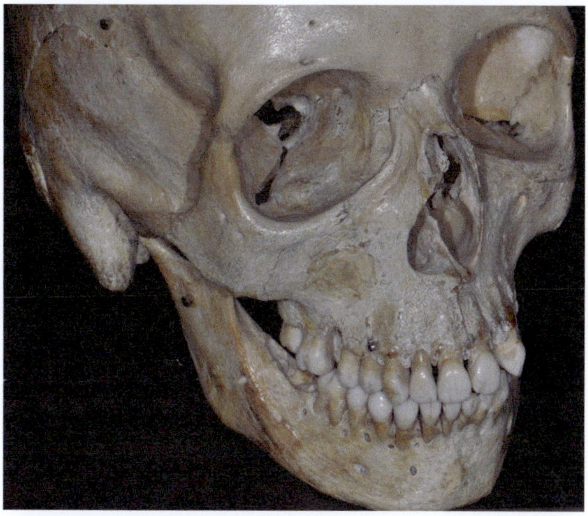

Fig. 7.1 Human skeletal model: 32 teeth with 30 upper dental roots and 22 lower dental roots. The pressure of natural selection has promoted highly efficient support in the posterior areas

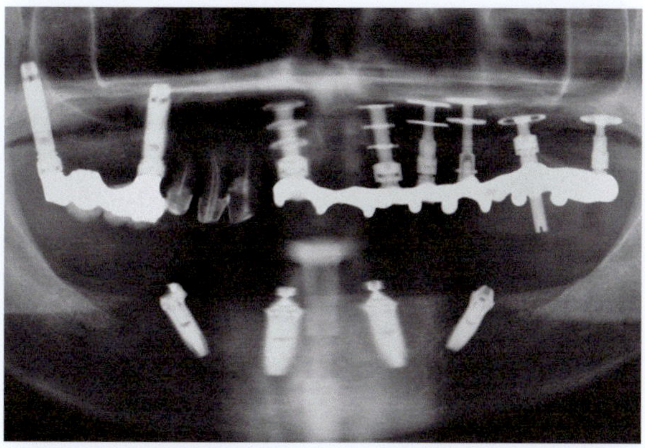

Fig. 7.2 Initial post-op panoramic radiograph of an "all-on-four" mandibular implant treatment

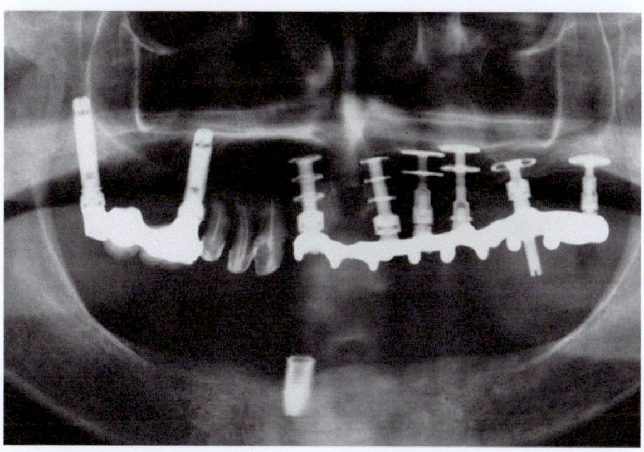

Fig. 7.3 Implant loss at 6 months. The upper maxillary rehabilitation placed in 1992 is still in service (26 years) (courtesy Dr Philippe Brenier)

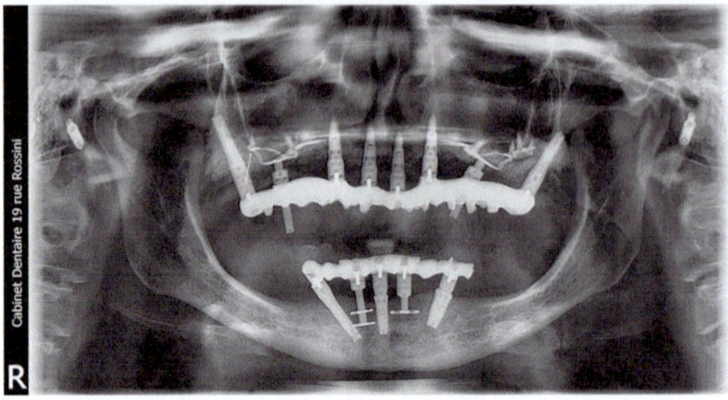

Fig. 7.4 Successful maxillo-mandibular rehabilitation (3 years post-op): basal and root-form implants were placed in the maxilla, and the mandible was restored using an all-on-five combination of root-forms and basal Diskimplants®. A reduced number of artificial roots may be acceptable in the mandible in elderly patients with decreased muscle tone

Fig. 7.5 Similar maxillo-mandibular rehabilitation: fixed, all-on-five mandibular restoration using root-forms (3 years post-op) and maxillary rehabilitation associating basal implants and pterygoid implants (10 years post-op)

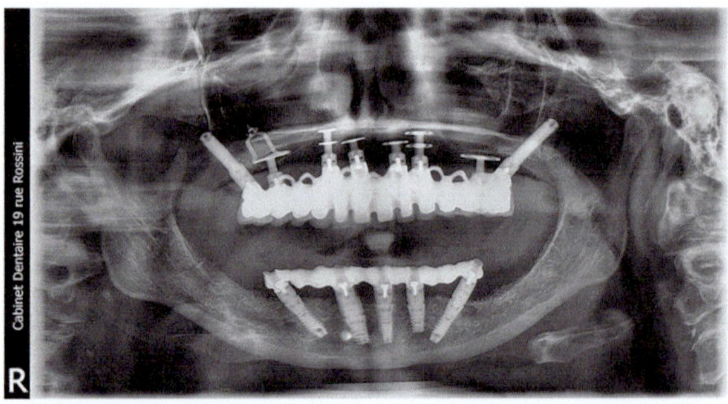

Fig. 7.6 Partially edentulous posterior mandible treated with two root-form implants to replace a lower molar on each side. Panoramic radiograph 2 years post-op

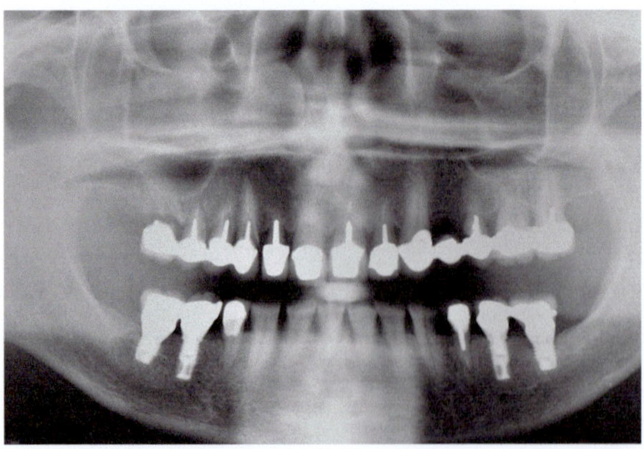

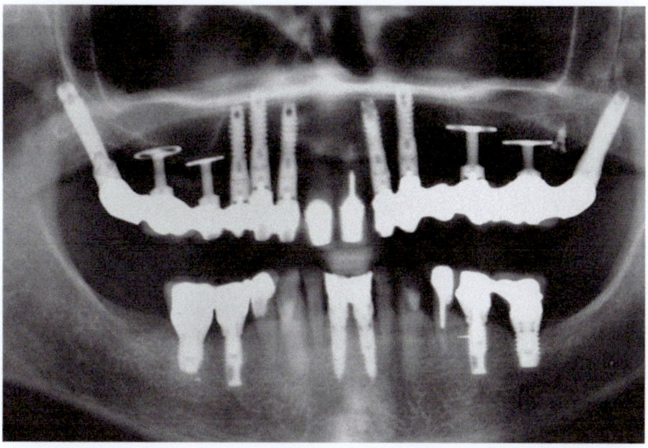

Fig. 7.7 Root-form and basal implants used for an immediate functional loading protocol to treat the upper right and upper left posterior maxilla. Panoramic radiograph after 24 years (2016). Same patient as Fig. 7.6

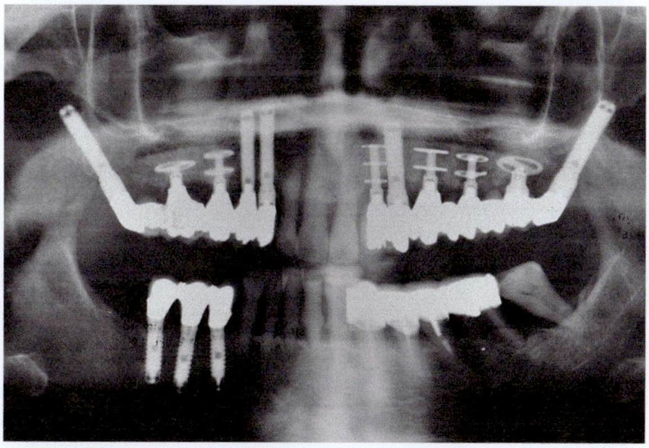

Fig. 7.8 Three root-form implants were installed in the posterior lower right mandible in 1988. In 1991, basal and root-form implants were installed in the posterior right and left maxilla (immediate functional loading protocol)

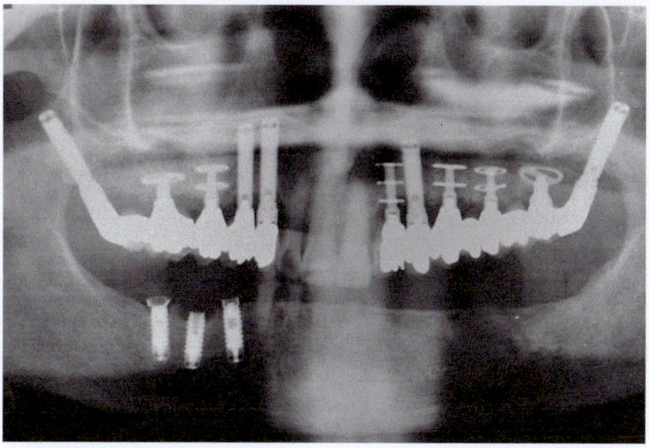

Fig. 7.9 In 2014, after 23 years of service, the same patient as in Fig. 7.8 broke the three lower root-form implants, probably due to loss of the lower left pontic and mechanical problems owing to fatigue at the crestal implant level. The internal hexagons were damaged as the result of fatigue and overload. A conventional full lower denture was made because the patient, now aged 89 years, did not want to undergo implant placement in the mandible

"All-on-a-Few" or "All-on-More"?

Reducing the number of implants has a number of advantages when managing complete edentulism:

- Easier and faster surgical procedure, hence shorter period of bone exposure.
- Impression taking and laboratory procedures are facilitated.
- Lower costs for patient, doctor, and dental laboratory.
- Placement of the prosthesis is easier, and retrieval, if necessary, is faster and less complicated.

Limitations

The "all-on-four" concept disregards the natural human model of root support (Fig. 7.1) (i.e., maxilla 16 teeth, 30 roots (including wisdom teeth); mandible 16 teeth, 22 roots (including wisdom teeth)) and is thus incompatible with long-term, reliable, and prudent full-mouth implant-supported rehabilitation. One of the major problems with "all-on-four" restorations on a limited number of implants is the need for a cantilever and reduced or absent tooth-to-tooth support in the second molar area, with all of the well-known mechanical consequences, discomfort, and occlusal and TMJ disorders.

Despite these drawbacks, an "all-on-five" rather than an "all-on-four" approach can be an option in selected clinical situations (Figs. 7.4 and 7.5) of complete edentulism. Partial edentulism can be a far more critical situation: the dental status can change drastically over time, and reduction of the number of implants can raise serious mechanical and biological problems.

Cantilevers

A 7–14 mm cantilever (one molar or two premolars) is generally accepted by the dental implant community, but not all patients are good candidates because this option raises potential biological and mechanical problems (screw loosening, fracture of prosthetic components, implant fracture, implant loss due to overload).

7.4 Diagnosis and Treatment Planning Sequence

First Appointment: Initial Patient Interview

- Patient preselection: listen to the patient's expectations.
- Inclusion/exclusion criteria at initial interview.
- Medical and dental history.

- Clinical examination (oral, gingival, dental, TMJ status).
- Photographs (AP, profile, smile).
- Radiographs.
- Presentation of treatment options.
- Discussion of alternative conventional treatments: GBR, autologous bone graft, etc.
- Basal dental implant option, number and location of basal dental implants, and risk/benefit analysis.
- Discussion of treatment timing, including pre-implant bone bed preparation (osseotensor)/immediate functional loading protocol or delayed loading (waiting period unloaded 6 months).
- Orthodontics if necessary.
- Prognosis; what solutions are available if problems (or even failure) occur?
- Estimated cost of the complete treatment, including the final prosthesis.
- Answer all questions the patient may have.
- Brief implant-oriented questionnaire for the patient's medical doctor and request for laboratory tests.
- Impression taken and imaging studies ordered if the patient agrees.

Second Appointment: Patient Interview and Treatment Planning (Figs. 7.10, 7.11, 7.12, 7.13, 7.14, 7.15, 7.16, 7.17, 7.18, 7.19, 7.20, 7.21, and 7.22)

Phobic patients must be detected at this point because they may require iv sedation or general anesthesia; patients with extremely atrophic jaws and/or complex situations may also necessitate special arrangements.

- Listen to the patient again; beware of unrealistic expectations.
- Inclusion/exclusion criteria reviewed at second interview.
- Analysis of all data collected (information provided by the patient's medical doctor).
- Analysis of laboratory tests, if any.
- Analysis of models in occlusion.
- Analysis of imaging studies (cone beam CT, stereolithographic model, etc.) — surgical guide 3D planning.
- Anticipate the esthetic aspect of the final basal implant-supported restoration (wax-up, mock-up).
- Initial treatment of any oral, gingival, and/or dental problems.
- Strategic extraction of unsalvageable teeth.
- Plan should failure occur.
- Answer any questions.
- Patient/doctor final decisions.
- Obtain informed consent (Table 7.1).

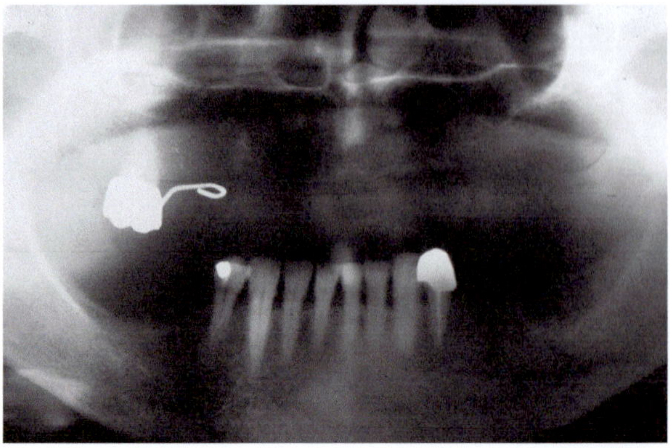

Fig. 7.10 Panoramic radiograph for initial treatment planning

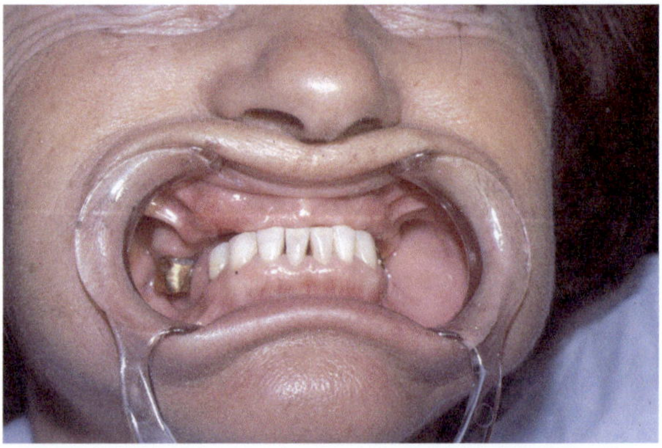

Fig. 7.11 Initial intraoral status (first appointment)

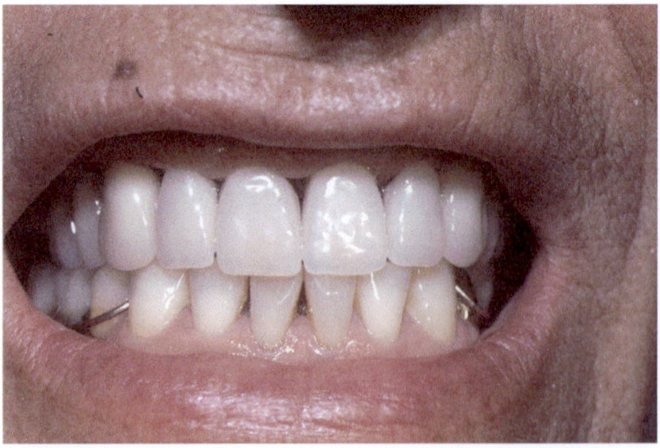

Fig. 7.12 New denture: verification of comfort, occlusion, speech, and trial cosmetic outcome

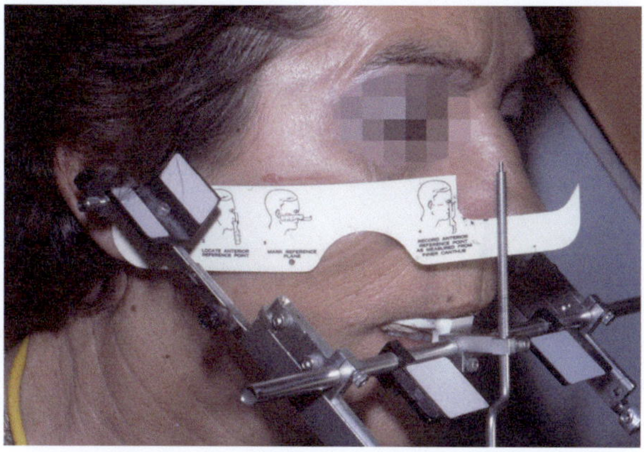

Fig. 7.13 New denture: registration of static and dynamic occlusions (third appointment)

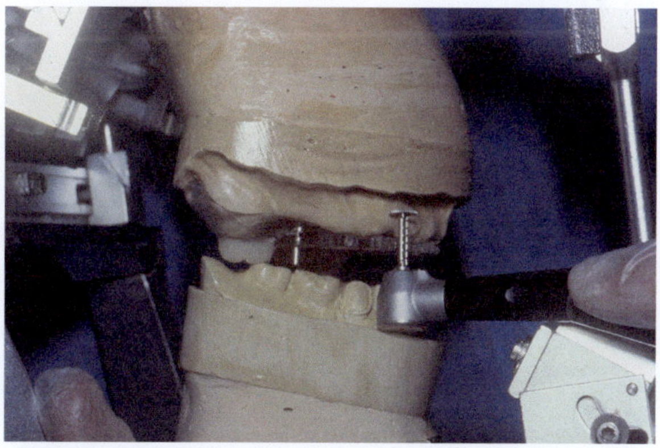

Fig. 7.14 Model mounted on a fully adjustable articulator (Denar, USA)

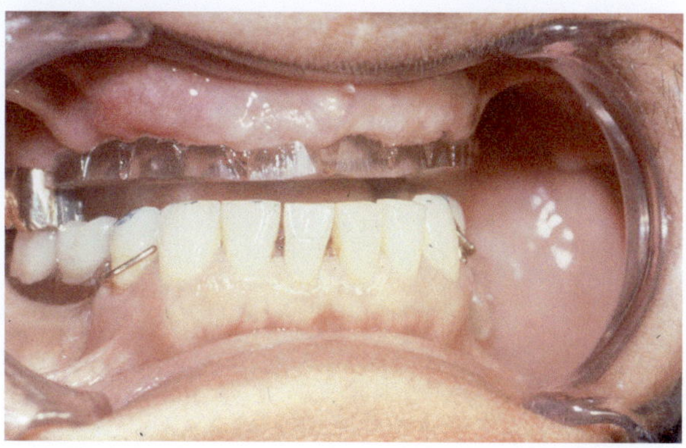

Fig. 7.15 Transparent surgical guide for basal implants

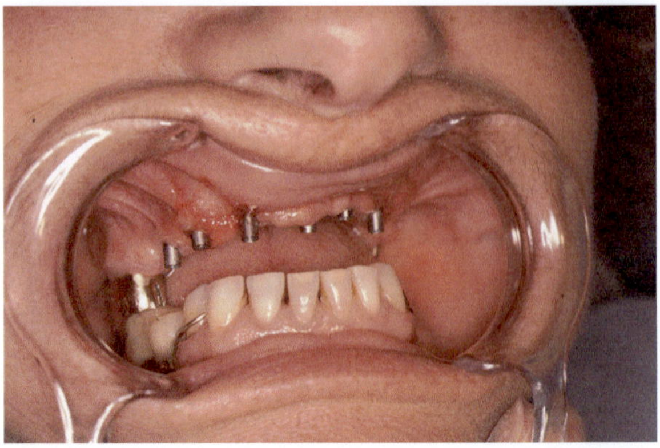

Fig. 7.16 Basal implant emergences placed in accordance with the surgical guide

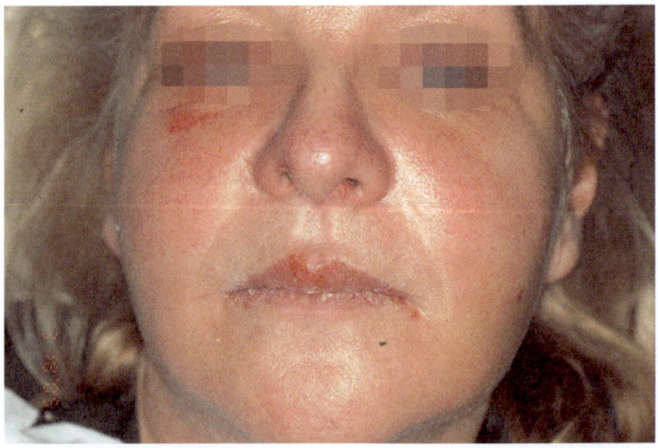

Fig. 7.17 Post-traumatic situation (car accident). Primary general and local healing must take place first, before any decision is made concerning implant placement

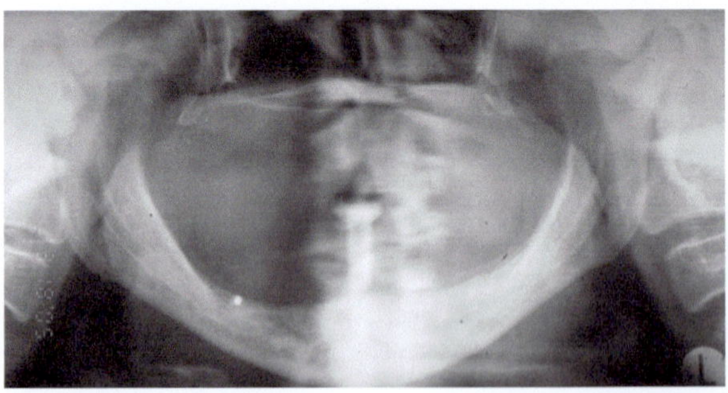

Fig. 7.18 Panoramic radiograph 2 months after a car accident (same patient as Fig. 7.17)

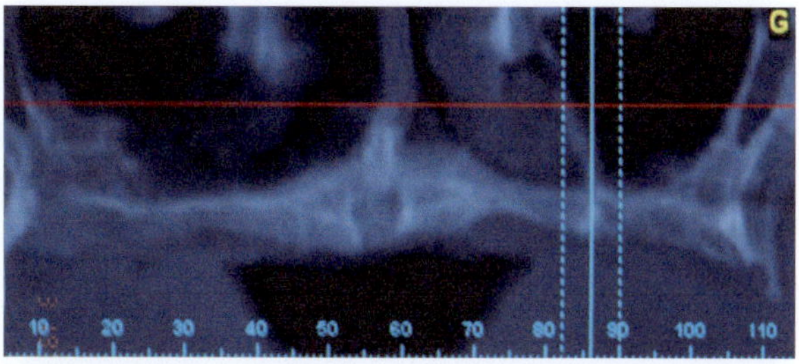

Fig. 7.19 Reconstructed CT panoramic view of the maxilla (same patient as Fig. 7.17)

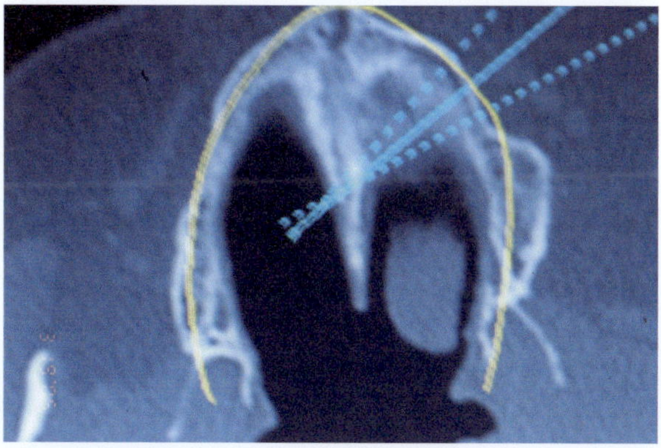

Fig. 7.20 Occlusal scan view (same patient as Fig. 7.17)

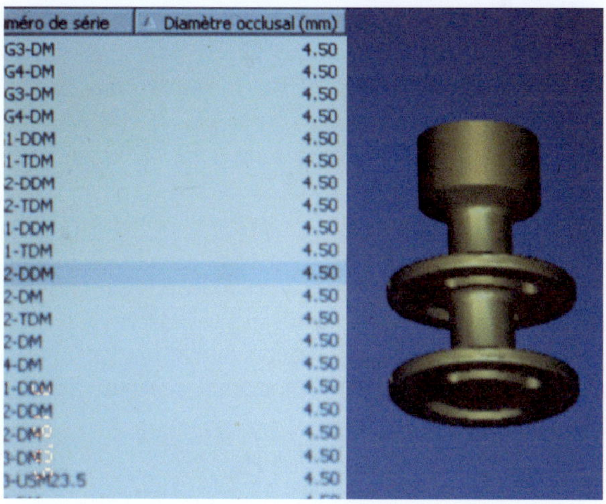

Fig. 7.21 Diskimplant® library (Materialise, SimPlant®, Dentsply)

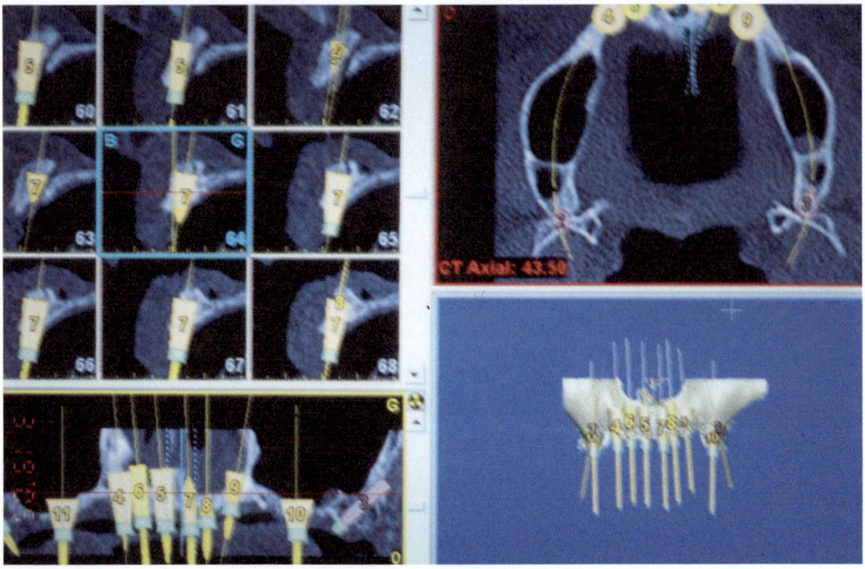

Fig. 7.22 3D simulation for basal implant placement

Pre-implantation Periodontal Surgery, When Required

Preoperative Botox, if Necessary (Heavy Bruxism)

Third Appointment: Bone Bed Preparation and Activation of the Patient's Stem Cells

- Osteogenic activation of the recipient bone bed is performed with a flapless approach under local anesthesia plus a flash of 2 g amoxicillin:
  - Manual osseotensors are used for the upper jaw (45–60 days before implant placement in type III or IV bone).
  - Rotary osseotensors are reserved for dense bone in the lower jaw (8–15 days before implant placement in type I or II bone).
- Extraction-implantation is possible at this appointment if conditions are favorable. If not, extraction with socket preservation should be followed by a waiting period of 45 days to 6 months before implants are installed. As extraction automatically induces an osteogenic response, the use of osseotensors is not necessary.
- Implant surgery modalities are explained to the patient, including pre-op and post-op recommendations.

Table 7.1 Model consent form for implant surgery, including basal implants (Diskimplants®) and anesthesia

Instructions to Patient

Please take this document home and read it carefully. Note any questions you might have. Bring this document back to our office at your next appointment, and the doctor will review it with you before you sign.

1. My doctor has explained the various types of implants used in dentistry, with and without prior bone grafting, including laterally inserted basal implants (Diskimplants® of various designs), and I have been informed of the alternatives to implant surgery for replacement of my missing teeth. I have also been informed of the foreseeable risks of those alternatives. I understand what procedures are necessary to accomplish the placement of implant(s) under the gum, in or on the bone, and the use of bone substitute material if necessary.
2. I have further been informed that if no treatment is elected to replace the missing teeth or existing dentures, the non-treatment risks include, but are not limited to:
   (a) Maintenance of the existing full or partial denture(s) with relines or remakes every 3–5 years or as otherwise may be necessary due to slow, but likely, progressive dissolution of the underlying denture-supported jaw bone.
   (b) Any present discomfort of chewing inefficiency with the existing partial or full denture may persist or worsen in time.
   (c) Drifting, tilting, and/or extrusion of remaining teeth.
   (d) Looseness of teeth, periodontal disease (gum and bone), possibly followed by extraction(s).
   (e) A potential jaw joint problem (TMJ) caused by a deficient, collapsed, or otherwise improper bite.
3. I am aware that the practice of dentistry, dental surgery, and oral implantology (including basal implantology) is not an exact science, and I acknowledge that no guarantees have been made to me concerning the success of my implant surgery, the associated treatment and procedures, or the postsurgical dental procedures. I am further aware that there is a risk that the implant surgery may fail, which might require further corrective surgery or the removal of the implant with possible corrective surgery associated with the removal. Such a failure and remedial procedures could also involve additional fees being assessed.
4. I understand that implant success is dependent upon several variables including, but not limited to, operator experience, individual patient tolerance and health, anatomical variations, patient home care of the implant, and the implant material and design. I also understand that implants are available in a variety of designs and materials, and the choice of the implant, including basal implants (Diskimplants® of various designs), is determined in the professional judgment of my dentist.
5. I have further been informed of the possible risks and complications of implant surgery, anesthesia, and the proposed drugs including, but not limited to, failure of the implant(s), inflammation, swelling, infection, discoloration, numbness (exact extent and duration unknown), inflammation of blood vessels, injury to existing teeth, bone fracture, sinus penetration, delayed healing, or allergic reaction to the drugs or medications used. No one has made any promises or given me any guarantee about the outcome of this treatment or these procedures. I understand that these complications can occur even if all dental procedures are performed properly.
6. I have been advised that smoking, alcohol, drug abuse, or sugar consumption may affect gum healing and may limit the success of the implant. Since there is no way to accurately predict the gum and the bone healing capacities of each patient, I know I must follow my dentist's home care instructions and report to my dentist for regular examinations as instructed.

Table 7.1 (continued)

7. I have also been advised that there is a risk that the implant(s) and/or implant-supported teeth may break, which may require additional procedures.
8. I authorize Dr. .... to perform dental services for me, including basal implants and other related surgery such as adding bone substitute material, bone grafting, and/or prior bone stimulation by osseotensors. I agree to the type of anesthesia that he/she has discussed with me, specifically (local) (IV sedation) or (general). I agree not to operate a motor vehicle or hazardous device for at least twenty-four (24) hours or more until fully recovered from the effects of the anesthesia or drugs given for my case.
9. If an unforeseen condition arises in the course of treatment that calls for the performance of procedures in addition to or different from that now contemplated, and I am under general anesthesia or intravenous sedation, I further authorize and direct Dr. .... or his/her associates or assistants of his/her choice to do whatever he/she/they deem necessary and advisable under the circumstances, including the decision not to proceed with the implant procedure.
10. I approve any modifications in designs, materials, or care, if my dentist, in his/her professional judgment, decides it is in my best interest.
11. To my knowledge, I have given an accurate report of my health history. I have also reported any prior allergic or unusual reactions to drugs, food, insect bites, anesthetics, pollens, and dust, blood or body diseases, gum or skin reactions, abnormal bleeding, or any other condition relating to my health or any problems experienced with any prior medical, dental, or other health care and treatment.
12. I authorize my dentist to take photos, X-rays, or any other visual aids of my treatment to be used for the advancement of implant dentistry in any manner my dentist deems appropriate. However, no photographs or other records that identify me will be used without my express written consent.
13. I realize and understand that the purpose of this document is to evidence the fact that I am knowingly consenting to the implant procedures, including basal implants (Diskimplants®), recommended by my dentist.
14. I agree that if I do not follow my dentist's recommendations and advice for postoperative care, my dentist may terminate the dentist-patient relationship, requiring me to seek treatment from another dentist. I realize that postoperative care and maintenance treatment are critical for the ultimate success of dental implants.
15. Questions I Have to Ask My Dentist:

–

–

–

16. I CERTIFY THAT I HAVE READ AND FULLY UNDERSTAND THE ABOVE AUTHORIZATION AND INFORMED CONSENT TO IMPLANT PLACEMENT AND SURGERY AND THAT ALL OF MY QUESTIONS, IF ANY, HAVE BEEN FULLY ANSWERED. I HAVE HAD THE OPPORTUNITY TO TAKE THIS FORM HOME AND REVIEW IT BEFORE SIGNING IT.

Dentist signature:
Witness signature:
Patient signature:
Witness signature:

Fourth Appointment: Basal Implant Placement

Basal implant installation is always a full-thickness flap procedure, and can be performed under:

- Local-regional anesthesia without oral sedation
- Local-regional anesthesia with oral sedation
- Local-regional anesthesia with iv sedation
- General anesthesia for complex cases and/or phobic patients

Follow-Up and Maintenance Explained in Detail to the Patient, Including the Importance of Oral Hygiene and Regular Verification of Occlusion

- 24 h after implant placement, at 1 week, 45 days, 6 months, and then annually

Immediate Functional Implant Loading, with Appropriate Explanation of Special Recommendations

When an immediate functional loading protocol is decided on, the prosthetic phase starts in the operating room as soon as surgery is completed. After meticulous suturing, an impression is taken and the occlusion is recorded. The fixed, transitional screw-secured prosthesis is installed 48–72 h later. A transpalatal bar is recommended for full-arch restorations of extremely atrophic maxillae. This bar can be removed 6–12 months later, after all implants have been checked individually. A soft diet must be respected for 45 days; only moderate forces must be applied for 6 months to the fixed appliance, which must be checked regularly.

Example of Specific Treatment Planning for Fully Edentulous Atrophic Jaws

- Evaluate the patient's general physical and mental status, paying particular attention to oral conditions (Figs. 7.23, 7.24, 7.25, 7.26, 7.27, and 7.28).
- Discuss the various treatment options, including bone grafting and/or basal implants with the patient.

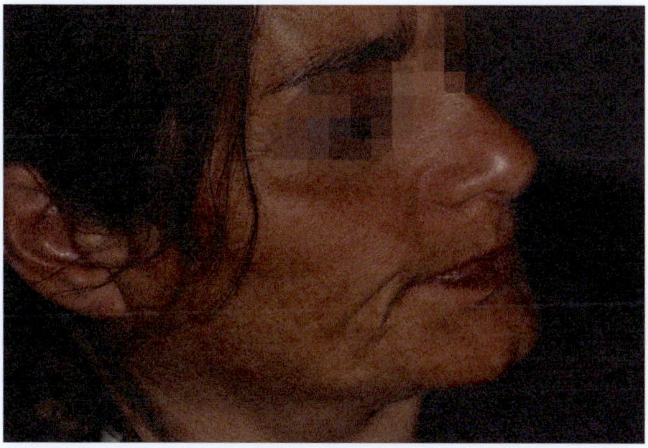

Fig. 7.23 Extraoral sagittal view of a 42-year-old patient with an atrophic jaw who requested a full-arch fixed implant-supported restoration. This patient had already experienced multiple implant failures and refused any bone grafting procedure

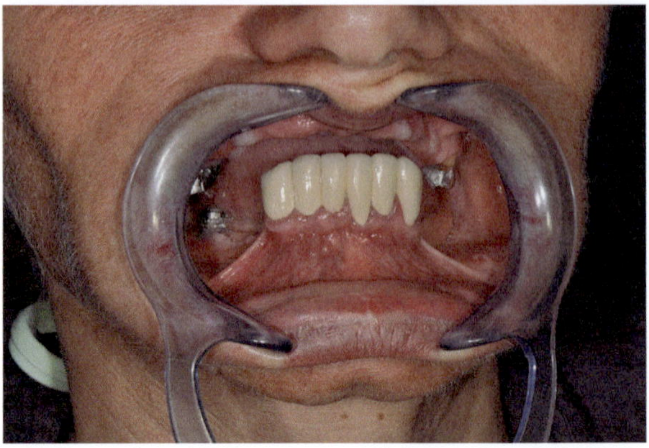

Fig. 7.24 Difficult intraoral mechanical conditions (same patient as Fig. 7.23)

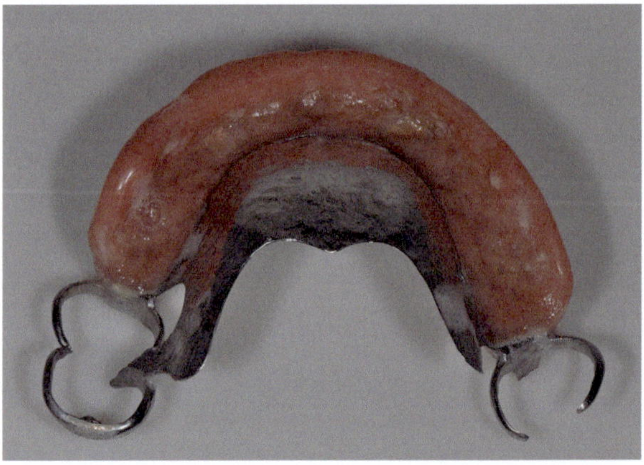

Fig. 7.25 Iatrogenic removable partial maxillary dentures aggravate continuous anterior bone resorption

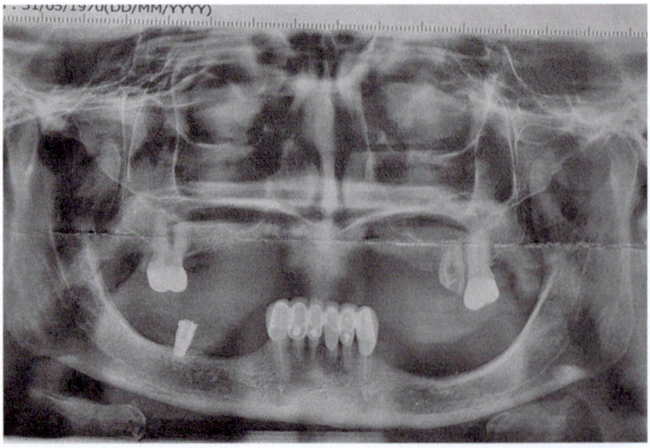

Fig. 7.26 The remaining upper molars have over-erupted in the mandibular area. Two posterior mandibular implants on both sides were lost 4 months after installation. Full removable lower and upper dentures were worn for 1 year after teeth extraction and implant removal

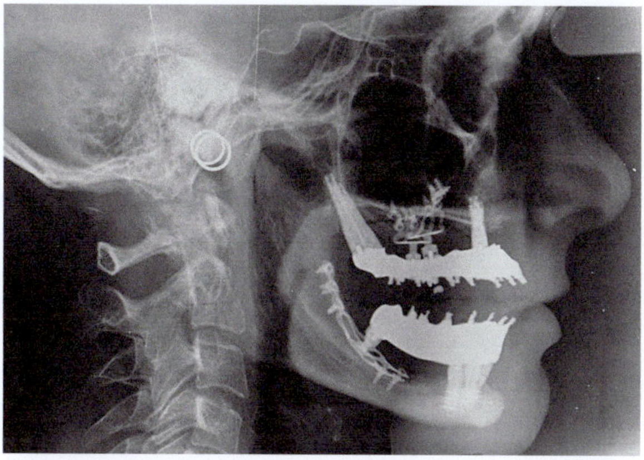

Fig. 7.27 Sagittal view after 1 year. Immediate functional loading procedure of a full-arch, implant-supported rehabilitation

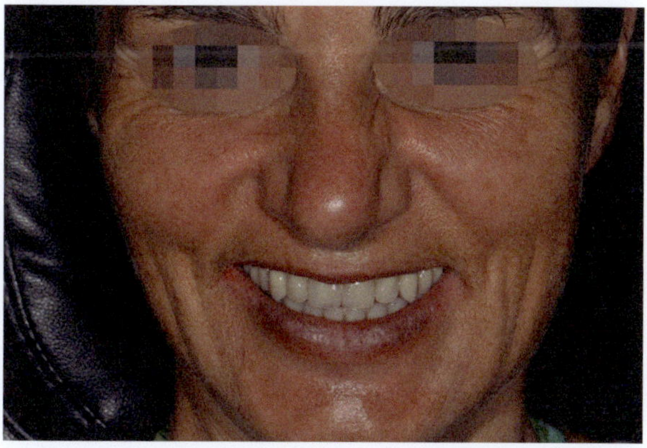

Fig. 7.28 Cosmetic aspect of the fixed, screw-secured rehabilitation on basal and root-form implants after 2 years (same patient as Fig. 7.23)

– Explain the difference between axial and basal implants. The discussion must also cover the total cost, the treatment timeline, the need to stop smoking for smokers, and the possible utility of preoperative Botox for heavy grinders and/or clenchers.

Atrophic Maxilla

For completely edentulous patients with severely atrophic maxillae who request bimaxillary implant-supported teeth, never begin with a fixed prosthesis of the lower jaw. Start by equipping the maxilla. Use a manual osseotensor to activate the future bone recipient bed 45–60 days before surgery. After the maxillary implants have been installed and equipped with an immediate fixed, screw-secured transitional functional denture, wait 1 year before installing implants in the lower jaw. Have the patient wear a removable lower denture for 6–9 months in order to reduce the mechanical stress on the eggshell-thin maxillary bone during the osseointegration process.

The patient in Figs. 7.23–7.28 was reluctant to undergo any prior bone grafting procedure and instead opted for basal implant-supported rehabilitation of both jaws. All remaining natural teeth were removed, and two full dentures were made in order to reestablish esthetics and occlusion. The patient had already lost root-form implants previously installed in the posterior mandible (Fig. 7.26). The bone was allowed to heal for 6 months. All implants were checked individually after retrieval of the screw-secured, fixed maxillary rehabilitation.

Explanation of the Two-Stage Submerged Implant Loading Protocol (Not Suitable for Fully Edentulous Patients)

If a delayed loading protocol is selected, the basal implants remain unloaded, completely covered over by the periosteum, for 4–6 months before the prosthetic phase is started. Patients must be told that a second procedure, performed under local anesthesia, will be required to uncover the implants and to install healing abutments and/or transgingival abutments, if necessary. The patient must be advised not to wear his or her partial removable denture during meals. Temporization must be respected in order not to compromise the outcome, especially when GBR is part of the procedure. When the implants are uncovered, osseointegration is checked, any necessary transgingival abutments are placed, and x-rays are taken to check the implant/abutment connection.

7.5 Implant Identification Card

Future generations of dentists will be responsible for managing the implants installed by their predecessors. Young practitioners and dental students should be informed of the potential risks of screw loosening, cement wear, implant body fracture, etc. They should also be taught the protocols for repair and rescue of existing implant-supported restorations and the means for return to a conventional denture with minimum damage, when necessary. Implant identification cards carried by patients are a simple means to help practitioners to recognize the wide variety of implants and components, and they facilitate contact with the patient's former dentist and implant manufacturers. This is particularly important for basal implants, which have specific criteria for determination of when such devices can be safely left in place or when they should be removed, and specific protocols for actual removal when necessary. Communication via the Internet greatly facilitates exchange of information about the patient's implant status.

Conflict of interest statement Gérard M. Scortecci is the inventor of the Diskimplant and holder of several associated patents that are exploited by the Victory company. He is an unpaid consultant to this firm and a minority shareholder in the company. No money was received from any of the companies mentioned in the book or from any of the companies whose products are mentioned.

Recommended Reading

1. Adell R, Lekholm U, Rockler B, Brånemark PI. A 15-year study of osseointegrated implants in treatment of the edentulous jaw. Int J Oral Surg. 1981;6:387–416.
2. Brunggenkate CM, Krekeler G, Kraïjenhagen HA, Foizik C, Nat P, Oesterbeek HS. Hemorrhage of the floor of the mouth resulting from lingual perforation during implant placement: a clinical report. Int J Oral Maxillofac Impl. 1993;8:329–34.
3. Rinaldi M, Ganz SD, Mottola A. Computer-guided applications for dental implants, bone grafting, and reconstructive surgery. St. Louis, MO: Elsevier; 2016.
4. Scortecci G, Meyere P, Zattara H, Doms P. Intra-oral applications in small bone volumes. Patient selection and long-term results. In: Laney W, Tolman D, editors. Tissue integration in oral, orthopedic and maxillofacial reconstruction. Philadelphia, PA: Quintessence; 1990. p. 350–5.
5. Scortecci GM, Misch CE, Benner KU, editors. Implants and restorative dentistry. London: Martin Dunitz; 2001.
6. Scortecci G, Misch C, Odin G, Binderman I, Sers L. Implantologie basale: approche chirurgicale conforme aux données actuelles avérées. La Tribune Dentaire. 2006;1(11):10–2.
7. Scortecci G, Odin G, Ferrari M. Crêtes mandibulaires hyperfines et hautes. Lettre de la Stomatologie. 2008;38:24–8.

Surgery

8

Gérard M. Scortecci and Guillaume Odin

8.1 Pre-implantation Procedures

Periodontal Surgery

Respect of the general principles of mucogingival and bone surgery, including alveolar bone preservation techniques, is obviously essential. The available bone volume must also be carefully preserved. After radiographic and topographic delimitation of the area destined to receive basal implants, the amount of attached gingiva must be analyzed. Both free and pedicle gingival grafts can be used to increase the height of attached gingiva. Whenever the territory next to the implant site allows, a laterally sliding flap is preferable.

Pre-implant procedures should include:

- Removal of plaque and calculus and correction of any overhanging restorations to avoid future plaque buildup
- Elimination of any purulent discharges that may not only compromise results but also increase the omnipresent risk of osteitis

G. M. Scortecci (✉)
University of Nice-Sophia Antipolis Medical School, Nice, France

New York University, New York, NY, USA

University of Southern California, Los Angeles, CA, USA

Private Practice, Nice, France
e-mail: scortecci@wanadoo.fr

G. Odin
ENT and Maxillo-facial Surgery Department, Institut Universitaire de la Face et du Cou, University of Nice-Sophia Antipolis Medical School, Nice, France
e-mail: odin.g@chu-nice.fr

© Springer Nature Switzerland AG 2019

G. M. Scortecci (ed.), *Basal Implantology*, https://doi.org/10.1007/978-3-319-44873-2_8

- Correction of all removable total or partial dentures, which irritate the soft tissues and hinder mucosal healing
- Correction of iatrogenic muscle insertions.

Constant muscle pull is one of the major sources of implant neck exposure and subsequent chronic pain and a starting point for peri-implantitis. Any muscle insertions lying close to the future point of implant emergence must be eliminated. When required, osteoplasty is generally performed at the time of surgery. If mucogingival corrections prove necessary after the implant-supported prosthesis is in place, conventional periodontal surgical techniques can be used to improve soft tissue management and the amount of keratinized tissue around the implant abutment.

Botox® Injections

This procedure can be helpful in patients with very powerful muscles. The masseter and temporal muscles must be injected on both sides 2 weeks before installation of basal implants. This prevents future overload and stress, especially when dealing with eggshell-thin maxillae and/or pencil mandibles.

Bone Bed Stem Cell Activation with Osseotensors (See Details in Chap. 5)

The use of bone matrix osseotensors (manual and/or rotary) is an integral part of all treatment plans. It improves initial bone conditions by promoting angiogenesis and osseogenesis 1 week to 45 days before basal implant surgery. This is particularly helpful before installation of tubero-pterygoid implants because a manual osseotensor can drastically improve D4 bone in the tuberosity; 45–60 days after osseotensor application, the bone callus obtained will have transformed into active D2 bone. The same procedure is used prior to basal implant placement in the sinus area.

In the mandible, when the bone is already dense, it is important to promote and/or increase the surrounding blood supply to improve closure of the soft tissue incision line. This is achieved by activating the periosteum with manual osseotensors (tunneling) 1 week before basal implant installation. In dense D1 bone in the mental sector, a rotary osseotensor must be used 1 week before surgery (a single impact per implant site).

8.2 Organizational Requirements (Figs. 8.1 and 8.2)

To reduce the risks of contamination, the operating room should be isolated from the rest of the dental office or clinic by two sets of doors and must be disinfected regularly. The air may be filtered or flow past an ultraviolet radiation device to reduce bacterial counts. Operating room equipment must include the specific instrument sets for axial and lateral osteotomy, general surgical instruments, and an appropriate assortment of implants in various lengths and diameters. The organizational advantages of a

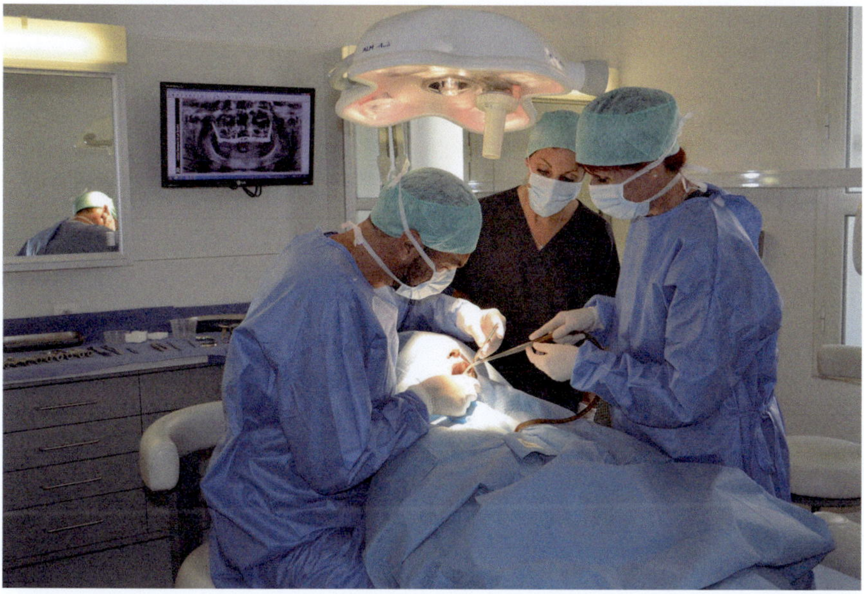

Fig. 8.1 Operating room dedicated to dental implant surgery. Trained team: the surgeon and two dental assistants are necessary to properly handle basal implantology

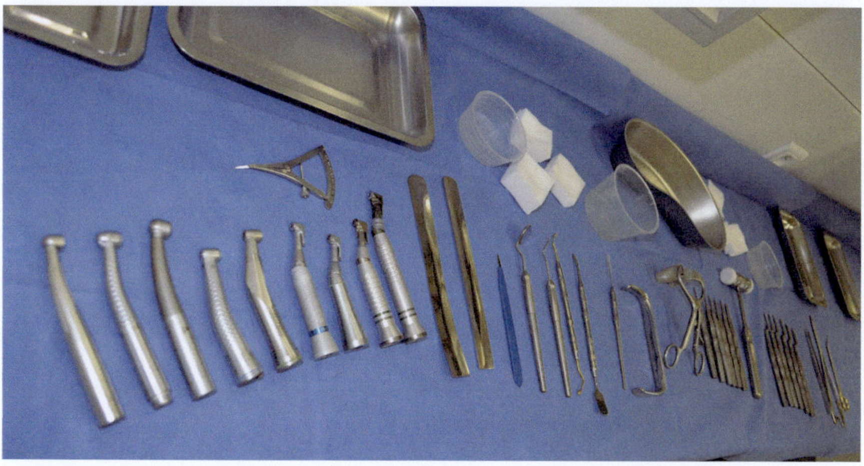

Fig. 8.2 Specific high-speed and low-speed handpieces and basal implant instruments

standardized instrument system suitable for the various implants envisaged, including extra "helper" implants, and a standardized operating protocol are obvious. Preservation of the sterility of surgical instruments between the time of autoclaving and placement in storage, as well as during storage in packs or trays, is paramount.

Before entering the operating room area, the surgeon and assistants must put on masks, gowns, gloves, caps, and special shoes or shoe covers. Likewise, draping isolates the future surgical site from other parts of the patient's body and from non-sterile operating room equipment. Availability of an intraoral digital imaging system in the operating room is extremely useful during the initial stage of lateral osteotomy. The angulation of the pilot cutter (dia. 5 mm) can be checked directly on the screen and corrected if necessary. A chairside digital periapical radiograph can be taken with the cutter inserted only partly into the buccal bone plate to check proper positioning.

8.3 Soft Tissue and Bone Management

Patient Preparation

Intraoral preparation consists in the use of 2% chlorhexidine. Cleansing is best achieved with a spray or jet lavage, with Ringer's solution and hydrogen peroxide serving as the primary media. Antiseptics such as Betadine® povidone-iodine may also be used. The patient's lips should be protected with Bepanthen® cream (Bayer) or vaseline. A flash of 2 g of amoxicillin is given 20 minutes preop. If the patient is allergic, three tablets of clindamycin 500 mg are administered.

Flap Elevation and Incisions

Exposure of the bone, the target organ of basal dental implants, requires meticulous elevation of full-thickness flaps of the soft tissues, including the periosteum, to ensure hemostasis, uncomplicated healing, an acceptable scar, and the preservation of essential vascular and nerve structures (e.g., palatal arteries, lingual and mandibular nerves). During surgery, saliva, bone debris, bacteria, and other contaminants are sucked into the inner workings of the handpiece. Maintaining the sterility of the handpiece and turbine is therefore essential.

Atraumatic soft tissue handling requires mastery of the scalpel technique. Skill in the use of interchangeable blades (no. 15 or no. 11) and soft tissue retractors is mandatory as is careful and atraumatic handling of the periosteum.

Bone is a bradytrophic tissue, and the mechanisms by which it compensates for a sudden disturbance in blood flow take time to become operative. Preservation of maximum blood supply during osteotomy and implant installation requires:

- Sharp incision of the soft tissue, including the periosteum, down to the bone crest
- Elevating (rather than scraping) the periosteum from the bone (a smoothly elevated, uninjured periosteal surface is a sign of atraumatic technique)
- Limiting the duration of exposure of the jaw bone
- Avoiding excessive temperature elevation by continuous profuse saline irrigation during the osteotomy and use of titanium cutters with a high cutting capacity
- Uncontaminated water and air.

Neglect in these areas can result in failure of an initially stable implant due to impaired blood supply, gradual loss of bone strength, and eventually mobilization of the implant.

8.4 The Diskimplant® System (Figs. 8.3, 8.4, 8.5, 8.6, 8.7, 8.8, 8.9, 8.10, 8.11, 8.12, 8.13, 8.14, 8.15, 8.16 and 8.17)

The wide range of disk diameters and heights along with multiple-disk and plate-form Diskimplants® allows achievement of bilateral cortical support in the vestibulo-lingual direction, even below the sinuses and above the mandibular

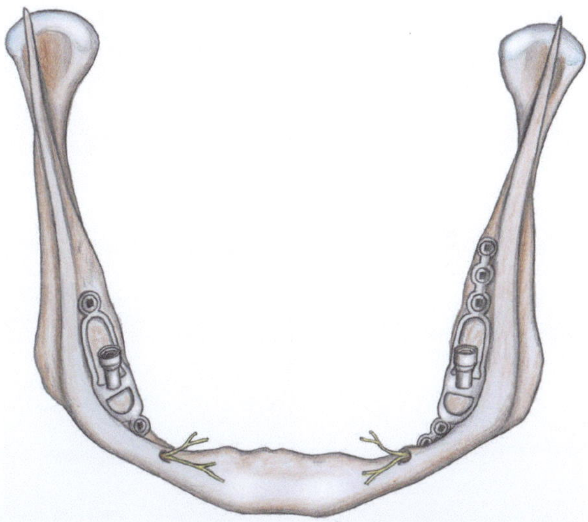

Fig. 8.3 Extremely atrophic dry mandible: difficult to graft, such cases can be more easily handled with plate-form Diskimplants® placed in the posterior sectors

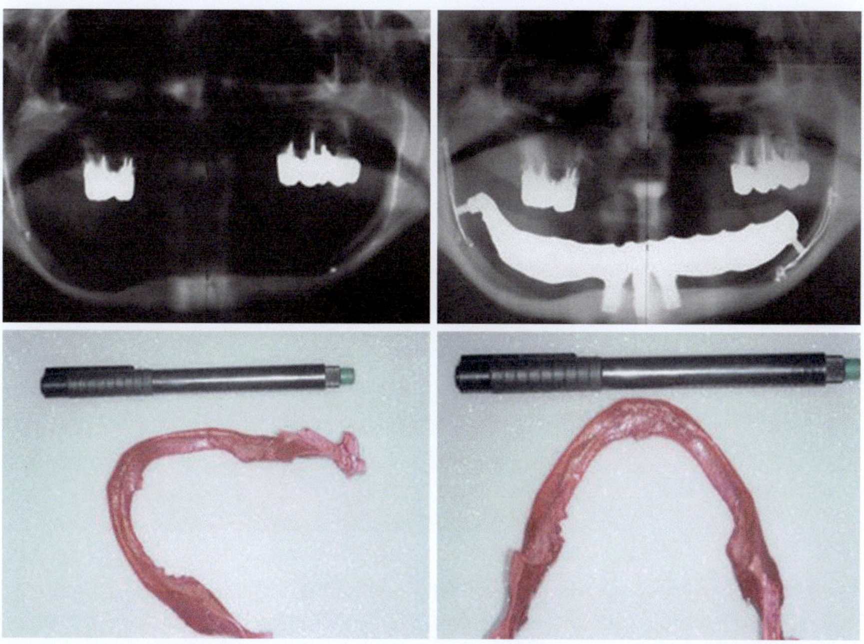

Fig. 8.4 Pencil mandible restored with plate-form Diskimplants® in the posterior regions and three root-form implants in the mental area

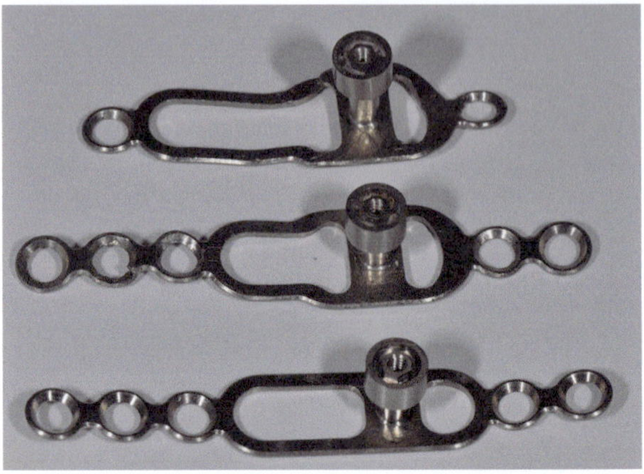

Fig. 8.5 Plate-form Diskimplants® of various dimensions to manage anatomic requirements

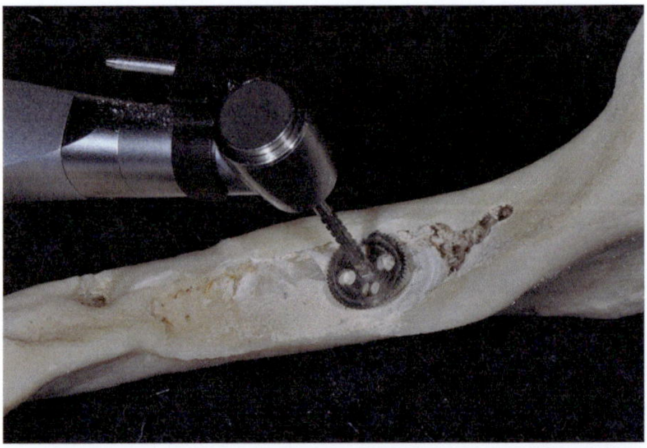

Fig. 8.6 Titanium cutter used under copious irrigation to prepare the recipient bone bed in this atrophic mandible

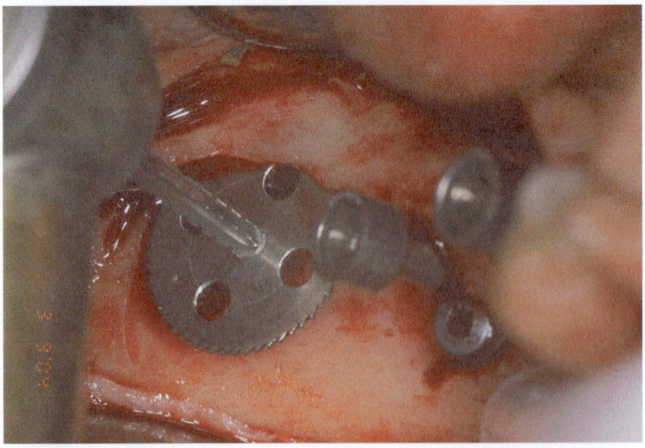

Fig. 8.7 A long internal lingual notch is prepared in order to laterally engage the plate-form Diskimplant®. Note the small bone opening 0.5 mm above the mandibular nerve

canal. The narrow shaft of the Diskimplant® allows passage through narrow ridges. Both submerged and non-submerged implant techniques can be used, depending on local bone anatomy, gingival thickness, and the type of edentulism.

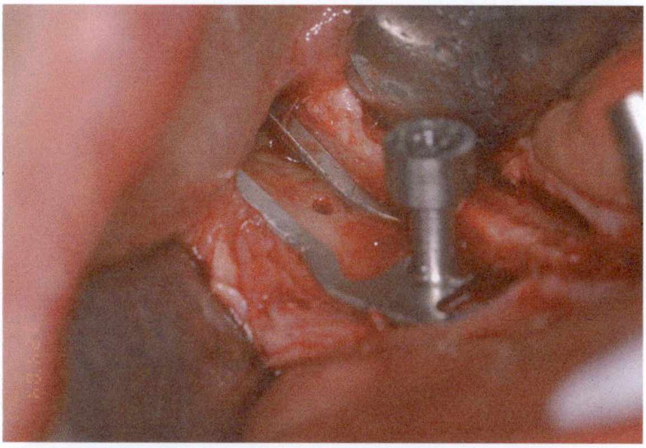

Fig. 8.8 The basal implant is gently tapped into the lateral lingual mandibular bony notch and then firmly screw-secured with 5-mm-long orthopedic screws in order to ensure absolute primary stability. When there is a risk of mandibular canal penetration, the surgeon must angle the screw lingually or buccally

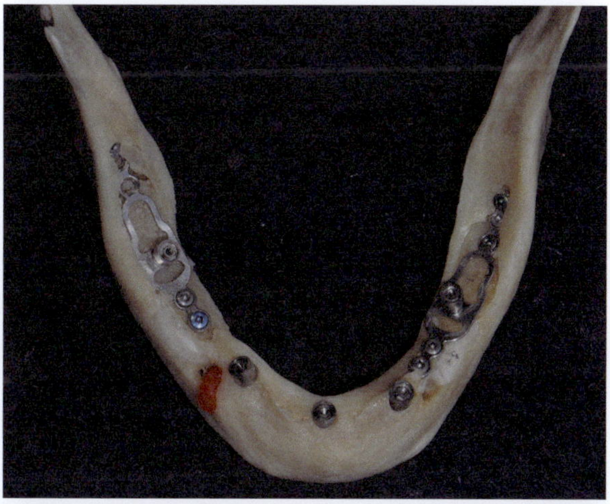

Fig. 8.9 The plate-form Diskimplant® must be intimately adapted to the recipient bone by tapping the implant base with a round-tipped seating instrument

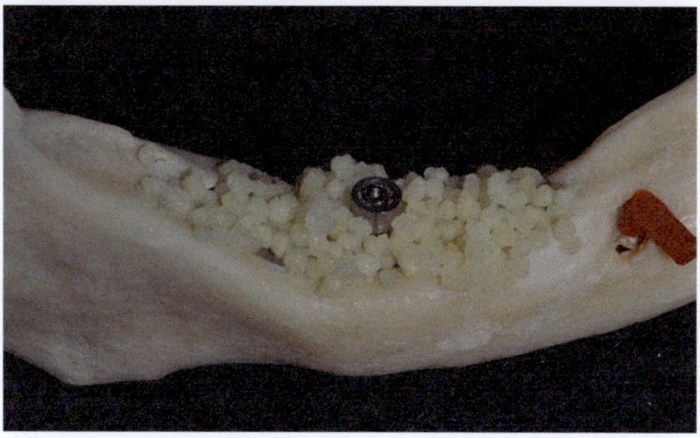

Fig. 8.10 Bone substitute material (CoreBone®, Interpore®, BioOss®, etc.) must completely cover the basal implant

The lateral osteotomy procedure minimizes technical bone loss at the crest level. Only the basal apical portion of the bone is of concern for primary Diskimplant® stability.

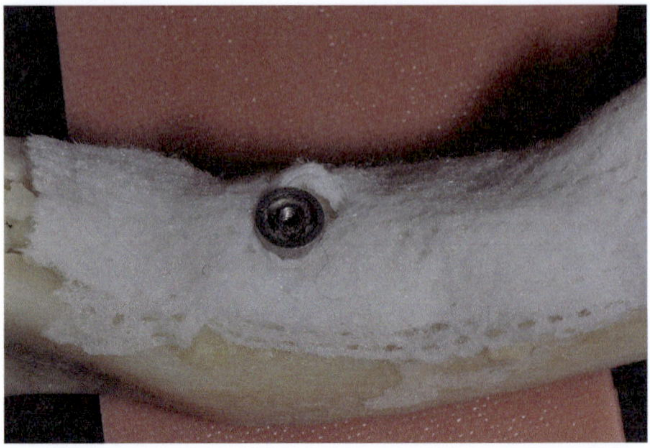

Fig. 8.11 An autologous PRF membrane is placed over the bone substitute material in order to hold it in place before suturing the full-thickness mucoperiosteal flap (4.0 suture)

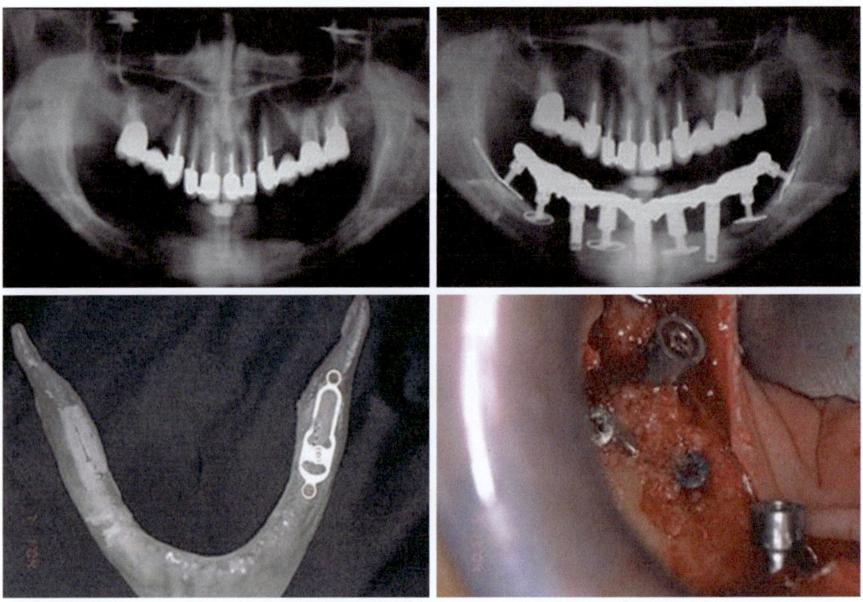

Fig. 8.12 Six months after failure of bilateral autologous bone grafts, correction was achieved with an immediate, screw-secured restoration on basal and root-form implants

Diskimplant® Emergence Profiles

Various generations of Diskimplants® with different emergence profiles have been developed since 1984:

- External thread (M2–0.40, then M2–0.25)
- Internal thread with an external hexagon (M2–0.25)

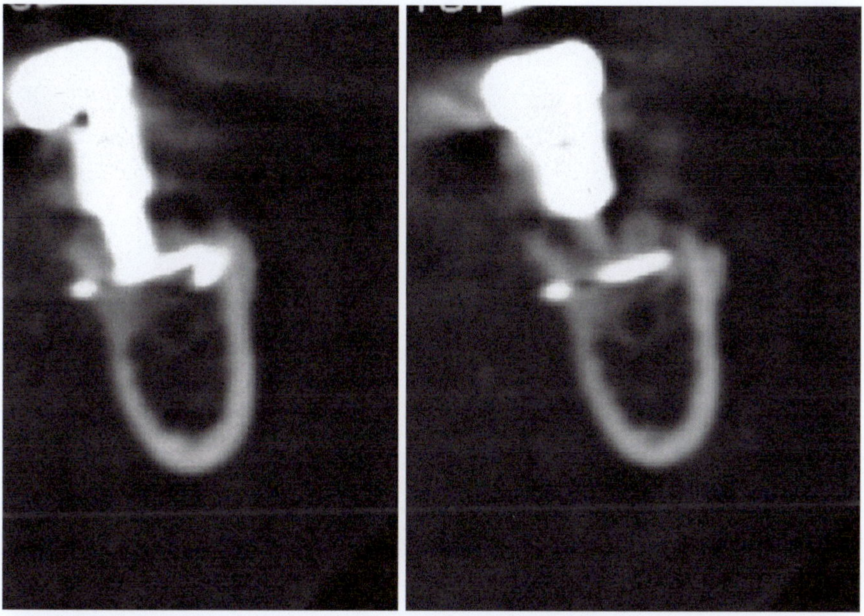

Fig. 8.13 Cone beam CT showing the posterior mandibular plate-form Diskimplant® 2 mm above the mental nerve

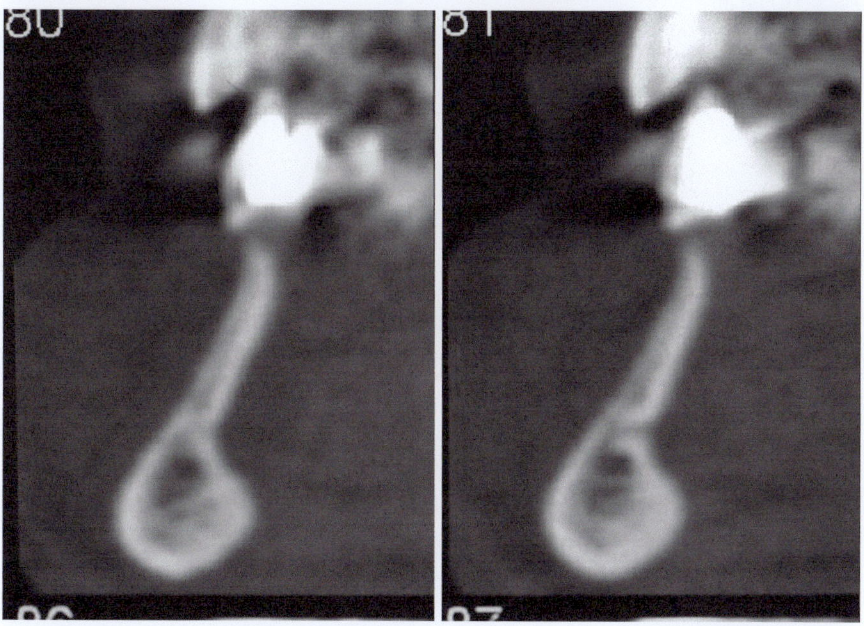

Fig. 8.14 Initial high knife ridge in the mental area (D1 bone)

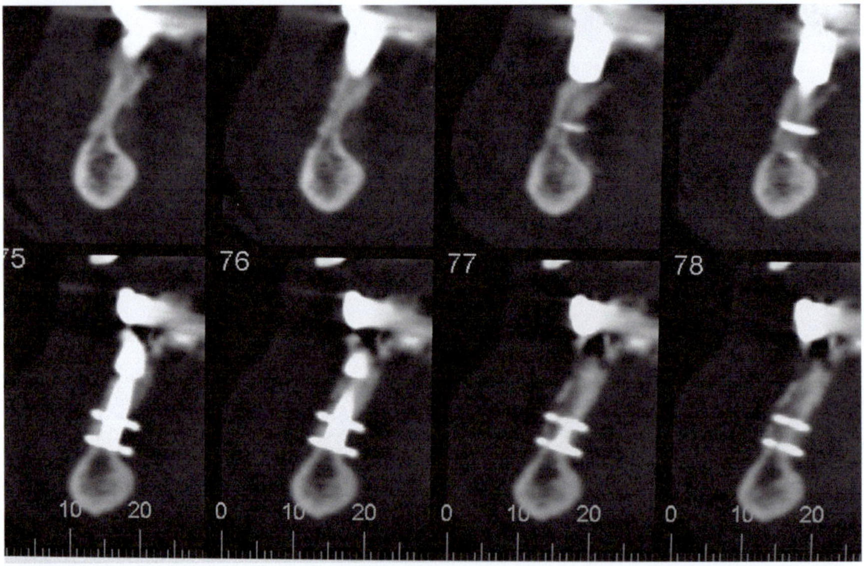

Fig. 8.15 Class III patient: sagittal view 48 hours post-op of a basal implant rehabilitation with an immediate loading protocol. Distal bone anchorage is mandatory to avoid a risky cantilever and ensure long-term success

Fig. 8.16 Front view of the same patient 10 years post-op (2007–2017)

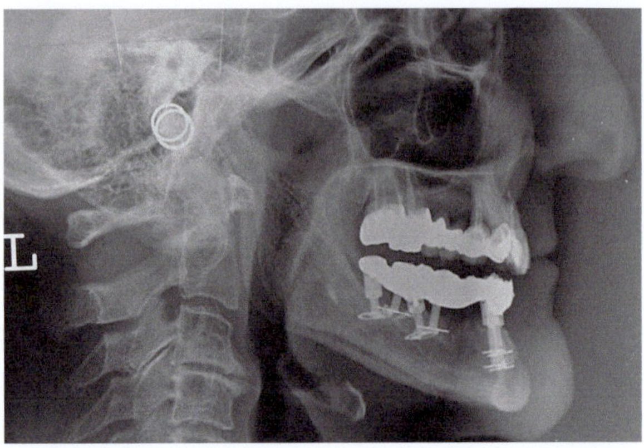

- Internal M1.4 thread with a Monobloc flat emergence profile (protected external hexagon plus Morse cone conical seal)
- Internal M2–0.40 thread with an internal octagon.

The characteristic features of current-day Diskimplants® include:

- A Monobloc crestal emergence identical to that of the Monobloc transgingival abutment originally developed for implants with an external hexagon. The cervical portion of the 3.5 mm high crestal cylinder is tapered slightly to form a

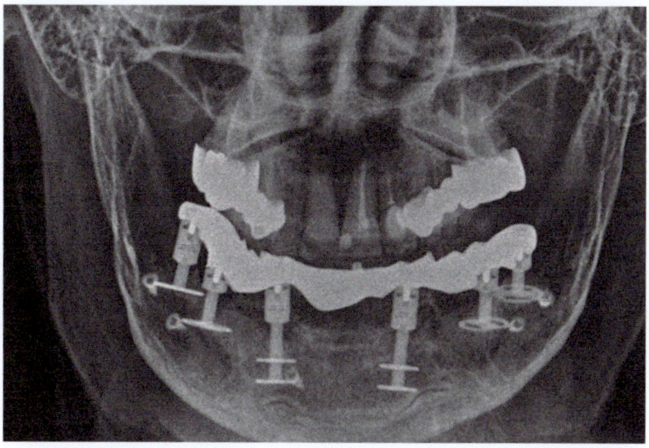

Fig. 8.17 Cone beam CT at 10 years: the double Diskimplants® are perfectly osseointegrated despite the thin knife ridge

0.5 mm inverted truncated cone; the smooth surface of the cylinder prevents plaque buildup and facilitates cleaning. This taper guarantees correct implant placement in the bone site and prevents the implant from moving out of position, thereby improving primary stability.

- A vertical cylindrical shaft, slightly larger in diameter (2.35 mm) than the vertical osteotomy created by the cutter.
- A horizontal circular or asymmetrical base, perpendicular at its center to the shaft, that allows the device to withstand occlusal forces and lateral forces in all directions. The symmetrical perforations in the base promote blood supply and osseointegration; bone ingrowth helps prevent rotation. The same is true for double- and triple-disk Diskimplants®.
- Plate-form Diskimplants® secured by mini orthopedic screws (5–6 mm) are used for severely atrophic jaws.
- Titanium cutters for lateral osteotomy to avoid polymetallism.

Armamentarium (Fig. 8.18)

The instruments required for Diskimplant® placement are as follows:

1. Titanium cutters of different lengths and diameters
2. High-speed handpiece (160,000 rpm) or air turbine set at ≥3 kgf/cm²/60 psi minimum
3. Scalpels (Bard-Parker® no. 15), resorbable and/or non-resorbable suture thread (000, 0000)
4. Periosteal elevators (medium and large)
5. Bone and gum scissors
6. Manual gum retractor, automatic retractor
7. Seating instruments (straight, curved, bayonet)
8. Surgical mallet
9. Needle holder

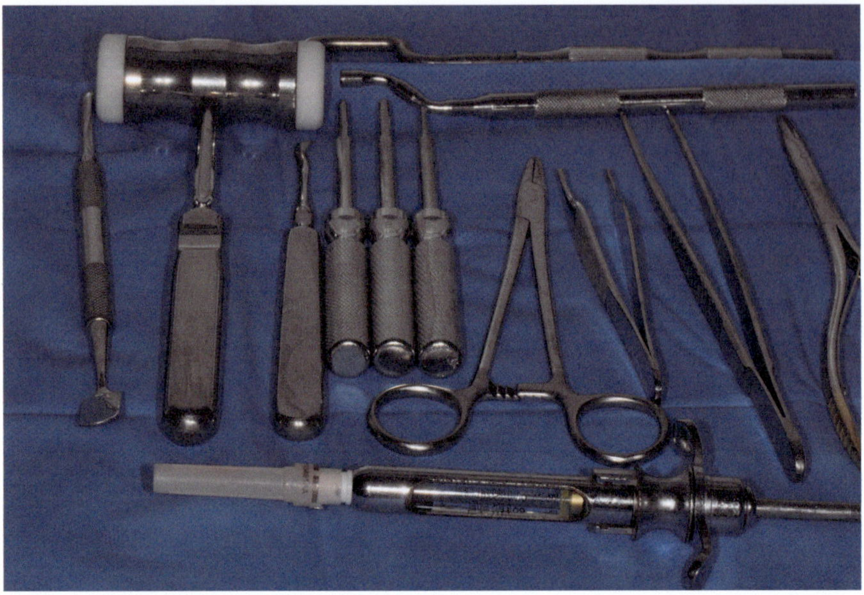

Fig. 8.18 Armamentarium for basal implant installation

10. Suture scissors
11. Self-tapping osteosynthesis screws for plate-form Diskimplants® and the corresponding screwdriver

8.5 Titanium Cutters for High-Speed Lateral Osteotomy

The specific instrument used for osteotomy, termed a "cutter," consists of a titanium shaft with cutting blades and a toothed circular base. These solid one-piece instruments, without any welds or added parts, allow precise lateral T-shaped osteotomy with sprays of water and air without risk of polymetal contamination. As it rotates, the cutter functions as a circular micro-saw that prepares the T-shaped implant lodging in a single step that lasts only several seconds. The microcanals on the wide circular cutter generate an aquaplaning phenomenon thanks to the copious irrigation; this promotes irrigation within the bone incision, thus preventing thermal injury.

The mechanical and biological qualities of these rotary titanium instruments optimize preparation of a bone recipient site corresponding exactly to the future implant:

- Continuous visual and tactile control
- No heat buildup
- No contamination by foreign metal particles (Diskimplants® and cutters are both manufactured of titanium)
- Minimal trauma
- Rapid surgical procedure

The cutter shaft adapts directly to all standard high-speed turbines and high-speed motor contra-angles (120,000 rpm); no special contra-angle is required. Turbines should be operated at ≥3 kg/cm^2 (60 psi) under copious irrigation plus lateral irrigation with saline solution. A turbine with a small head is necessary for narrow passages between natural teeth. Air turbines are preferable: despite their high speed, their extremely low torque considerably limits the Joule effect. High-speed contra-angles with micromotors are recommended for dense mandibular bone under copious irrigation. Titanium cutters are reusable and should be sterilized in an autoclave. The number of uses (maximum 10) depends on wear of the cutter teeth. Brand-new titanium cutters should be used for dense mandibular bone, whereas previously used cutters are suitable for soft maxillary bone.

Titanium cutters are available in different diameters, heights, and shape for osteotomy corresponding to the intended Diskimplant®, itself selected according to the bone anatomy. Each cutter diameter corresponds to a Diskimplant of identical diameter (the cutter is slightly smaller in dimension than the implant to ensure primary stability when the implant is impacted into the bone). For example, a diameter 9 mm cutter is used to install a 9 mm diameter Diskimplant®. Double-disk and triple-disk cutters exist for double- and triple-disk Diskimplants®. The distance between two cutting disks on multi-disk cutters is always 3 mm. A cutter with a diameter smaller than that of the intended implant can be used first to verify correct positioning; the site is then enlarged with a cutter corresponding to the implant diameter.

8.6 Specific Instruments for Critical Areas

In order to pass close to very high teeth, it may be necessary to prolong the turbine cutter by using an Orthoroad extender (Orthoroad, Paris) (Figs. 8.19 and 8.20). When the dimensions of the handpiece prevent passage between two teeth, either an L series cutter can be used with an extender or a mini-head high-speed handpiece set at ≥3 kgf/cm^2 can be utilized.

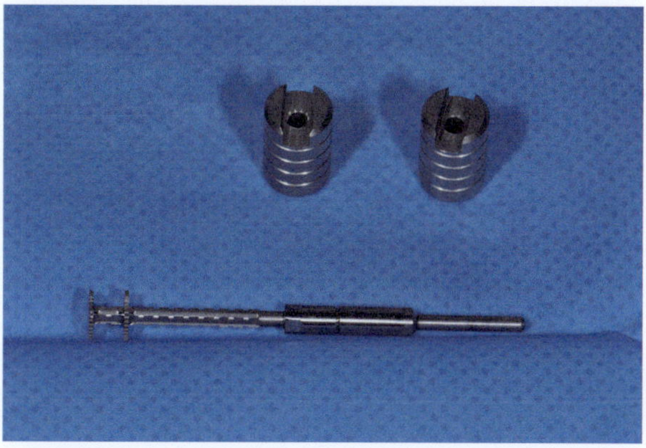

Fig. 8.19 Cutter extenders for high-speed turbines are helpful for lateral osteotomies in narrow spaces

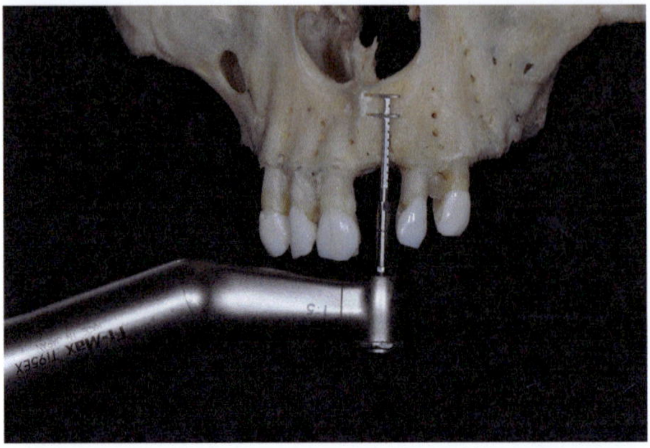

Fig. 8.20 An extender for cutters mounted on a high-speed handpiece facilitates lateral osteotomy between teeth

Prior to use, operation of the cutter must always be checked outside of the mouth after mounting on a high-speed contra-angle or air turbine. The irrigation system must also be verified. If the turbine or contra-angle is damaged, or if the cutter shaft is bent, the patient may be injured.

8.7 Osteotomy Procedure

Proper planning of the implant position at the outset is essential. Lateral osteotomy allows direct visual control of bone penetration and tactile awareness of passage from one cortical plate to the other. An appropriate surgical guide should be used when necessary. The high-speed air turbine or contra-angle handpiece must be gently guided laterally, without exerting excessive pressure to avoid the cutter from becoming blocked in the bone or bent. Diskimplant® cutters are designed to control the drilling speed: if the operator exerts too much pressure manually, the turbine stops automatically. As soon as the pressure lessens, bone cutting resumes. After the cutter has begun to cut the horizontal groove in the bone, the high-speed handpiece cannot deviate from its trajectory along this plane because the upper and lower surfaces of the cutter are perfectly smooth. Once the cutter shaft enters the bone, the instrument is automatically "piloted" by the disk's guide surfaces. Care must be taken to orient the shaft osteotomy vertically, taking prosthetic requirements into consideration (parallelism, axis of insertion, etc.).

When the treatment plan calls for installation of several Diskimplants® next to one another, the osteotomies must be offset slightly to avoid creating a bone block fracture. The full-thickness mucoperiosteal flap should be protected by holding a large, rigid plastic suction tip firmly against the bone plate. The cutter must always remain in this "safety box" during osteotomy. In certain cases, a transparent surgical guide with an open lateral window can be prepared on the study model mounted in occlusion and used for initial lateral osteotomy. An ultrasonic surgical generator (Piezotome, Acteon) may prove useful for initiation of the lateral osteotomy, which should be completed by the use of a calibrated cutter.

Special Precautions During Lateral Osteotomy

- For Diskimplants®, a small lateral cut is first made in the cortical bone with a 5 mm diameter cutter. This cutter can be left in place in the initial cut to radiographically verify correct positioning (2 mm above the mandibular canal, for example) before continuing with a larger diameter cutter. If need be, the position of the cut can be modified (higher, lower, to one side). A piezotome may prove useful for the posterior mandible.
- The soft tissues, periosteum, and mandibular nerve must be protected by firmly holding a large plastic suction tip against the buccal or lingual bone plate when using a cutter.
- For the mandible, start with a 5 mm diameter cutter (single or double disk), and then use the final cutter (7 or 9 mm diameter). In soft maxillary bone, it is better to use a 7 or 9 mm cutter directly.
- A brand-new cutter guaranteeing optimum cutting performance should always be used for dense cortical bone.

Cylindrical Monobloc Diskimplants® (Figs. 8.21, 8.22, 8.23, 8.24 and 8.25)

Elevation of both lingual (or palatal) and buccal full-thickness flaps permits visualization of the moment when the cutter reaches and starts to enter the opposite cortical plate. This allows avoidance of injury to the periosteum.

If part of the implant protrudes outside of the bone after Diskimplant® installation, it can be left as a graft holder for autogenous bone chips that have been collected in situ or for placement of a non-resorbable biomaterial such as autologous dentin, BioOss®, CoreBone®, Ivory®, Interpore®, and/or a PRF membrane (Figs. 8.26, 8.27 and 8.28). The full-thickness flaps are then sutured passively. For single-tooth replacements in the esthetic zone, an Invisalign®-like removable temporary should be used during a waiting period of 6 months (Figs. 8.29 and 8.30).

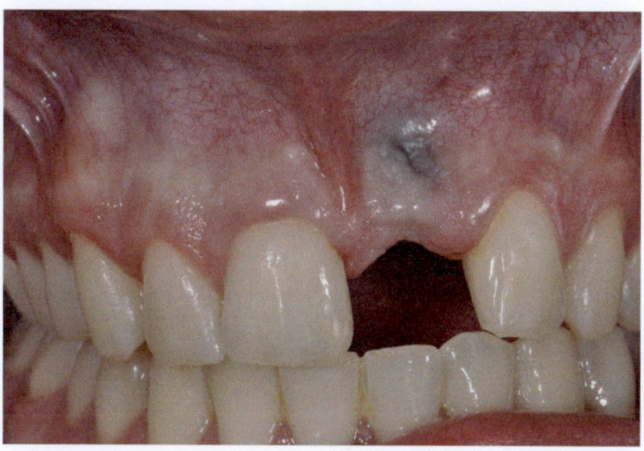

Fig. 8.21 Typical situation for single-tooth replacement using either root-form dental implants with prior bone grafting or immediate placement of basal implants (double Diskimplants®)

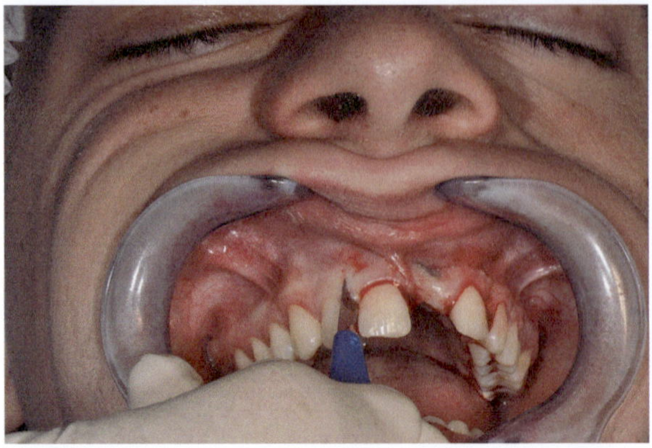

Fig. 8.22 Angulated soft tissue incision including the two adjacent teeth

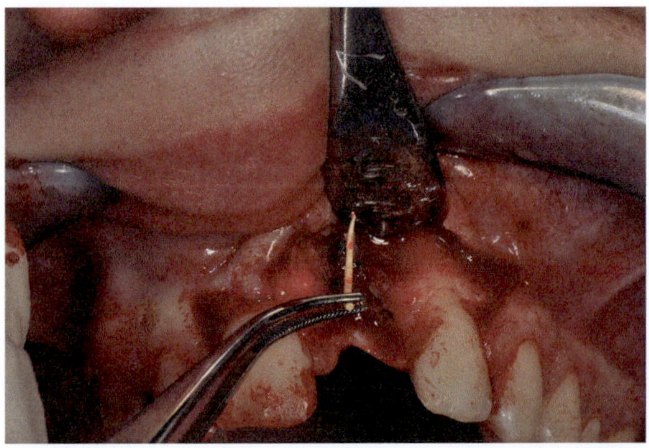

Fig. 8.23 A full-thickness flap is elevated; a gutta-percha root canal filling trapped in the bony defect caused the recurrent fistula

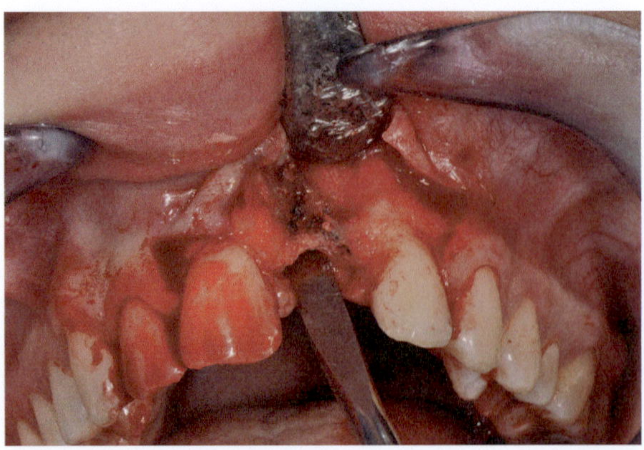

Fig. 8.24 Very little bone remained after removal of the foreign body; only the palatal plate remains intact

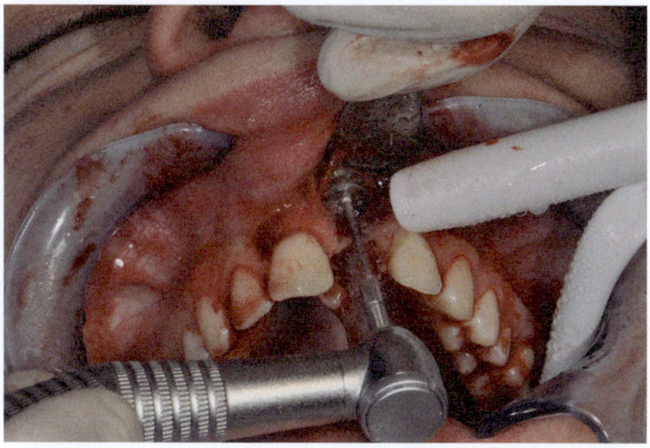

Fig. 8.25 This patient refused a bone graft but accepted basal implant treatment (7G5-DDM double Diskimplant®). Lateral osteotomy was performed under copious irrigation

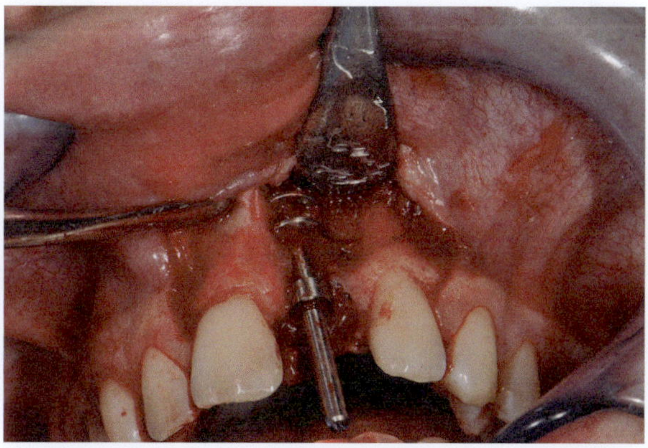

Fig. 8.26 A double Diskimplant® was inserted laterally and absolute primary stability was checked

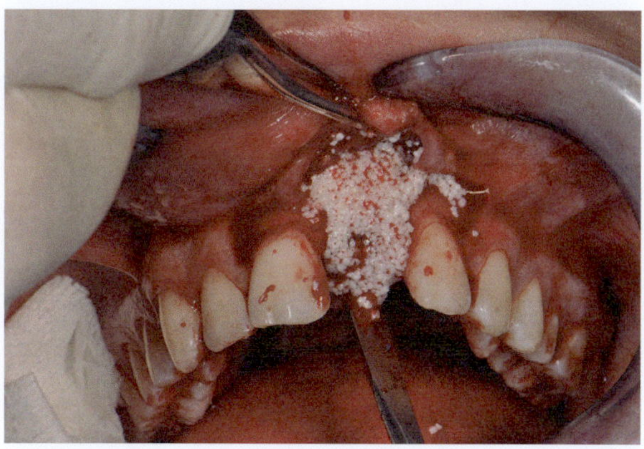

Fig. 8.27 Full coverage with bone substitute material and PRF

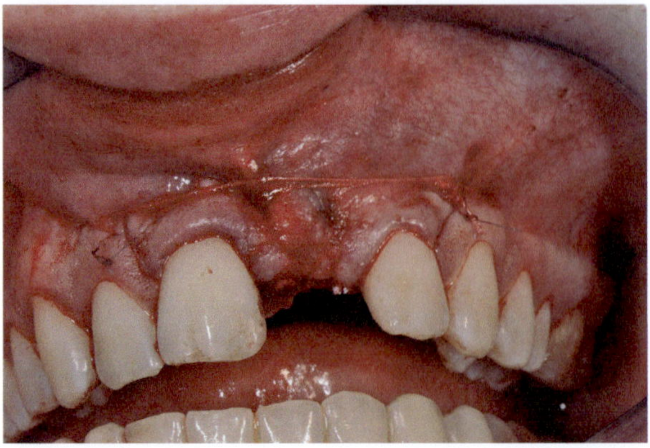

Fig. 8.28 After a high horizontal internal periosteal incision, the full-thickness flap was passively sutured with 4/0 Glycolon® suture material

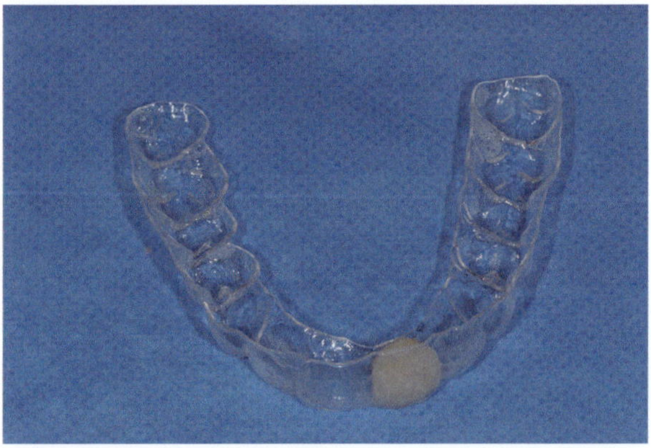

Fig. 8.29 An Invisalign®-like temporary template was made with commercial teeth and left in place for 6 months

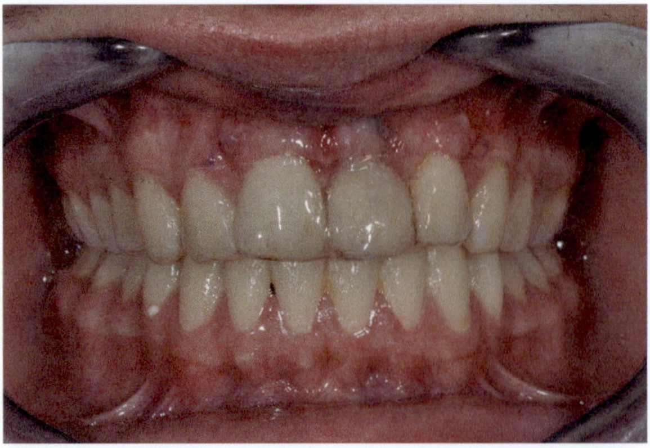

Fig. 8.30 The temporary appliance must not injure the implanted area. At 6 months post-op, a titanium/composite tooth was screw-secured onto the double Diskimplant®. Healing at 1 week post-op. Complete submerged technique. Second surgery at implant exposure 6–7 months later

Asymmetrical Monobloc Diskimplants®

Depending on the planned direction of insertion, a cutter corresponding to the larger or the smaller diameter is used (e.g., a ø7 mm or ø5 mm cutter for a Diskimplant® with a 7 × 5 mm rectangular base). Mesio-distal preparation of the osteotomy is achieved using a discrete back-and-forth movement of the corresponding cutter (single-, double-, or triple-disk cutter corresponding to the future implant). This slightly enlarges the vertical shaft cut, permitting a gentle press fit of the Diskimplant® using a surgical mallet and an appropriate implant-seating instrument (Fig. 8.31). The Monobloc emergence profile can be installed at bone level or just above (Fig. 8.32). A small diamond-coated wheel bur can be used to create an appropriate crestal bone housing if needed. Protruding disks should be covered with a bone substitute material (BioOss®, Ivory®, CoreBone®, Dentin Grinder® graft, etc.) and PRF (Figs. 8.33 and 8.34). The full-thickness flaps (lingual/palatal and buccal) must then be sutured passively (Fig. 8.35).

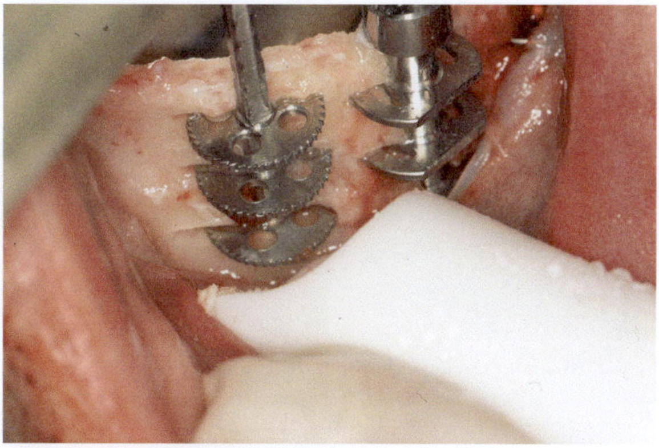

Fig. 8.31 Knife ridge (D1 bone) in the mental area: lateral osteotomy for installation of a triple Diskimplant® that must engage the lingual plate

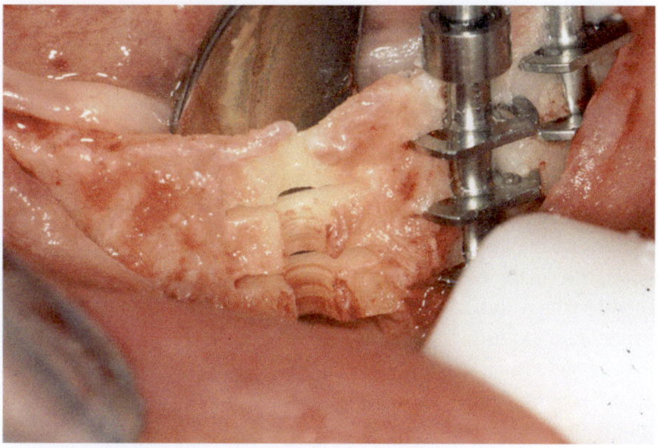

Fig. 8.32 The vertical cortical bone wall of the lingual plate must be preserved, otherwise the entire bone height and the Diskimplant® can be lost

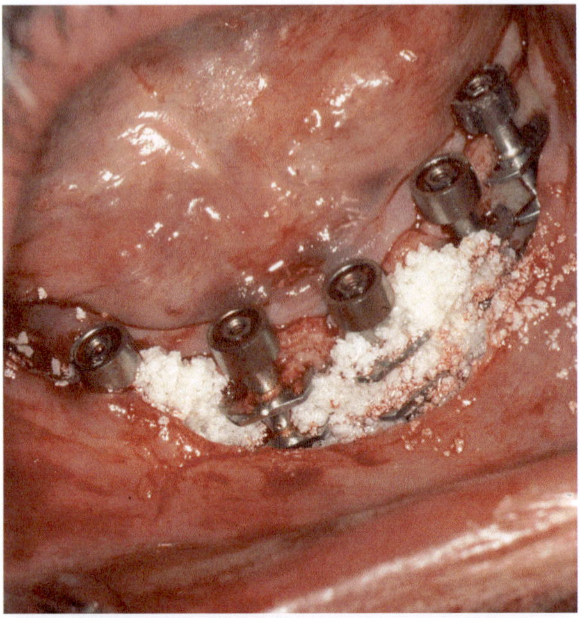

Fig. 8.33 The protruding portion of the triple Diskimplant® must be completely covered by bone substitute material. Adding an orthopedic screw (diameter 2 mm, length 5 mm) after Diskimplant® installation is sometimes useful because absolute primary stability is mandatory

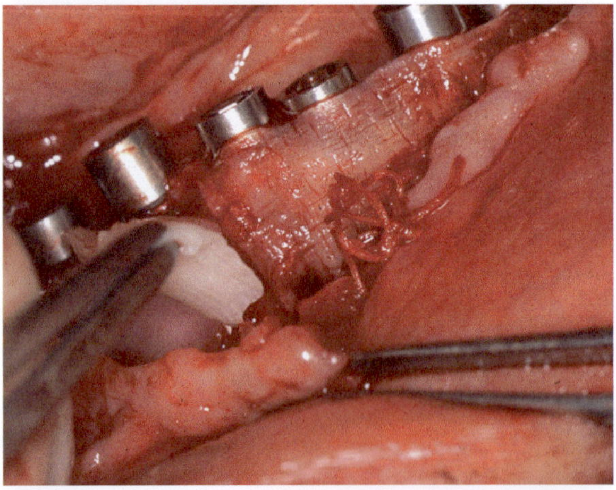

Fig. 8.34 PRF membranes are placed over the bone substitute material to hold it in place

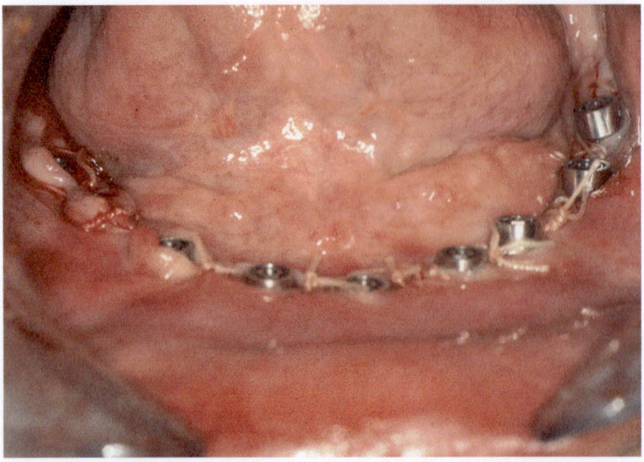

Fig. 8.35 Release of the periosteum using a horizontal incision allows passive suturing of the full-thickness flap. An immediate loading procedure with a fixed, screw-secured bridge is mandatory

Plate-Form Diskimplants® with Osteosynthesis Screws (Figs. 8.36, 8.37, 8.38, 8.39, 8.40, 8.41, 8.42, 8.43, 8.44, 8.45, 8.46 and 8.47)

Plate-form Diskimplants® must always be rendered endosseous; they must not remain subperiosteal. This can be achieved by inserting the plate in a lateral bone cut and covering it with a bone substitute material and PRF, or, when preparation of a bone notch is not feasible, by simply covering it with a non-resorbable bone substitute material (BioOss®, Interpore®, CoreBone®, Synthograph®, or equivalent) plus autologous PRF membranes using GBR technology. The periosteum and/or Schneiderian membrane (for plate-form Diskimplants® secured on the zygomatic process) should always be kept at a distance from the plate to avoid future exposure with time due to the pull of masticatory muscles. The plate portion of the basal Diskimplant® must always remain in intimate contact with the bone bed. A round-tipped seating instrument and a surgical mallet should be used to gently shape the titanium plate to the bone crest.

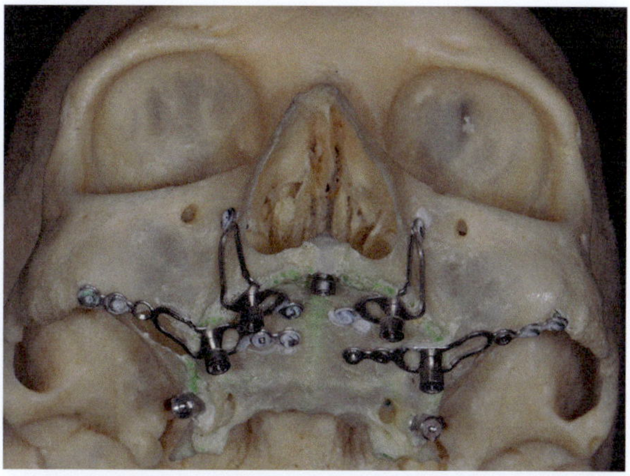

Fig. 8.36 Atrophic dry maxilla with basal implants inserted on the major maxillary buttresses

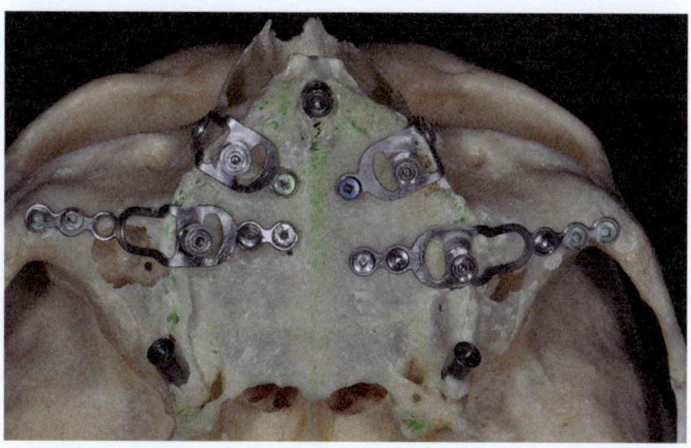

Fig. 8.37 Occlusal view of basal implants firmly screw-secured in the remaining dense bone. The wide base of the plate-form Diskimplant® (43 × 9 mm) provides reliable support for a fixed, screw-secured prosthetic appliance

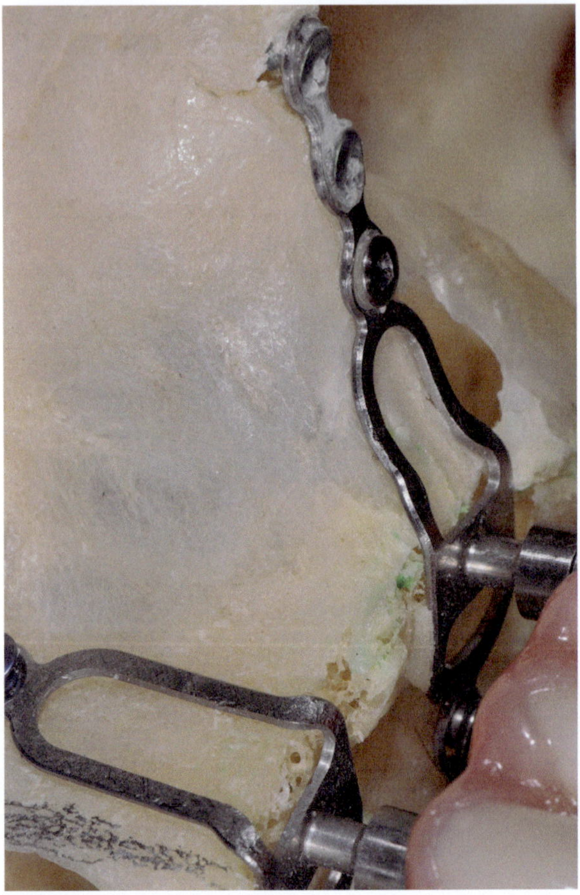

Fig. 8.38 Closeup view of basal implants in close contact with the recipient bone site

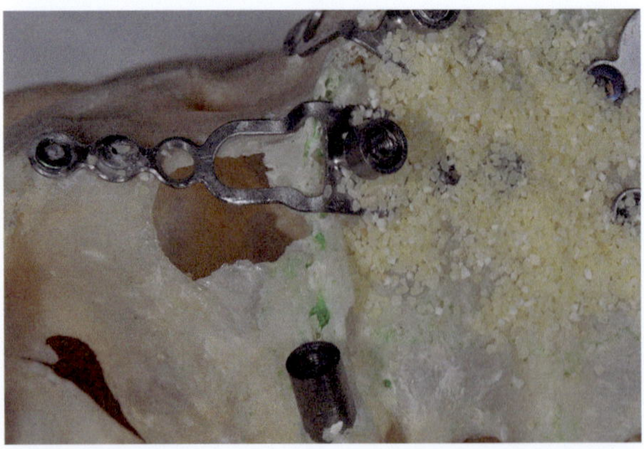

Fig. 8.39 The zygomatic Diskimplant® spans an oro-antral communication

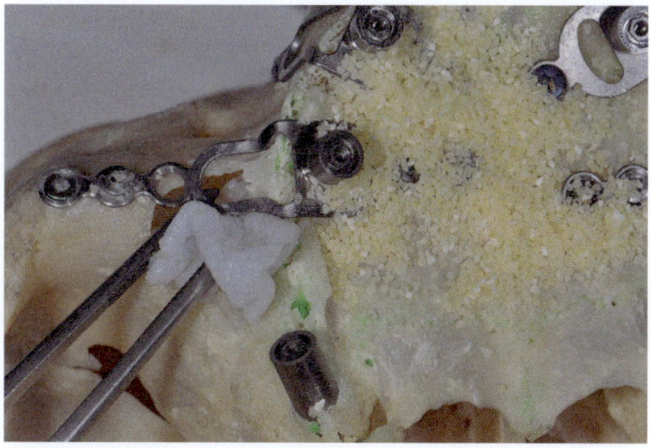

Fig. 8.40 The sinus membrane must be elevated using PRF membranes

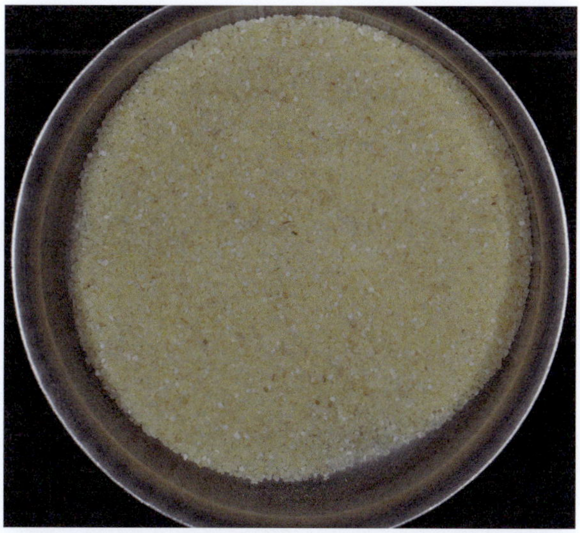

Fig. 8.41 Bone substitute material is used to cover the entire area

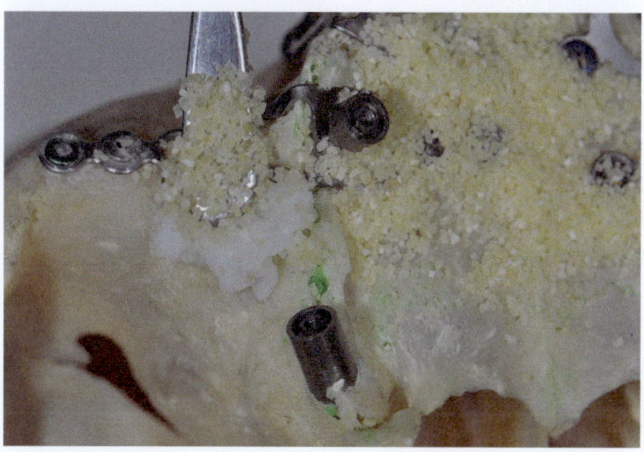

Fig. 8.42 Bone substitute material is placed over the PRF membranes in order to close the lateral opening in the sinus wall

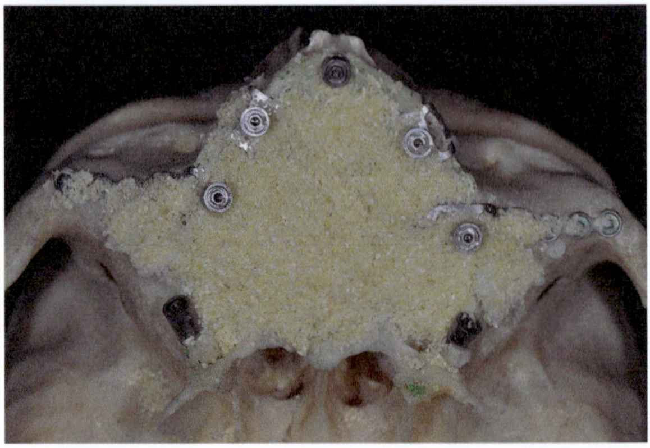

Fig. 8.43 Bone substitute material must cover the entire area; no portion of the basal plate should remain exposed

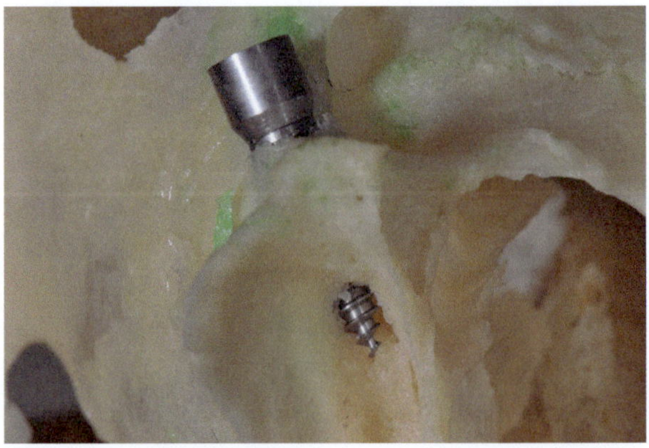

Fig. 8.44 Fratex® implant firmly anchored in the pterygoid bone

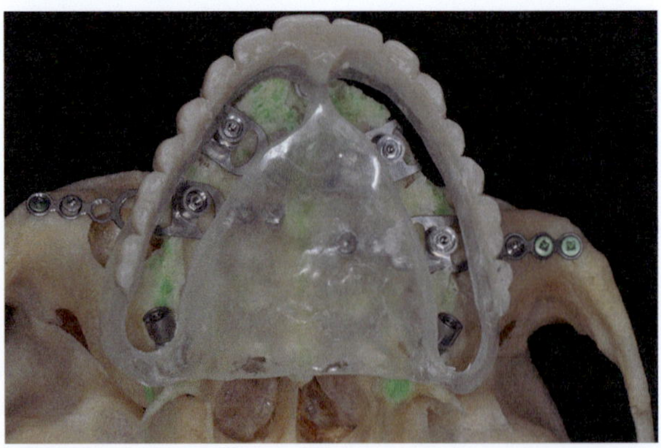

Fig. 8.45 A transparent surgical guide made with the full upper denture can be helpful for basal implant installation

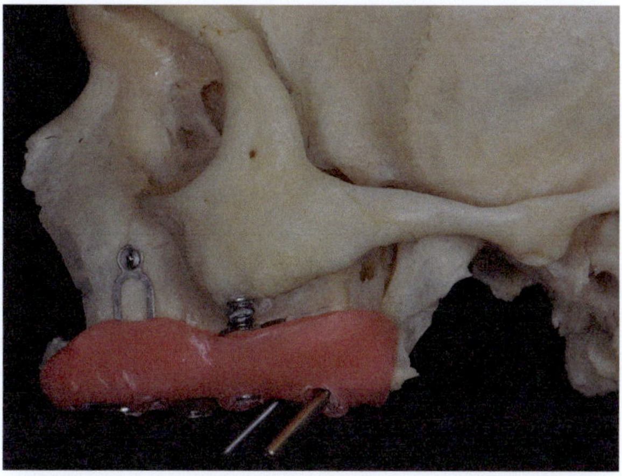

Fig. 8.46 In atrophic jaws, distal anchorage in the major skeletal buttresses is mandatory. A tubero-pterygoid root-form implant can be angled at 45° without problem because its flat emergence profile makes it easy to screw-secure the fixed prosthesis

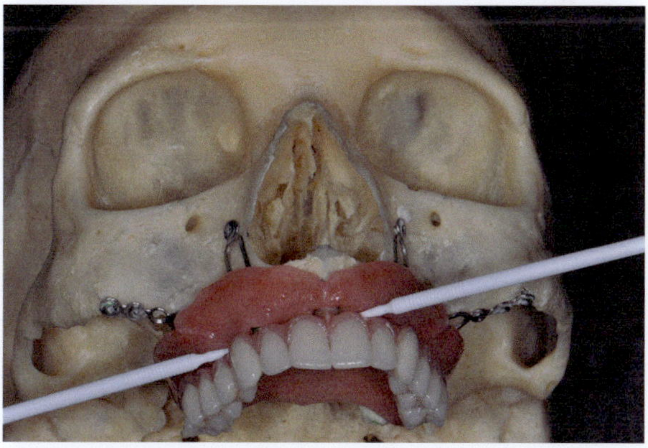

Fig. 8.47 Screw-secured prosthesis in place with space for maintenance and easy cleaning

- Mandible: The recipient bone bed is first flattened with a 7 or 9 mm diameter cutter. Whenever possible, a notch should be prepared in the bone to anchor the plate on the lingual or buccal aspect of the recipient bone site.
- Maxilla: Use a 7 or 9 mm diameter cutter, depending on the dimensions of the basal implant selected. In the zygomatic area, prepare a cut passing completely through the crest or simply flatten the surface for placement directly on the crest. If the sinus is effracted, push the membrane away with PRF membranes and bone substitute material, then install the wide plate-form Diskimplant®. Firmly secure the implant to the zygomatic process and the palatal maxillary bone with 2 to 5 mini orthopedic screws (5 or 6 mm in length, diameter 2 mm).

In the canine pillar area, the plate must always be bent at a 90° angle. A lateral osteotomy is prepared at the crestal level.

8.8 Diskimplant Placement at Bone Level

Implant placement at bone level is recommended when using a submerged approach. When very little bone height is available (as is most often the case in basal implantology), the desired bone level can be obtained artificially by GBR with an autologous bone graft and a biomaterial plus a PRF membrane at the time of basal implant installation. The basal implant provides a "tent" effect for GBR. Any protruding part of the Diskimplant® must be covered over by bone substitute material and soft tissue, then sutured without tension. A scalpel technique or soft brushing can be used to release the periosteum in order to gain soft tissue coverage and permit passive flap closure. Osteogenic activation of the periosteum with bone matrix osseotensors is indicated several weeks before implant installation and GBR in order to increase local blood supply and thereby avoid flap necrosis.

8.9 Indications for Transgingival Abutments

Transgingival Monobloc abutments with a smooth, machined surface are used to manage the peri-implant soft tissue compartment. These 3.5 mm high, cylindrical titanium components (ref. PLM-3.5) raise the emergence of the implant from an intragingival bone level to a paragingival or supragingival position. This facilitates hygiene and eliminates the need to re-intervene on the transmucosal "biological zone." A stable biological link is created between the titanium abutment and the surrounding mucosa (connective tissue and epithelium). Guidelines for the use of transgingival abutments for screw-retained and cement-retained restorations are given in Table 8.1.

The emergence profile of the PLM-3.5 abutment is identical to that of Diskimplants®. This simplifies the prosthetic phase because the same components can be used (impression copings, analogs, etc.). The use of a specially designed driver for abutment installation (ref. PP) allows a "no touch" procedure, just as for implant placement. These cylindrical abutments can be placed:

1. Immediately after implant installation, in order to augment the initial tissue volume at the emergence by creating a "tent effect" when the flap is closed. Release of the periosteum and use of GBR with a biomaterial and PRF are necessary.
2. At reentry, in order to maintain the full-thickness flap and increase the amount of attached vestibular gingiva.

Table 8.1 Guidelines for use of transgingival abutments

Soft tissue thickness	Procedure
<4 mm	Single-tooth restoration directly on the implant. No abutment is required
≥4 mm	Place one cylindrical titanium Monobloc abutment (PLM-3.5, h 3.5 mm) on top of the implant
≥7 mm	Use two cylindrical titanium Monobloc abutments placed one on top of the other

Transgingival Abutment Installation

After placing the PLM-3.5 abutment on the implant using the abutment driver (ref. PP) mounted on a handpiece, tighten it with a mini hollow hex driver (ref. CHMM). A digital or conventional periapical radiograph should be taken perpendicular to the implant, before taking the impression, to make sure that the transgingival abutment is seated correctly. Tighten the abutment to 10–15 Ncm with a manual torque wrench. Depending on gingival thickness, a cover screw or a 3-mm-high healing abutment should be installed to avoid soft tissue closure while the prosthesis is fabricated. In esthetically demanding areas, the abutment should be slightly shorter than the gingival thickness to anticipate tissue retraction. For example, if the gingival thickness at the Diskimplant emergence is 4 mm, place one Monobloc abutment. If the gingival thickness is <4 mm, no abutment is required; the prosthesis can be prepared directly on the implant.

8.10 Immediate Loading of Basal Implants

For over 40 years, endosseous root-form dental implants have been placed routinely using a two-stage procedure, in accordance with Brånemark's original philosophy. Histomorphometric data, however, indicate that much earlier loading is compatible with osseointegration. This can be attributed at least in part to improved implant designs with greater retentiveness that reduce micromotion to such a degree that bone regeneration is possible even with immediate loading. Osseointegration can be obtained with both approaches provided absolute stability is achieved.

Immediate Functional Loading of an Atrophic Edentulous Maxilla Using Basal Implants (Figs. 8.48, 8.49, 8.50, 8.51, 8.52, 8.53, 8.54, 8.55, 8.56, 8.57, 8.58, 8.59, 8.60, 8.61, 8.62, 8.63, 8.64, 8.65, 8.66, and 8.67)

Following IV sedation or local-regional anesthesia, full-thickness buccal and palatal periosteal flaps are elevated to completely expose the edentulous maxillary bone up to the two tubero-pterygoid processes, the nasal floor, and the two zygomas.

The density of the tuberosity is checked manually using a manual osseotensor. Two pterygoid Fractal® implants must be installed first to generate strong reliable and absolutely stable bony anchorage for the immediate loading procedure. These implants (total length 20 or 23 mm, including the Monobloc emergence crestal cylinder) can be screwed into place (self-tapping) or gently "press-fit" (tapped at the end of insertion) for better primary stability (Fig. 8.53). Should a problem occur, an unstable pterygoid implant can be removed and the defect filled in with bone substitute material. The full denture is then put back in place; after a 3- to 6-month waiting period, another attempt can be made to equip the eggshell-thin maxilla. To pursue the surgery without having first ensured strong initial distal bone anchorage in the tubero-pterygoid area would put the patient at risk, which is unacceptable as many patients in this situation have already experienced implant and/or bone graft failures.

After successful placement of the two pterygoid implants (Fig. 8.55), a lateral osteotomy is prepared (1.5 mm bone depth, just under the sinus floor) using a 9 mm diameter cutter (Figs. 8.56 and 8.57). Two plate-form Diskimplants® are then firmly anchored on the zygomatic process and the palate using mini orthopedic screws.

The two plate-form Diskimplants® for installation on the two canine pillars are shaped at an angle of 90°. A 9 mm cutter is used for lateral bucco-palatal osteotomy in order to prepare an endosseous bed at the crest level. The basal canine implant is

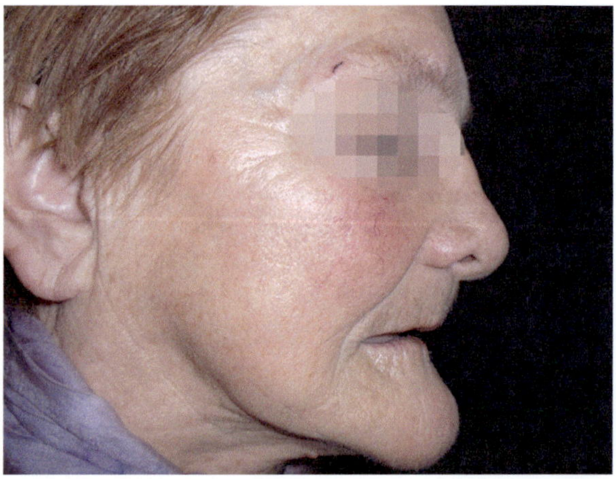

Fig. 8.48 Facial aspect of an elderly patient with atrophic jaws

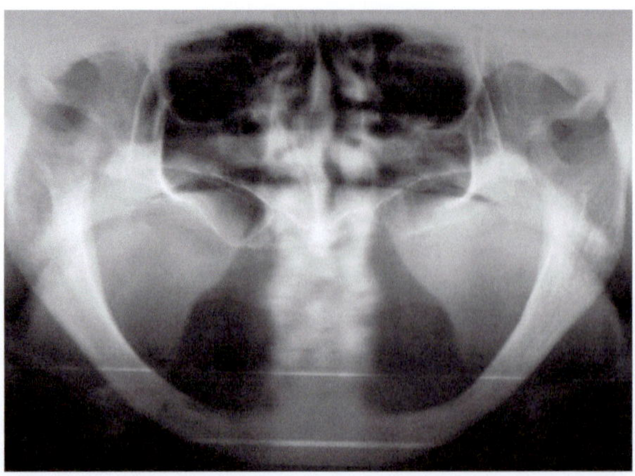

Fig. 8.49 Panoramic view 45 days before implant installation. Osseotensor application was performed under local anesthesia

inserted in such a way that the vertical loop borders the vertical maxillary nasal bone wall. The orthopedic mini screws are then screwed into the palatal bone and the canine bone. Installing the basal implant close to the vertical nasal wall eliminates the risk of injury to the infraorbital nerve (Figs. 8.58 and 8.59).

Intimate contact with the recipient bone bed is completed by gently tapping the plate-form Diskimplants® with a seating instrument (Fig. 8.60). All exposed portions must be entirely covered buccally and palatally with a bone substitute material and PRF.

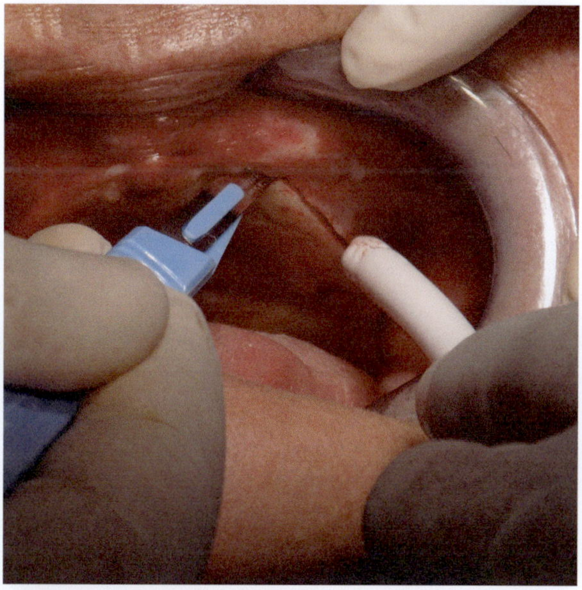

Fig. 8.50 Crestal incision line for full-flap elevation

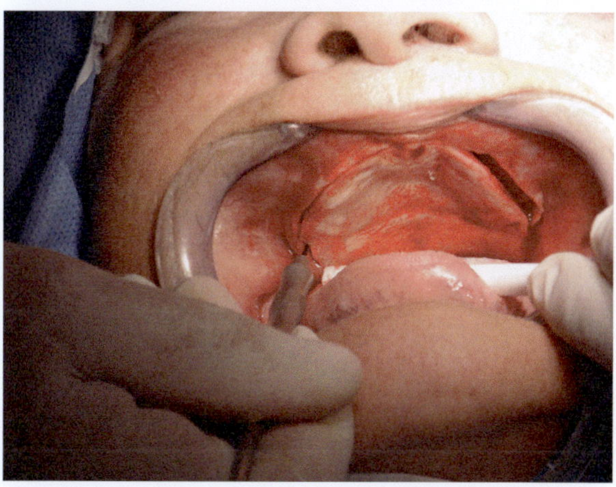

Fig. 8.51 A manual osseotensor is always used to verify the bone density in the tubero-pterygoid area before starting osteotomy with a pterygoid pilot drill

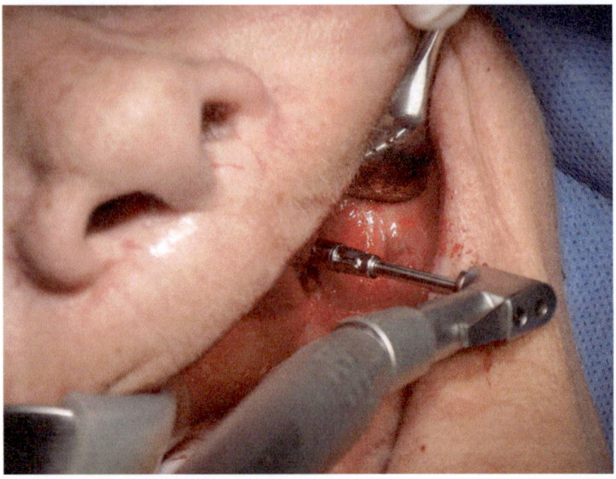

Fig. 8.52 Low-speed placement of a self-tapping tubero-pterygoid Fractal® implant (19 mm in length)

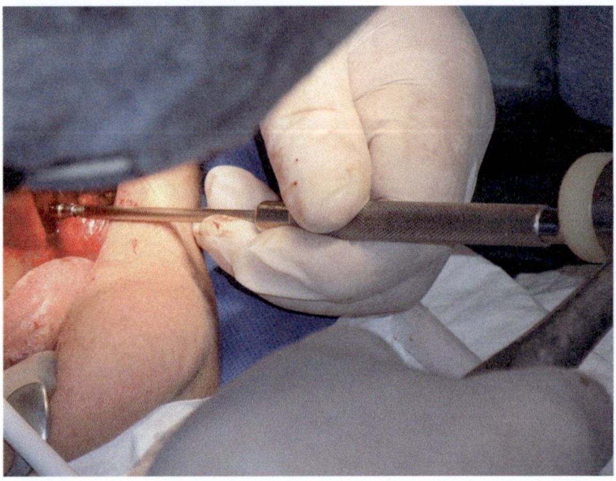

Fig. 8.53 Final seating is achieved by tapping the implant through the pterygoid processes

A high horizontal incision to release the buccal periosteum allows complete closure of the grafted area without tension. This can be improved by using a palatal poncho flap (Figs. 8.61 and 8.62) and 2/0 and 4/0 sutures. An impression is taken and the occlusion is recorded using the existing full denture. This step is performed in the surgical room just after suturing. A highly rigid, screw-secured prosthesis is installed 48 hours post-op (Fig. 8.63). Six months later, the fixed bridge is retrieved and a cone beam CT scan is taken (Fig. 8.64). A frontal view shows the bone-anchored basal implant and the mini orthopedic screws in the zygomatic area

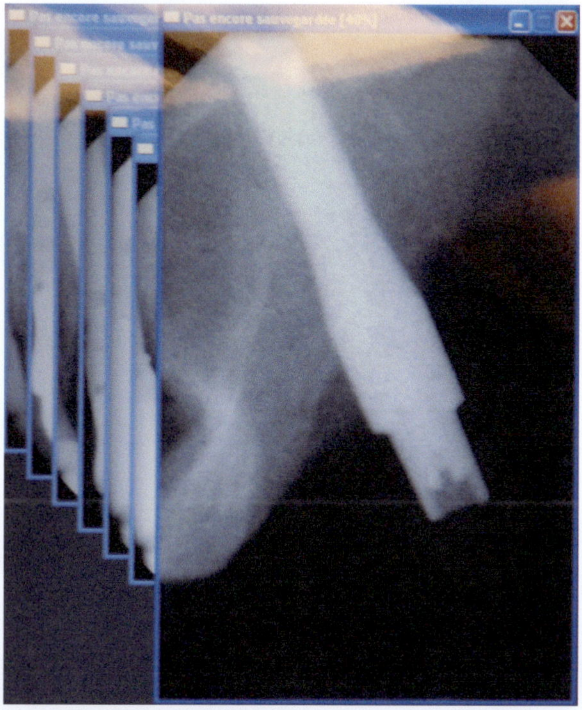

Fig. 8.54 Peroperative digital radiograph for verification of proper implant positioning

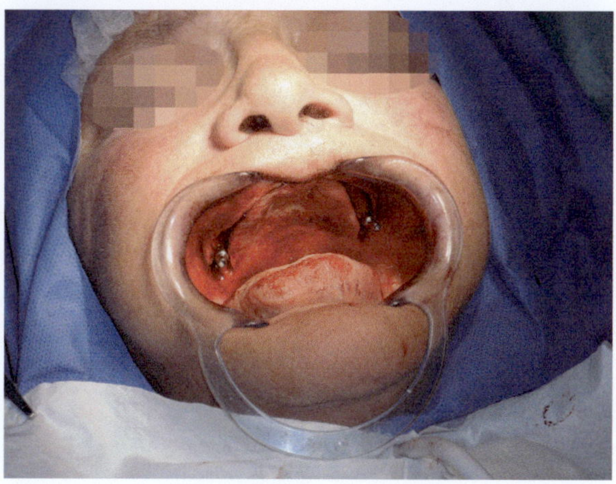

Fig. 8.55 The two pterygoid implants should be installed first. Should a problem occur (improper positioning, absence of initial absolute stability, etc.), it is easy to remove the implant, graft, put back the full denture, and make a new attempt 3 months later

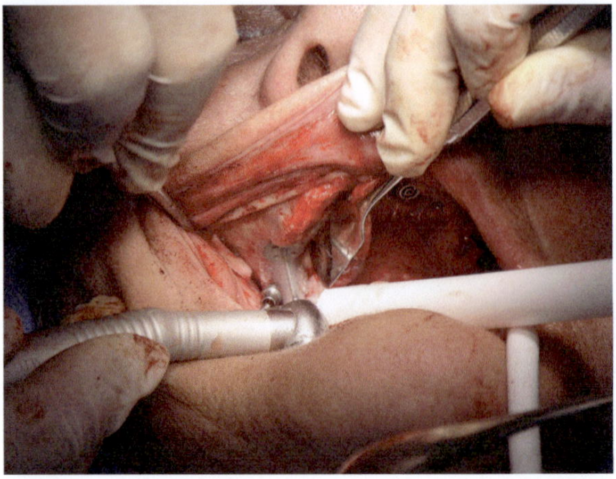

Fig. 8.56 Lateral osteotomy at a bone depth of 1.5 mm, just beneath the sinus floor. If there is a small sinus opening, PRF and bone substitute material should be packed in before placing the zygomatic Diskimplant®

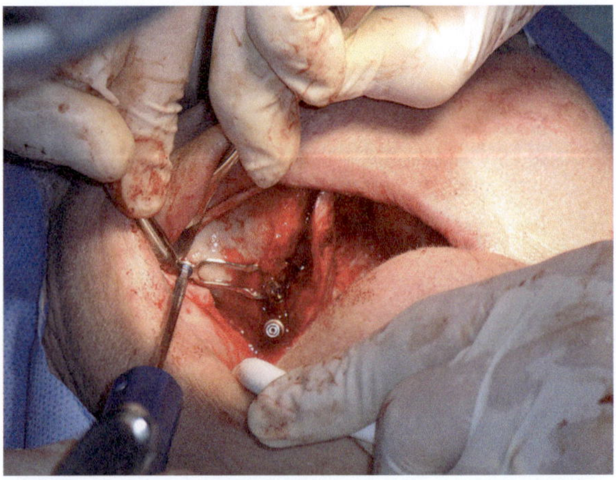

Fig. 8.57 Zygomatic implant in place in the crestal bone cut and firmly screw-secured both to the palate and the zygomatic process

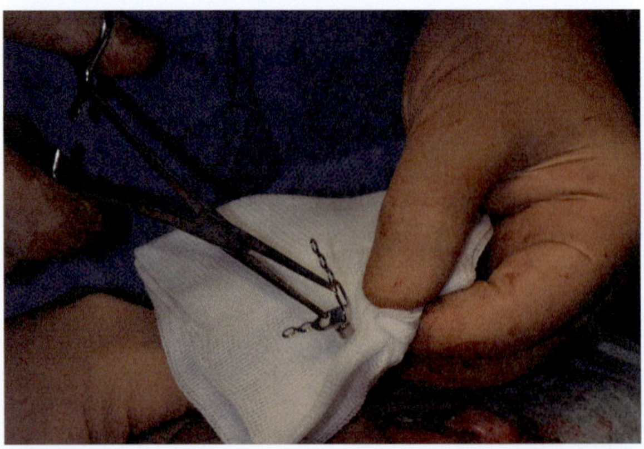

Fig. 8.58 Plate-form Diskimplant® shaped at 90° for installation on the canine pillar

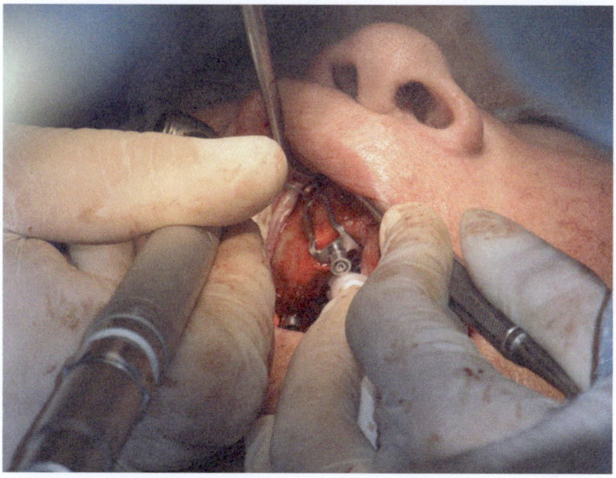

Fig. 8.59 The basal implant is screw-secured to the canine pillar, adjacent to the nasal rim, and to the palatal plate

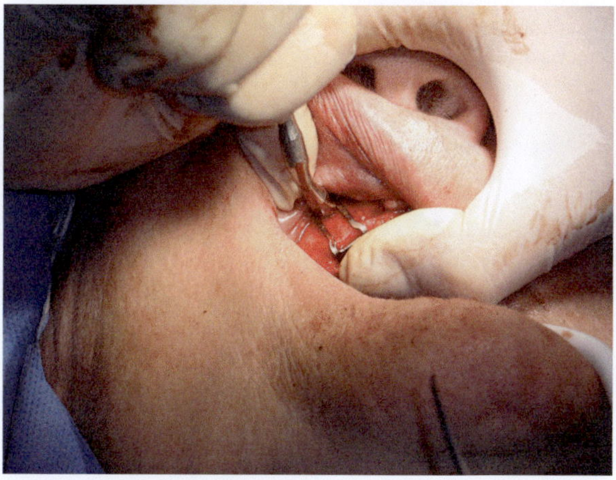

Fig. 8.60 The Diskimplant® is adapted to the anatomy of the canine pillar by tapping it with a round-tipped seating instrument

(Fig. 8.65). All implants are checked individually to make sure they are clinically and radiologically osseointegrated, without pain, micromovement, or inflammation. In this example, both sinuses appear healthy (Fig. 8.66), and the patient was satisfied with the final cosmetic outcome (Fig. 8.67). In highly challenging situations such as patients with a history of implant and bone graft failure, a molar-to-molar transpalatal bar is advisable. This bar can be removed 6 to 9 months later, after osseointegration has been achieved.

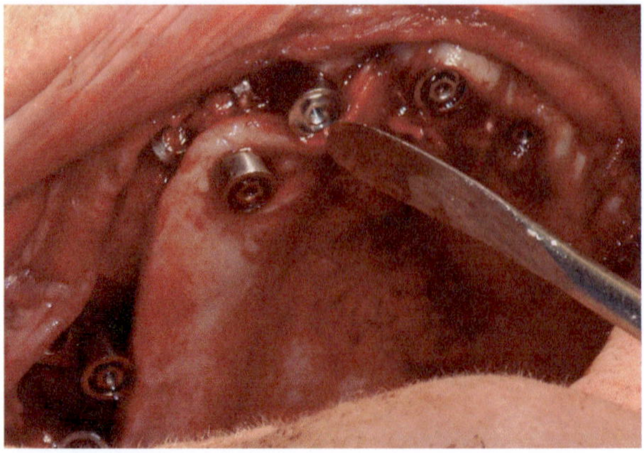

Fig. 8.61 Full-thickness flap repositioned using the "poncho" technique

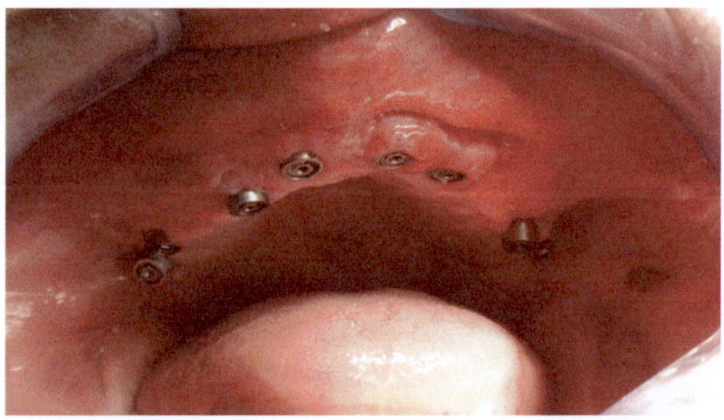

Fig. 8.62 Soft tissue healing one week post-op. The immediate, screw-secured fixed bridge was retrieved for suture removal

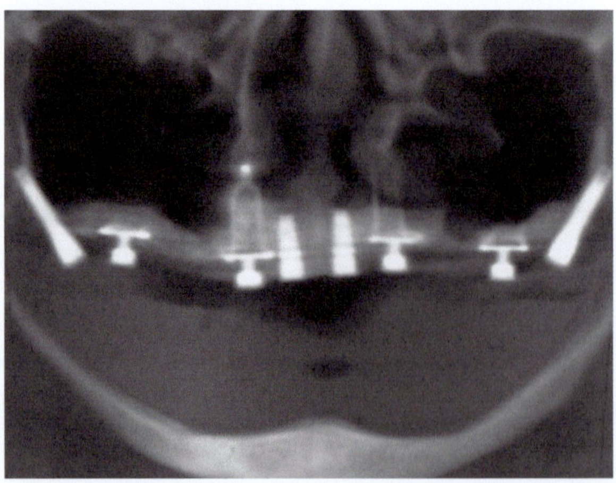

Fig. 8.63 Cone beam CT panoramic view at 6 months. A bone gain is visible compared to the initial status

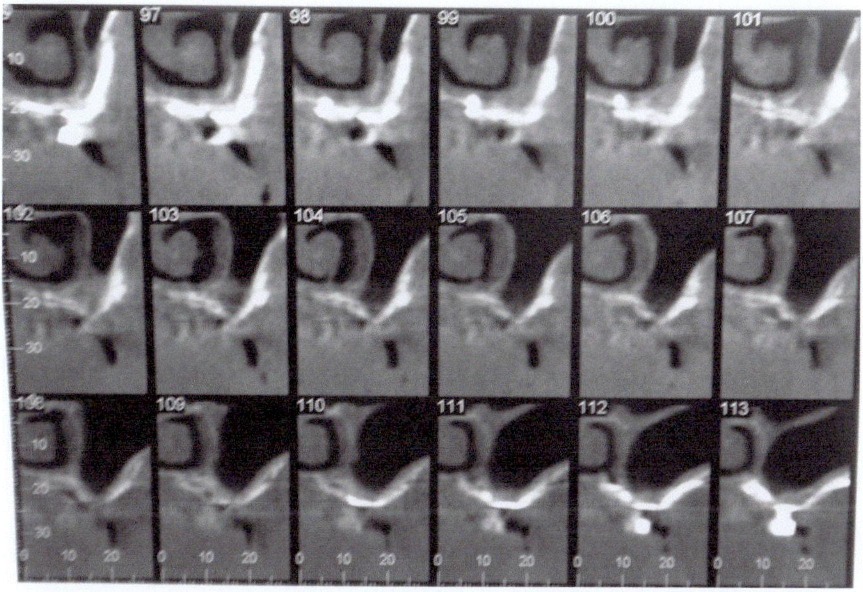

Fig. 8.64 Cone beam CT view of a basal implant screw-secured onto the canine pillar and zygomatic process

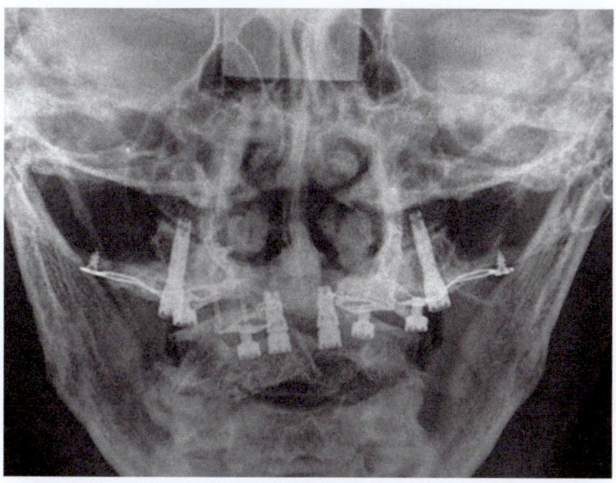

Fig. 8.65 Front view of the full implant rehabilitation of an atrophic maxilla (2-year check-up). The fixed bridge was unscrewed to allow individual assessment of all implants. The zygomatic plate-form implant and the pterygoid root-form implant are clearly visible. Both sinuses are healthy

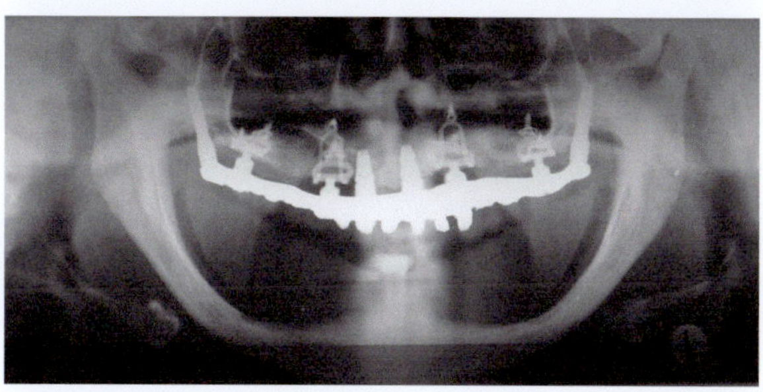

Fig. 8.66 Panoramic view with the fixed bridge in place 2 years post-op

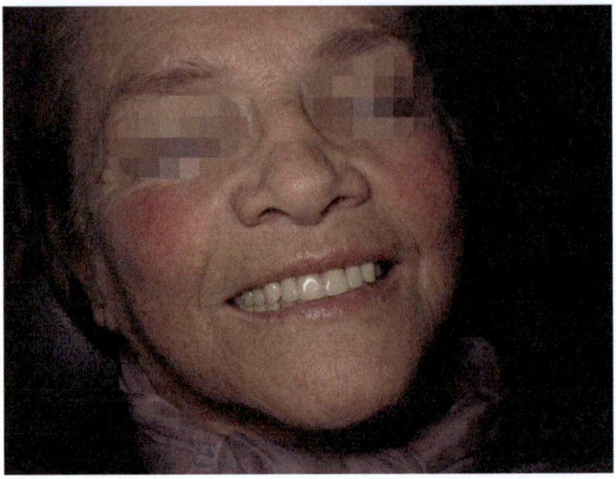

Fig. 8.67 Final cosmetic outcome (same patient as Fig. 8.48)

8.11 Delayed Loading of Basal Implants

A submerged technique, where the basal implant is left covered by the gingiva for healing purposes, is the recommended procedure for single-tooth replacements and rehabilitation of partial edentulism with Diskimplants®. In such situations, GBR is always associated with implant installation in order to protect and increase the initial bone volume. When bone quality can be considered excellent or good, a waiting period of approximately 6 months is necessary for the maxilla and 4 months for the mandible. Longer healing periods (9 months) are required for bone of lesser quality. Implants can be lost with the submerged approach because of the iatrogenic effect of the removable appliance worn during the healing phase. Insufficient space between the implanted area and the opposite dental arch can also become a problem, even if the patient does not wear a provisional denture. If local conditions allow use of a fixed appliance on the remaining natural teeth during temporization, this is the preferred option. A free inter-arch space of at least 4 mm is mandatory. When less space is available, the patient may accidentally chew on the sector and subsequently open the incision line, expose the bone, contaminate the GBR, and ultimately mobilize the Diskimplant®.

8.12 Postoperative Instructions for Patients

A control visit is usually scheduled the day after surgery. The following recommendations should be followed after implant placement to ensure adequate healing.

1. Place ice packs over the surgical area (20-minute applications), starting right after the operation and continue for 24 hours.
2. *Do not* rinse your mouth or brush the surgical site during the first 48 hours after the operation.

3. Starting 48 hours after surgery, gently rinse your mouth with a single-dose saline solution after each soft meal. Begin gentle gingival cleaning with Dakin Cooper solution on a cotton swab (toothbrushes and interdental tips are forbidden). *Do not* use the Dakin Cooper solution as a rinse or mouthwash.
4. If nasal bleeding occurs, *do not* blow your nose vigorously. Block the bleeding nostrils with packed cotton.
5. If bleeding begins in the surgical area, apply gentle pressure to the area by biting on a roll of gauze for 20 minutes. If the bleeding does not stop, please contact Dr. ….
6. Use an elevated headrest or an extra pillow for the first two nights after the operation.
7. Stay on a liquid and soft diet for the first 3 weeks after the operation. *Do not* smoke or consume alcoholic beverages during the first week.
8. *Do not* practice any violent physical activity until complete relief of postoperative symptoms. In particular, avoid diving or swimming under water.
9. *Do not* wear your removable denture until it has been relined (this applies only to delayed loading protocols).
10. Carefully follow the directions for any prescribed medications.
11. If you have any questions or any problems arise concerning your operation, please contact Dr. ….

Conflict of interest statement Gérard M. Scortecci is the inventor of the Diskimplant and holder of several associated patents that are exploited by the Victory company. He is an unpaid consultant to this firm and a minority shareholder in the company. No money was received from any of the companies mentioned in the book or from any of the companies whose products are mentioned.

Recommended Reading

1. Aaboe M, Schou S, Hjørting-Hansen E, Helbo M, Vikjaer D. Osseointegration of subperiosteal implants using bovine bone substitute and various membranes. Clin Oral Implant Res. 2000;11(1):51–8.
2. Adell R. Clinical results of osseointegrated implants supporting fixed prostheses in edentulous jaws. J Prosthet Dent. 1983;50:251.
3. Adell R, Lekholm U, Rockler B, Branemark PI. A 15-year study of osseointegrated implants in the treatment of the edentulous jaw. Int J Oral Surg. 1981;10:387–416.
4. Albrektsson T. Direct bone anchorage of dental implants. J Prosthet Dent. 1983;50:255.
5. Allen WL, Evans HR. Subperiosteal and mandibular bone plate implants: a comparison and presentation of criteria used. Implantologist. 1984;3:19.
6. Ansel A, Galmiche F, Menetray D, Stenger A. Quand l'implantologie devient un élément essentiel de l'arsénal therapeutique à disposition de l'omnipraticien pour réussir ses cas complexes dans le but de recouvrer l'esthétique tant revendiquée par nos patients. Implant Dent. 2013:5–17.
7. Ansel A, Menetray D, Cotten P, Stenger A. Atrophies maxillaires et technique Diskimplant. Implantologie basale: «mode d'emploi». Implantologie. 2010:19–33.
8. Bessade J, Scortecci G. L'implantologie basale: La troisième voie. Implantologie Les 10 points clés novembre. 2005.
9. Branemark PI, Zarb GA, Albrektsson T. Tissue-integrated prostheses: Osseointegration in clinical dentistry. Chicago: Quintessence; 1985.

10. Cotten P, Carmona D. Mandibule et maxillaire à forte résorption osseuse. Extractions, implantations totales, mise en charge immédiate. Technique Diskimplant: Implantologie. février; 2007. p. 7–27.
11. Donsimoni JM, Dohan D. Les implants maxillo-faciaux à plateaux d'assise. Concepts et technologies orthopédiques, réhabilitations maxillo-mandibulaires, reconstructions maxillo-faciales, réhabilitations dentaires partielles, techniques de réintervention, méta-analyse. 1ère partie: concepts et technologies orthopédiques. Implantodontie. 2004;13(1):13–30.
12. Donsimoni JM, Bermot P, Dohan D. Les implants maxillo-faciaux à plateaux d'assise. Concepts et technologies orthopédiques, réhabilitations maxillo-mandibulaires, reconstructions maxillo-faciales, réhabilitations dentaires partielles, techniques de réintervention, méta-analyse. 2ème partie: rehabilitations maxillo-mandibulaires. Implantodontie. 2004;13(1):31–41.
13. Donsimoni JM, Dohan A, Bermot P, Dohan S, Scortecci G, Dohan D. Implantologie basale: concepts, techniques et applications cliniques. EMC. 2005:1–39.
14. Donsimoni JM, Dohan A, Gabrieleff D, Dohan D. Les implants maxillo-faciaux à plateaux d'assise: 3ème partie: reconstructions maxillo-faciales; Les implants maxillo-faciaux à plateaux d'assise: concepts et technologies orthopédiques, réhabilitations maxillo-mandibulaires, reconstructions maxillo-faciales, réhabilitations dentaires partielles, techniques de réintervention, méta-analyse. Implantodontie. 2004;13(2):71–86.
15. Donsimoni JM, Gabrieleff D, Bermot P, Dohan D. Les implants maxillo-faciaux à plateaux d'assise; Concepts et technologies orthopédiques, réhabilitations maxillo-mandibulaires, reconstructions maxillo-faciales, réhabilitation dentaires partielles, techniques de réintervention, méta-analyse. 4ème partie: réhabilitations dentaires partielles. Implantodontie. 2004;13(2):139–50.
16. Donsimoni JM, Gabrieleff D, Bermot P, Dohan D. Les implants maxillo-faciaux à plateaux d'assise; Concepts et technologies orthopédiques, réhabilitations maxillo-mandibulaires, reconstructions maxillo-faciales, réhabilitations dentaires partielles, techniques de réintervention, méta-analyse. 5éme partie: techniques de réintervention. Implantodontie. 2004;13(2):207–16.
17. Donsimoni JM, Gabrieleff D, Bermot P, Dohan D. Les implants maxillo-faciaux à plateaux d'assise; Concepts et technologies orthopédiques, réhabilitations maxillo-mandibulaires, reconstructions maxillo-faciales, réhabilitations dentaires partielles, techniques de réintervention, méta-analyse. 6ème partie: une méta-analyse. Implantodontie. 2004;13(2):217–28.
18. Dougnac-Galant D. Apport de l'implantologie basale dans les reconstructions implantaires fixes: une alternative aux greffes osseuses ? Implantologie. 2007;février:55–61.
19. Ham JW, Patterson SS, Healey HJ. An evaluation of handpiece sterilization for periapical surgery. J Oral Surg. 1970;28:35.
20. Juillet JM. Three-dimensional implants – development and evaluation. Oral Implantol. 1974;4:527.
21. Marcelat R. Intérêt des implants pterygoïdiens dans la stratégie d'évitement des sinus maxillaires. Implant Dent. 2014;(février):53–60.
22. Monin JC, Monin A. De la mastication en prothèse implanto-portée. Implant Dent. 2009;(novembre):71–6.
23. Odin G, Balaguer T, Savoldelli C, Scortecci G. Immediate functional loading of an implant-supported fixed prosthesis at the time of ablative surgery and mandibular reconstruction for squamous cell carcinoma. JOI. 2010;XXXVI(3):225–30.
24. Odin G, Misch CE, Binderman I, Scortecci G. Fixed rehabilitation of severely atrophic jaws using immediately loaded basal disk implants after in situ bone activation. JOI. 2012;XXXVIII(5):611–6.
25. Odin G, Petitbois R, Cotten P, Philip P. Distraction osteogenesis using bone matrix osteotensors in ectodermal dysplasia: a case report. Implant Dent. 2015;24:612–9.
26. Odin G, Petitbois R, Scortecci G. Soulevé de sinus et ostéotenseur: le Fractal Lift. Lettre de la Stomatologie. 2009;44(novembre):4–11.
27. Odin G, Scortecci G, Levratto F, Morin L. Techniques avancées en implantologie basale chirurgico-prothétique. Stratégie Prothétique. 2011;11(3):1–10.

28. Odin G, Sevalle M, Scortecci G. La révolution ostéogénique. Chirurgien-Dentiste de France. 2009;1398(2009):49–52.
29. Petitbois R. L'implant à plaque: une révolution en implantologie basale. Alpha Omega News. 2008;120(octobre):11–2.
30. Petitbois R. Réhabilitation et implantologie basale à la suite d'un échec chez une patiente présentant une atrophie sévère des maxillaires. Information Dentaire. 2017;24(14 juin 2017):16–22.
31. Petitbois R, Arrius-Oppo JM. Intérêt de l'implant Fratex en présence de crêtes fines. Implantologie. 2011;(mai):53–9.
32. Petitbois R, Arrius-Oppo JM. Soulevé de sinus et ostéotenseur: le Fractal Lift. Taux de succès sur une période de 2 à 6 ans. Implantologie. 2014;(novembre):25–33.
33. Petitbois R, Monsarrat P, Papeleux C. Implant Fractal. Taux de succès sur une période de 1 à 3 ans. Implantologie (février); 2010. p. 5–10.
34. Scortecci G. Immediate function of cortically anchored disk-design implants without bone augmentation in moderately to severely resorbed completely edentulous maxillae. J Oral Implantol. 1999;25(2):70–9.
35. Scortecci G, Misch CE, Benner KU. Implants and restorative dentistry. London: Martin Dunitz; 2001.
36. Scortecci G, Misch C, Binderman I, Philip P. Intérêt des ostéotenseurs matriciels en implantologie. De l'observation clinique à l'innovation thérapeutique. Implantologie février. 2009:5–17.
37. Scortecci G, Morin L. Implantologie basale et nouvelles technologies. Lettre de la Stomatologie. 2014;61(mars):22–4.
38. Scortecci G, Odin G. Diskimplant à plaque basale ostéosynthésée. Surmonter les situations complexes. 2008;120(octobre):18–20.

Prosthodontics 9

Gérard M. Scortecci, Laurent Morin,
Isabelle Morin, and Fabio Levratto

9.1 Laboratory Techniques and Implant-Supported Restorations [1–11]

The laboratory steps that require special equipment and experience are usually delegated to a commercial dental laboratory familiar with basal implant prosthodontic procedures. The dentist should clearly define his expectations and inform the technicians of the specific prosthetic components and materials required.

Regardless of whether the laboratory procedures are performed in the dental office or in a commercial dental laboratory, the dentist must supply high-quality clinical work and explicit written and oral instructions. Inadequate impressions, misfit of transfer impression copings and machined analogs, unrealistic implant-supported constructions due to poor implant positioning, casts, and jaw relation records should be returned to the dentist with an explanation of why they are unacceptable. If instructions are not clear or are insufficient, clarification should be obtained from the dentist before proceeding. The specific components and materials requested by the dentist must be used, even if they are not "customary" laboratory

G. M. Scortecci (✉)
University of Nice-Sophia Antipolis Medical School, Nice, France

New York University, New York, NY, USA

University of Southern California, Los Angeles, CA, USA

Private Practice, Nice, France
e-mail: scortecci@wanadoo.fr

L. Morin · I. Morin
Laboratoire Arcade, Nice, France
e-mail: contact@arcade-laboratoire.com

F. Levratto
Laboratoire Levratto, Monaco, Principality of Monaco
e-mail: levrattocolori@monaco.mc

© Springer Nature Switzerland AG 2019

G. M. Scortecci (ed.), *Basal Implantology*, https://doi.org/10.1007/978-3-319-44873-2_9

procedures. The dentist has complete responsibility for the patient's treatment and must carefully check the quality of all laboratory work. Unacceptable work must be returned to the laboratory with a detailed description of all deficiencies. This allows the laboratory technician to progress on his own learning curve with basal implant-supported prosthodontics. Transfer of information over the Internet between the dental office and the dental laboratory greatly facilitates the prosthetic phase.

9.2 Flat Emergence Connection (Fig. 9.1)

All Diskimplants®, Monobloc Fractal® implants, and the Monobloc transgingival abutment feature the same flat emergence profile (Monobloc concept) patented by the author in 2000. A combination of three elements, a flat joint and an external hexagon protected by a cylindroconical seal (Morse cone), this emergence ensures a passive fit even in an angulated and/or divergent position.

Prosthetic options for Monobloc implants include:

- Prolongation with a Monobloc transgingival abutment in case of gingival thickness over 3.5 mm
- Direct screw retention of the prosthetic element to the implant
- Hex abutment posts for cement-retained prostheses
- Ball attachments
- Locator®/Equator® option
- Telescope
- Castable plastic copings for single-tooth replacements and multiunit bridges.

When a Diskimplant® is installed in a sector with thick gingiva (>3.5 mm), addition of a Monobloc transgingival abutment (height 3.5 mm) at the moment of surgery may be helpful for bone height augmentation and soft tissue management. This abutment can be removed ulteriorly should gingival retraction occur. The fit between the abutment and the Diskimplant® must be checked immediately after the abutment has been seated. Even a small gap means that the impression will be inaccurate, the prosthesis will not seat properly, and the forces from the superstructure will not be optimally transferred to the implant. This may lead to screw loosening or fracture of the abutment screw or the implant body itself.

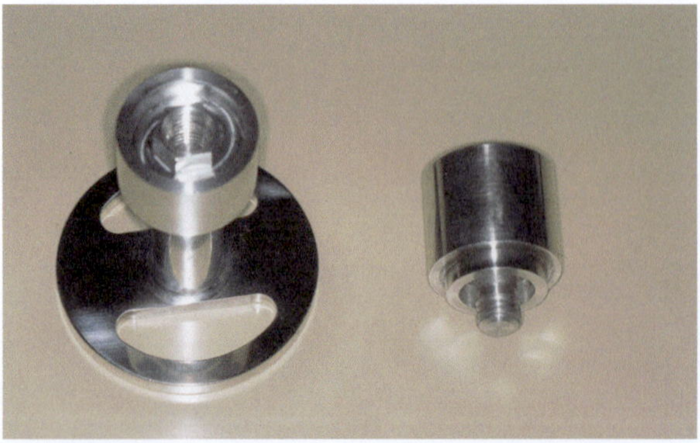

Fig. 9.1 Diskimplant® with a Monobloc flat emergence profile and a transgingival Monobloc abutment (same profile)

Small misfits can best be detected using periapical or intraoral digital radiographs that provide high geometric resolution at a low radiation dose. The X-ray beam is directed at a right angle to the longitudinal axis of the implant. The incident beam must be parallel to the upper surface of the implant and the opposing surface of the abutment: even small deviations can prevent visualization of a clinically significant gap. Panoramic images are recommended for abutment verification when intraoral radiographs are difficult to obtain (patients with edentulous atrophic jaws) or when anatomic conditions render intraoral films insufficient; they are particularly helpful for assessment of extensive rehabilitations and full-arch restorations.

9.3 Impression Techniques (Figs. 9.2, 9.3 and 9.4)

Diskimplants® use the same prosthetic components as Monobloc Fractal® root-form implants that have the same flat emergence profile. Conversion abutments with the Monobloc emergence profile also exist for root-form bone-level Fractal® implants with an internal octagon emergence. This considerably reduces the number of components required, thereby simplifying procedures when basal implants and root-form implants are combined.

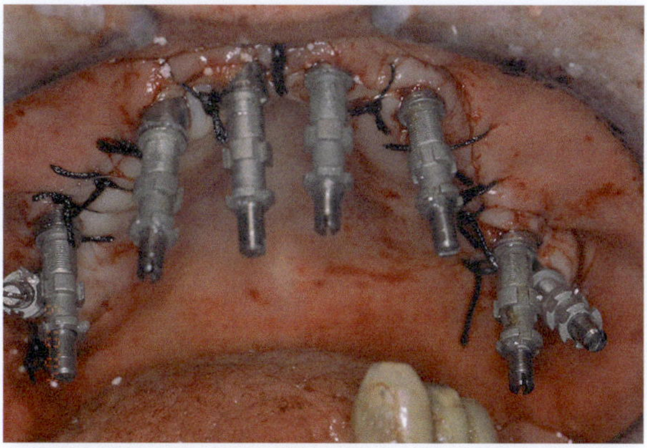

Fig. 9.2 Impression copings in place. Even though the pterygoid implant is angled 45°, the flat emergence profile makes it easy to take the impression

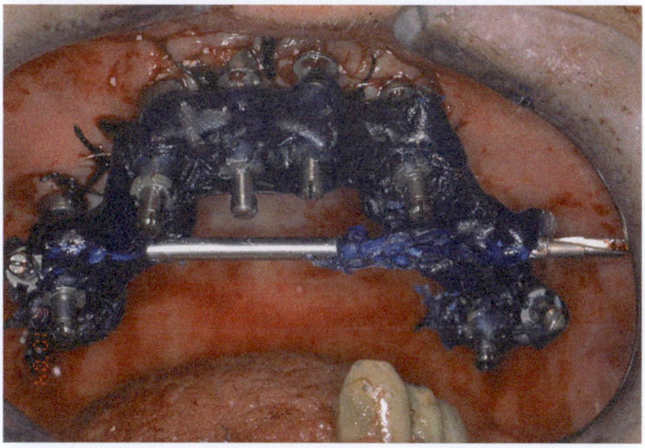

Fig. 9.3 Impression copings connected with Luxabite®. A transpalatal bar is used to prevent distorsion of the impression

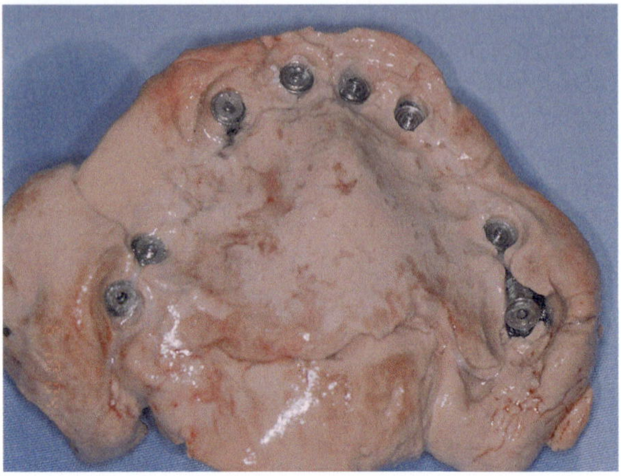

Fig. 9.4 Impression taken with heavy silicone, no tray required

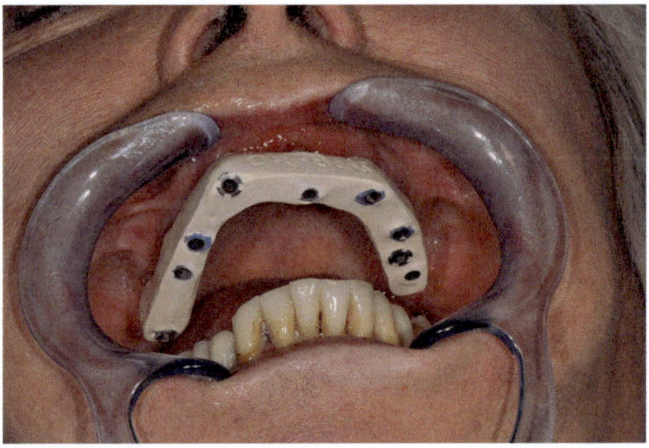

Fig. 9.5 A plaster impression is used to validate absolute passive fit

Except in certain clinical situations such as a reduced buccal opening, an open impression tray and pick-up-type titanium impression copings are recommended.

- For partial restorations (bridges), pick-up-type titanium impression copings (for abutments or implants) connected together with Luxabite® resin are used with an appropriate open impression tray. The same cylindrical analog is used for transgingival Monobloc abutments, Diskimplants®, and Monobloc Fractal® implants.
- For completely edentulous patients, a pick-up impression can be taken without an impression tray. All of the titanium impression copings must be firmly connected together with Luxabite®. The procedure for the mandible is similar. For the maxilla, a transpalatal bar from molar to molar is necessary to avoid distorsion.
- Use of a plaster rim to check accuracy is highly recommended (Fig. 9.5).

9.4 Transfer of Interarch Relationships and Recording of Occlusion (Figs. 9.6, 9.7 and 9.8)

There are three major clinical situations:

1. Fully edentulous patients
   This is a critical step in prosthetic rehabilitation for long-term implant success. After the impression is taken, a first interarch relationship is recorded using a direct hard silicone bite or the existing full denture relined with silicone. This allows the dental technician to prepare a rigid, screwed-to-implant occlusal resin rim with six anterior commercial teeth and a posterior wax block in order to recheck the occlusion.

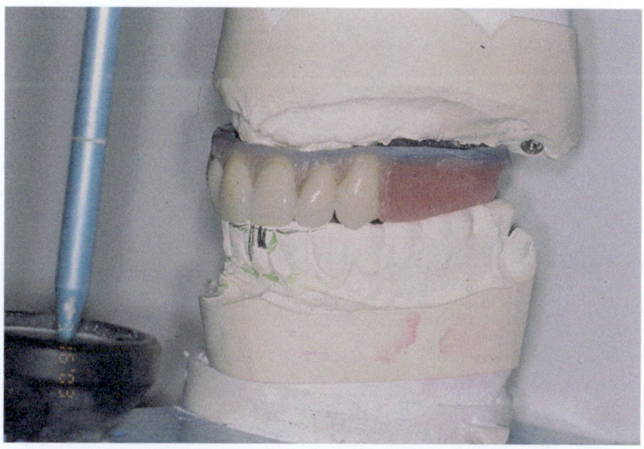

Fig. 9.6 Screw-secured, acrylic/titanium occlusal rim with six commercial front teeth for evaluation of occlusion and cosmetics

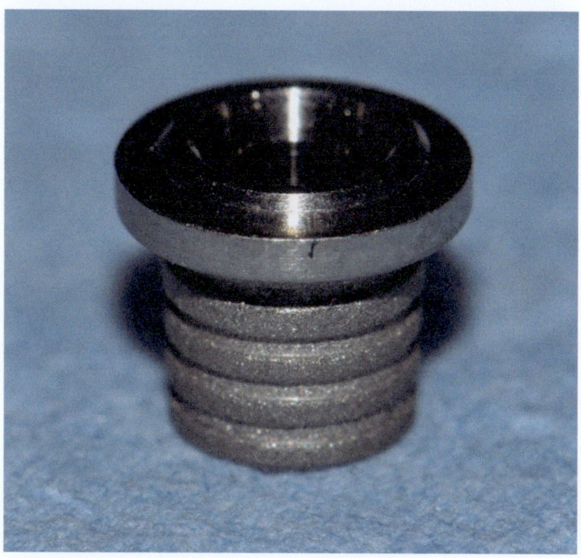

Fig. 9.7 Titanium flat emergence bonding cylinder to be glued into the framework of the fixed prosthesis

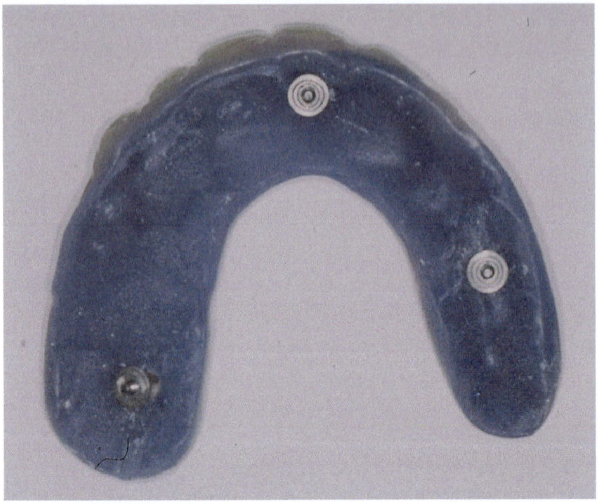

Fig. 9.8 Internal view of the screw-secured bite appliance

2. Partially edentulous patients; this group can be subdivided into two categories:
   - Patients who still have some reliable natural teeth in occlusion. A silicone bite, Luxabite®, or Beauty Pink® hard wax can be used to give a reliable interarch relationship to the dental lab.
   - Patients without any opposing natural teeth in occlusion. In this case, a screw-secured occlusion rim must be made by the dental lab to record the interarch relation.
3. When a patient already has a screw-secured-to-implant transitional prosthesis, this appliance can serve as a transfer using the pick-up impression technique.

9.5 Fabrication of Transitional and Final Prostheses (Figs. 9.9, 9.10, 9.11, 9.12, 9.13, 9.14, 9.15 and 9.16)

Screw-Secured Fixed Restorations (Figs. 9.17, 9.18, 9.19, 9.20, 9.21, 9.22, 9.23, 9.24, 9.25, 9.26, 9.27, 9.28, 9.29, 9.30, 9.31, 9.32, 9.33, 9.34, 9.35, 9.36, 9.37, 9.38, 9.39, 9.40, 9.41, 9.42, 9.43, 9.44, 9.45, 9.46, 9.47, 9.48, 9.49, 9.50 and 9.51)

- Pick-up impression taken with titanium impression copings. For delayed loading procedures, the impression and occlusion are taken 4–6 months after implant placement. For the immediate loading protocol, the impression is taken immediately after surgery, and a transitional, fixed screw-secured titanium/resin restoration is installed 24–72 h post-op.
- Occlusion, phonation, and esthetics are then checked.
- 6 months later, a new pick-up impression is taken with the transitional prosthesis or new impression copings. The wax-up and mock-up are checked and the final prosthetic restoration is then completed. If full zirconia is selected (Zirkonzahn),

machined titanium bonding cylinders are glued into the full zirconia prosthesis and screw-secured directly to the implant(s) or to the transgingival abutments.
- Follow-up and maintenance: 1 month, 3 months, and 6 months after restorative treatment (and yearly thereafter).

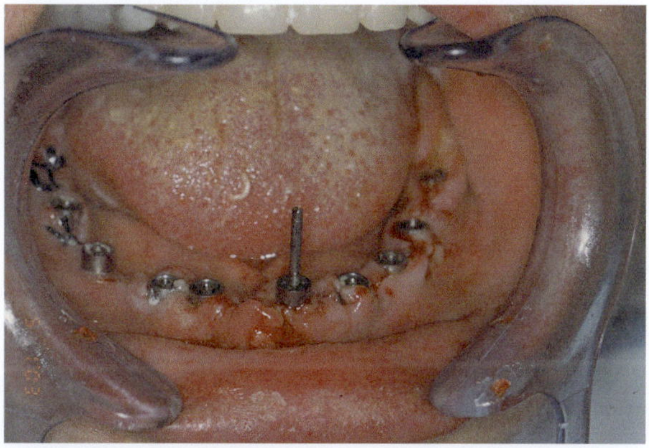

Fig. 9.9 A positioning screw allows easy placement of the bridge to be screw-secured on the flat emergence profiles

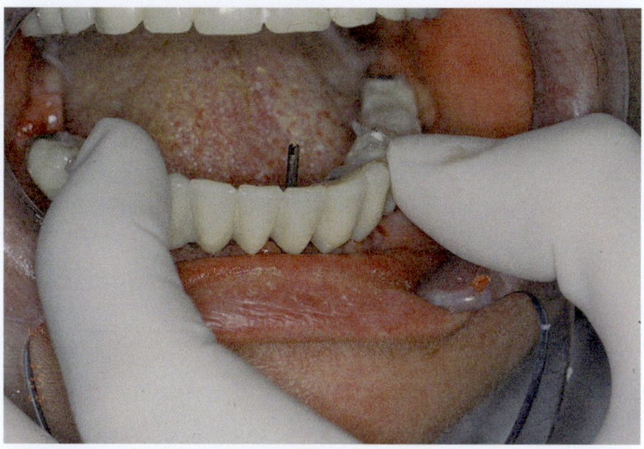

Fig. 9.10 Placement of the lower fixed-to-implant prosthesis. The positioning screw holds the bridge in place during the screwing procedure

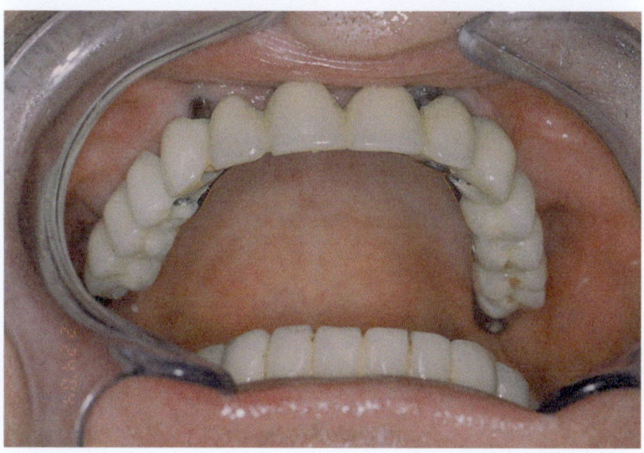

Fig. 9.11 Cobalt-chromium frames with resin teeth: screw-retained full maxillo-mandibular restoration. Immediate functional loading protocol

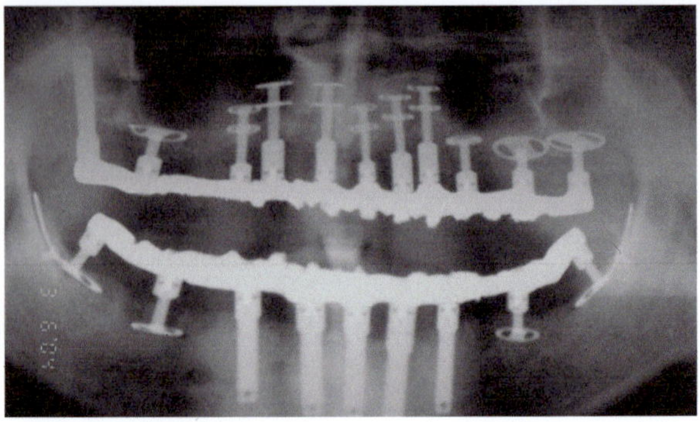

Fig. 9.12 Panoramic view at 1 year

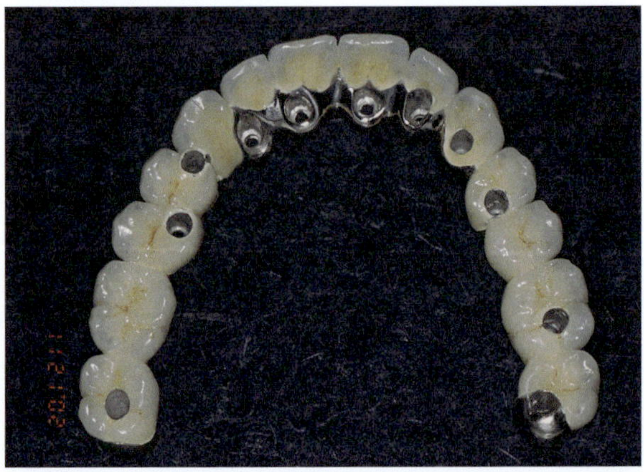

Fig. 9.13 After 1 year of function with the transitional bridge, the final ceramic-baked-to-metal bridge was made

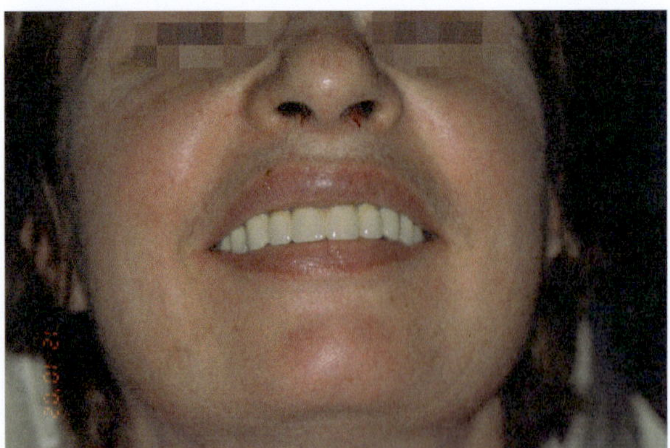

Fig. 9.14 The transitional bridge was used to transfer information

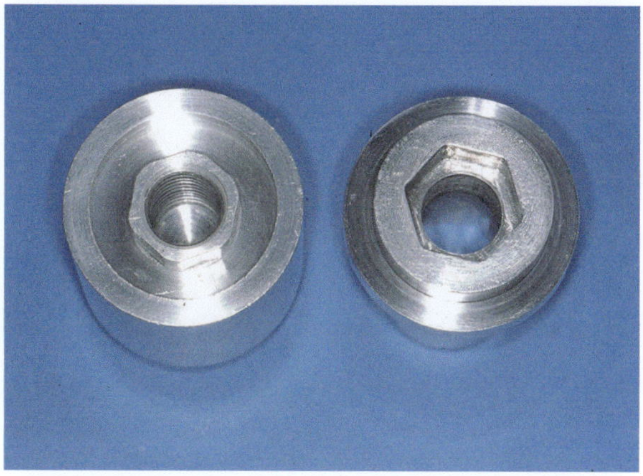

Fig. 9.15 Occlusal view of the flat emergence Monobloc analog and the corresponding abutment for a single tooth

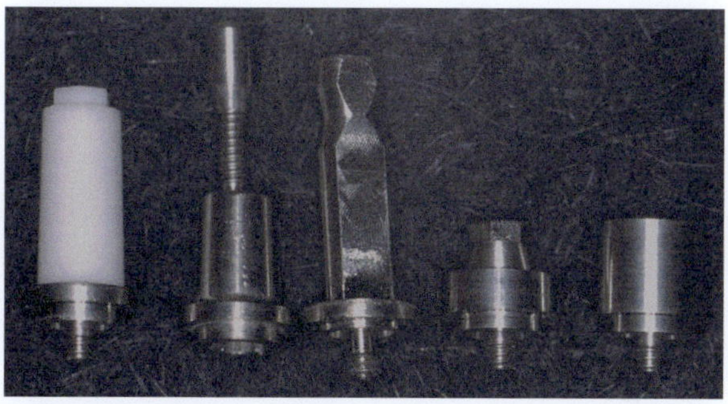

Fig. 9.16 Various options are available for the flat emergence profile

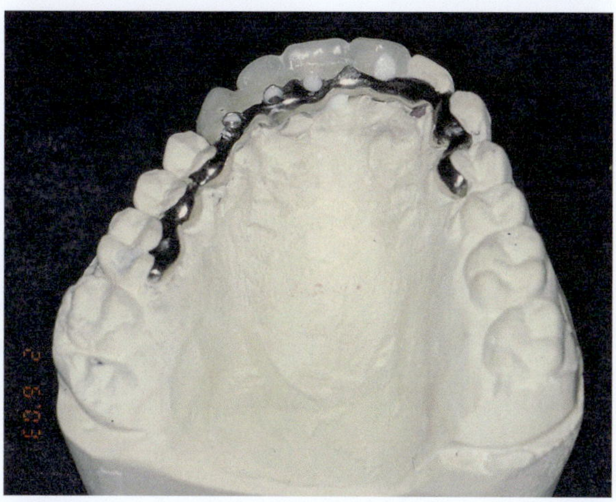

Fig. 9.17 Anterior Maryland bridge screw-secured to four implants (immediate functional loading)

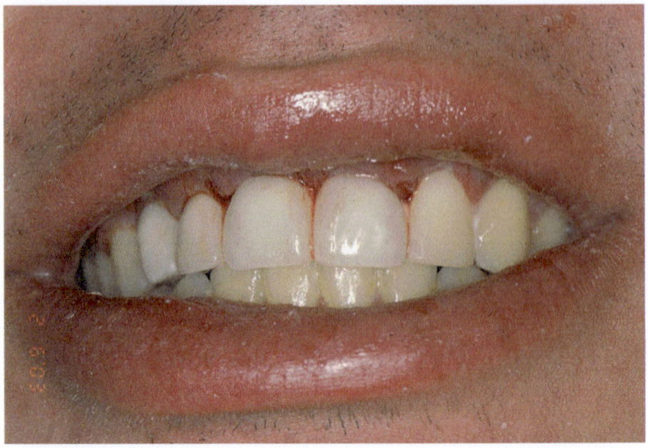

Fig. 9.18 Cosmetic aspect 48 hour post-op

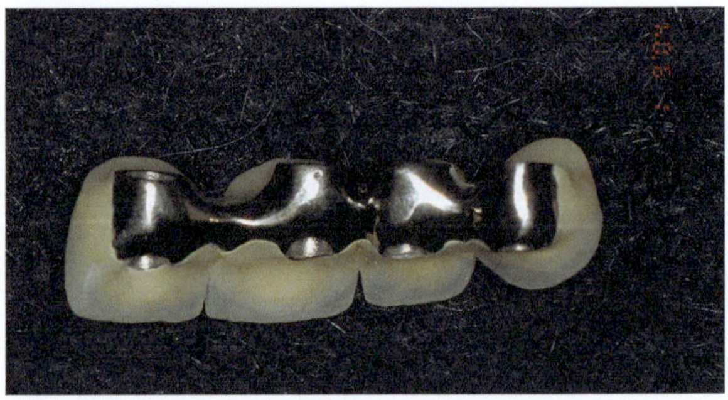

Fig. 9.19 The Maryland extensions were cut and removed after 6 months. Each implant was checked individually

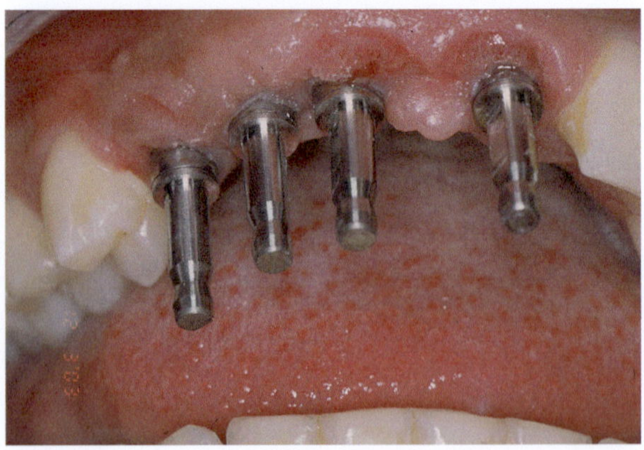

Fig. 9.20 "Pop-in" impression copings in place for a hydrocolloid impression for the final prosthesis

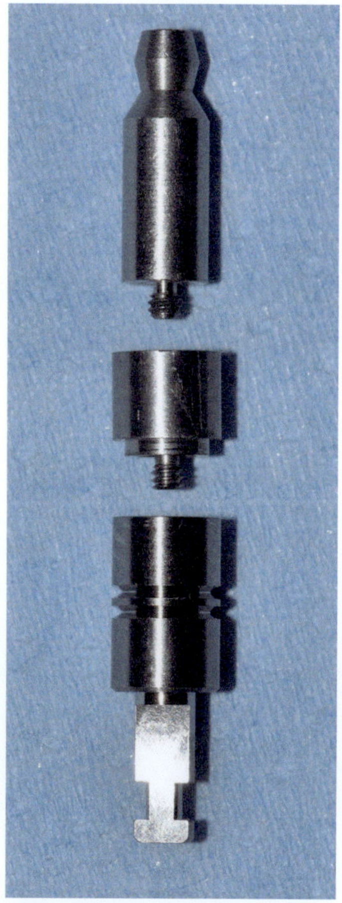

Fig. 9.21 In order to give the dental laboratory the actual situation in the mouth, the impression coping must be connected to the transgingival abutment that is screwed onto the analog

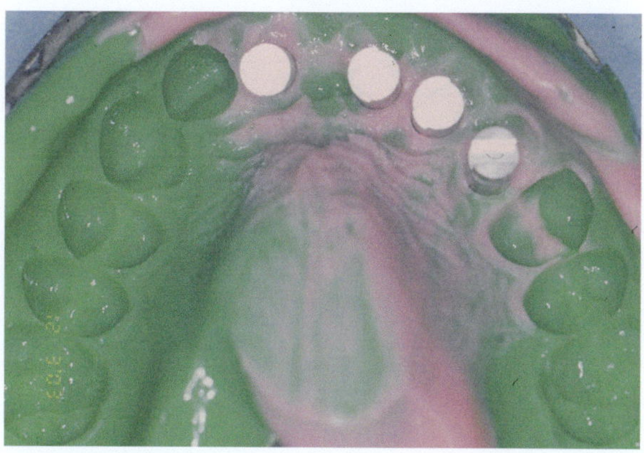

Fig. 9.22 The assembly is "popped" back into the hydrocolloid impression

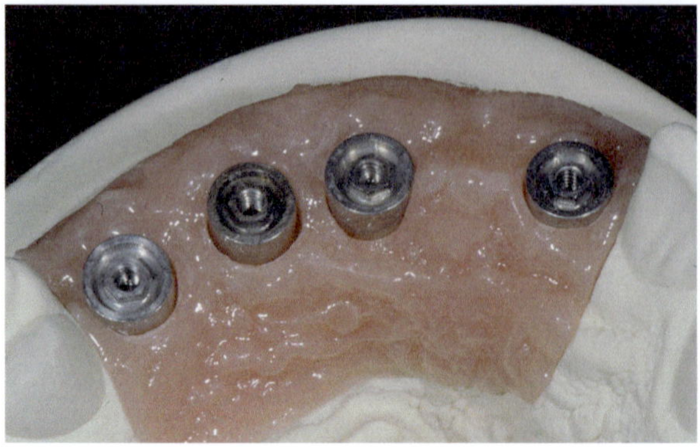

Fig. 9.23 Master model with pink silicone gingiva

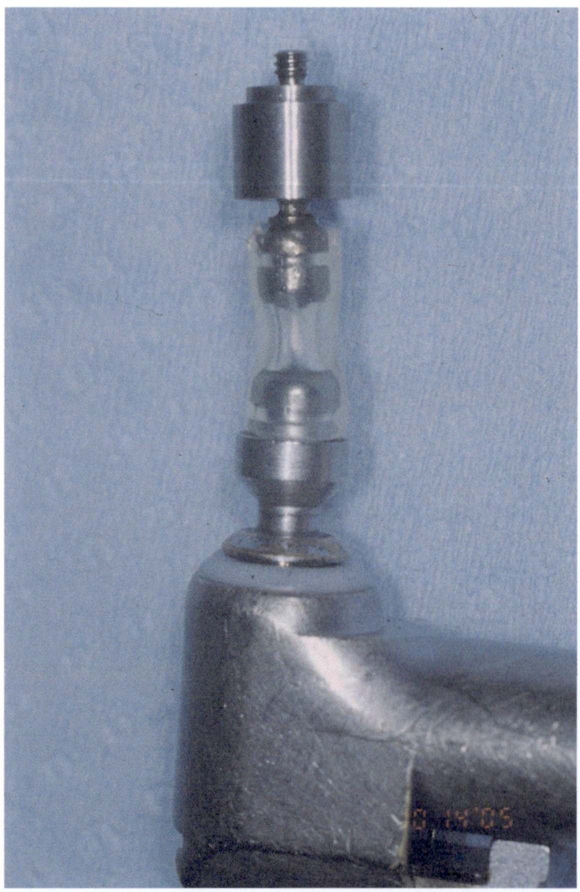

Fig. 9.24 Transgingival abutment installation with an abutment driver

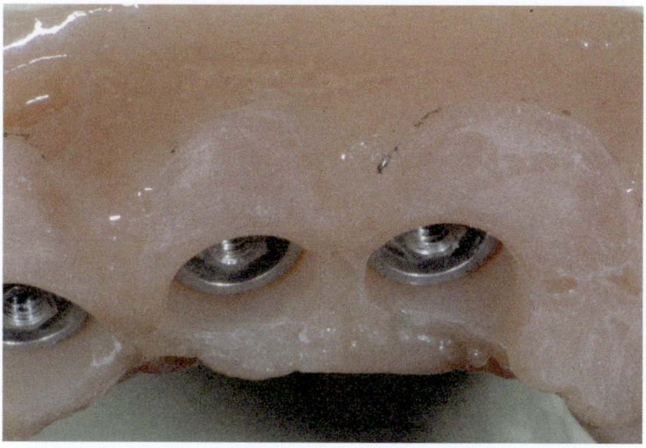

Fig. 9.25 Transgingival abutments are removed from the analogs that have the same emergence profile as the implants

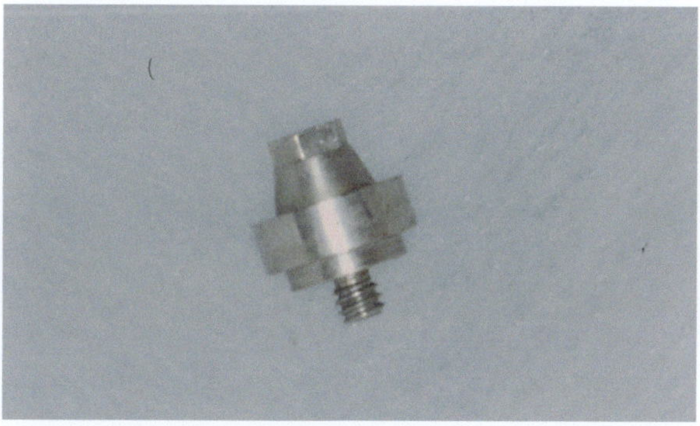

Fig. 9.26 Selected multiunit abutment

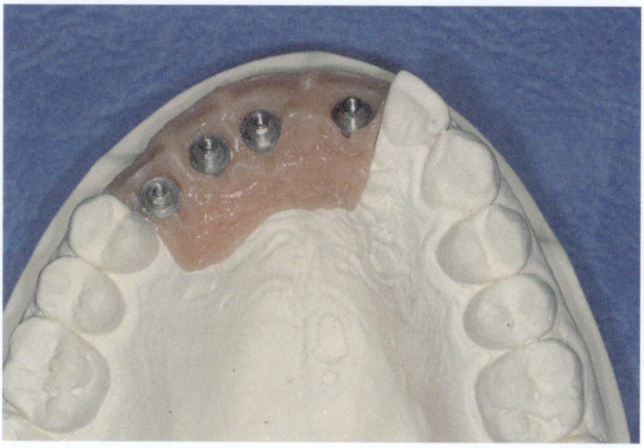

Fig. 9.27 Multiunit abutments positioned on the implant analogs

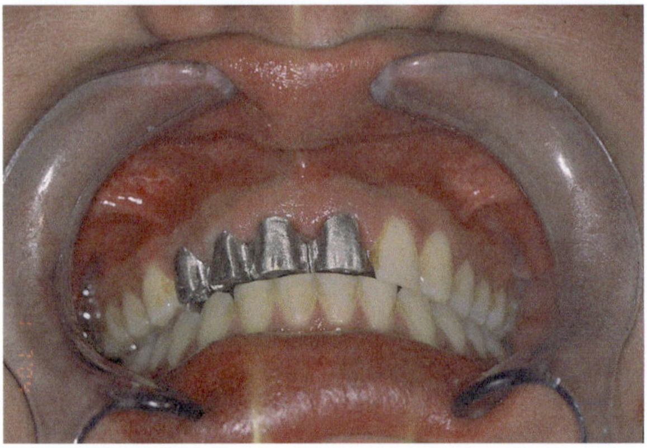

Fig. 9.28 Trial of the framework prepared for secondary bonding

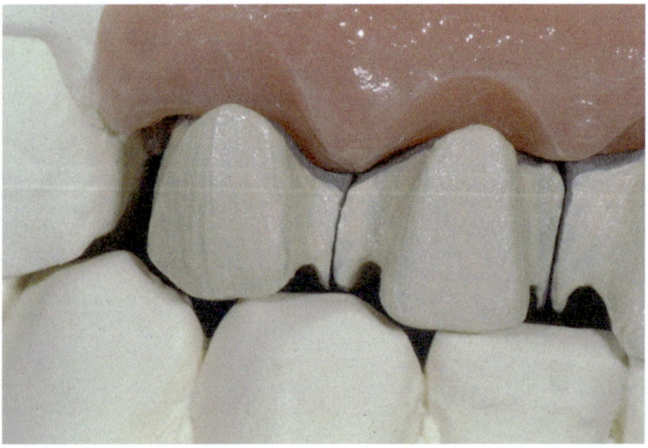

Fig. 9.29 Opaque in place

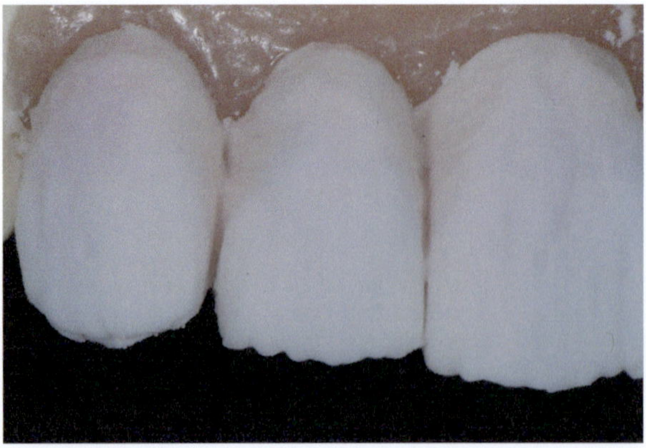

Fig. 9.30 Ceramic mounted

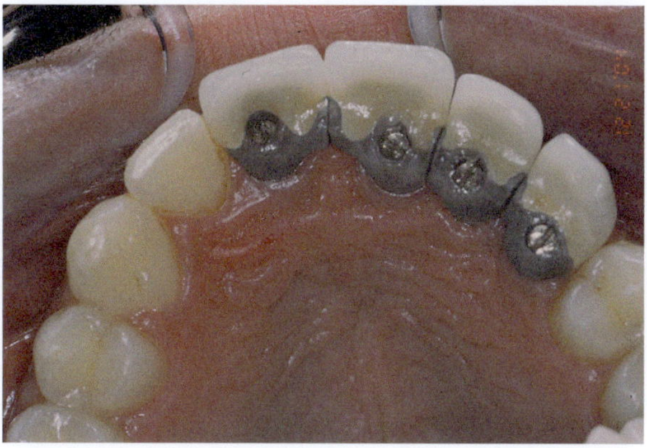

Fig. 9.31 Intraoral verification

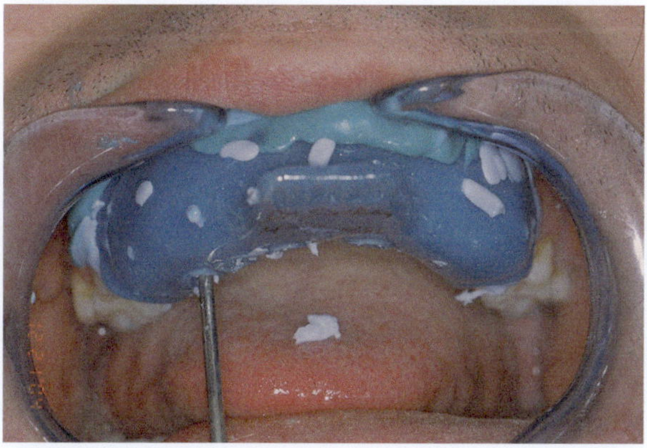

Fig. 9.32 Silicone impression

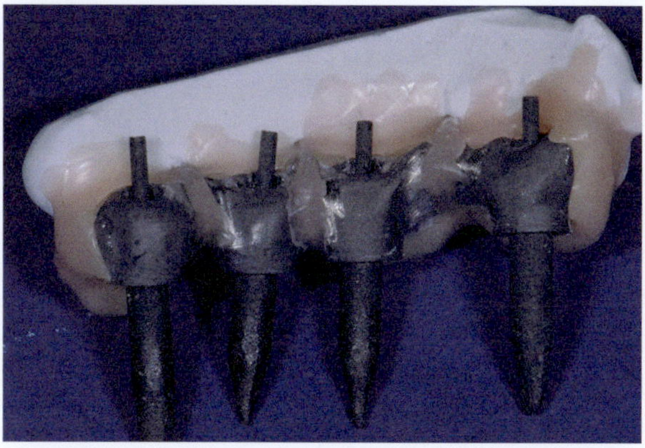

Fig. 9.33 Ceramic-baked-to-gold with secondary welds (gold)

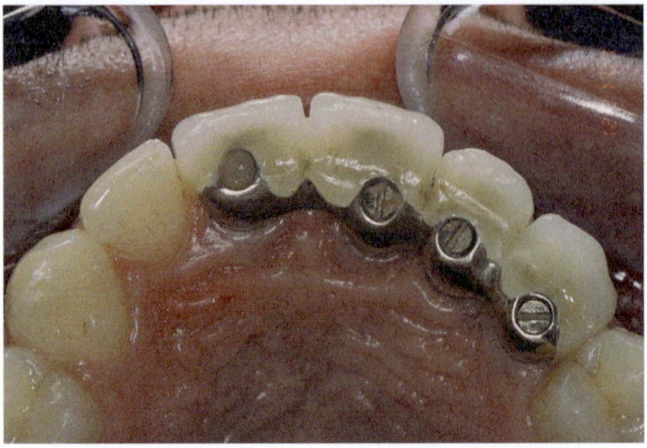

Fig. 9.34 Palatal view of the final screw-secured prosthesis

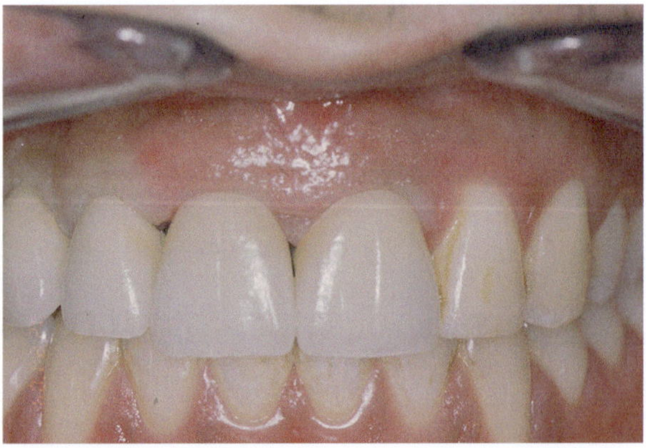

Fig. 9.35 Cosmetic aspect

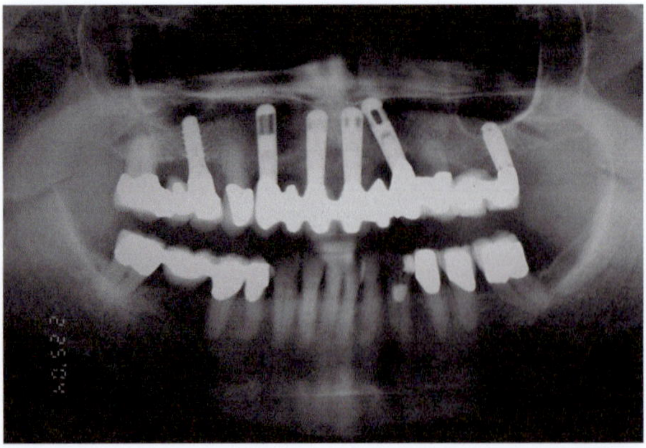

Fig. 9.36 Fractured teeth and implant on the upper left side

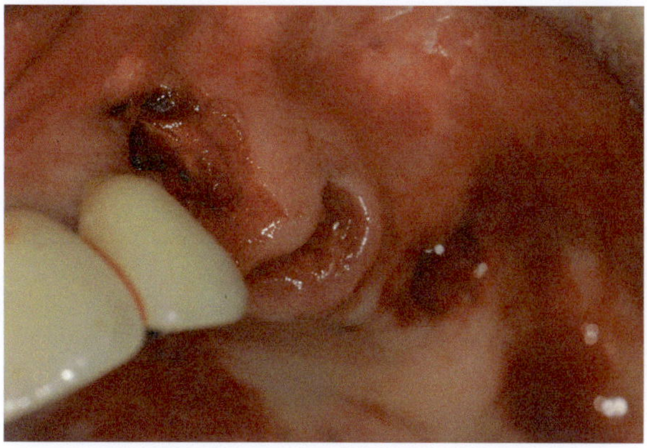

Fig. 9.37 Intraoral aspect of the defect

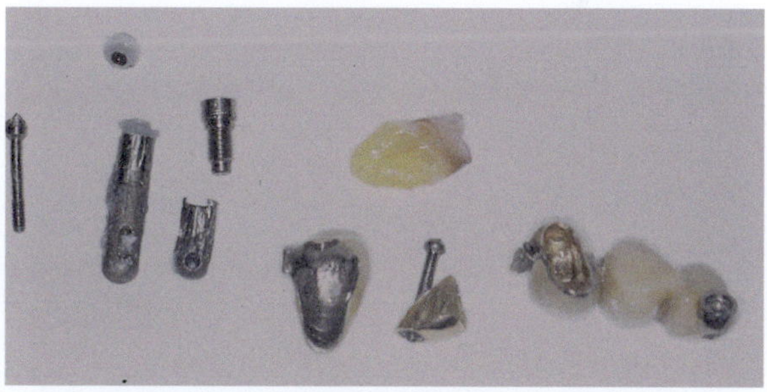

Fig. 9.38 The fractured elements were removed

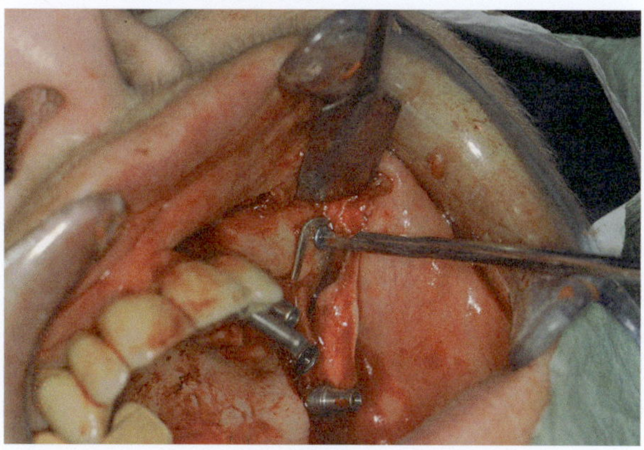

Fig. 9.39 Immediate installation of a screw-secured plate-form basal implant on the zygoma

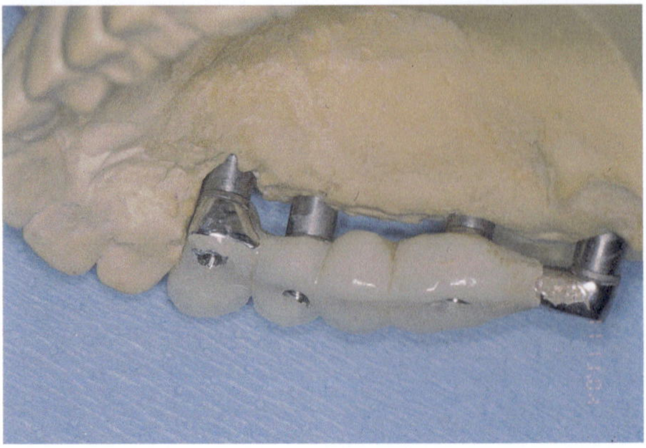

Fig. 9.40 Immediate functional screw-secured fixed bridge. One year post-op, the gingiva had retracted, and the transgingival abutment had to be removed

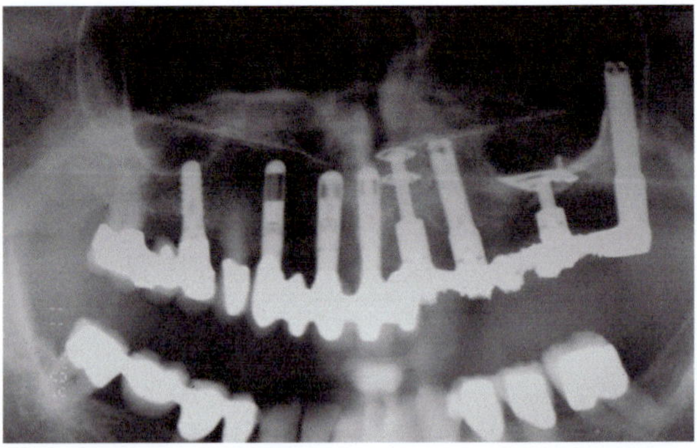

Fig. 9.41 Panoramic radiograph 1 year post-op. The sinuses are clear

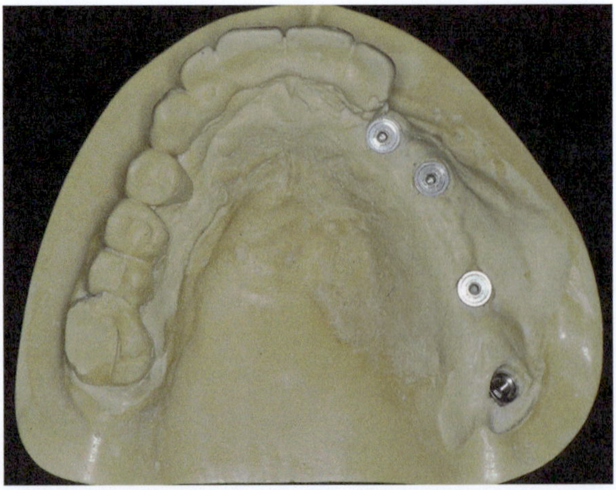

Fig. 9.42 Master model: the Monobloc analogs with their flat emergence profile can be seen after removal of the transgingival abutments

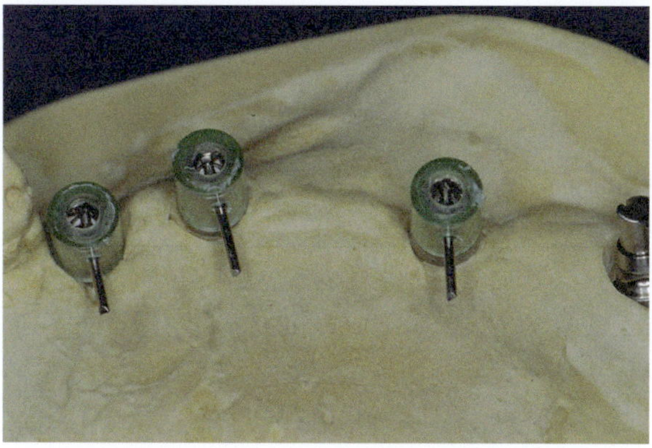

Fig. 9.43 Preparation for a cemented prosthesis on three implants and screw retention on the pterygoid implant

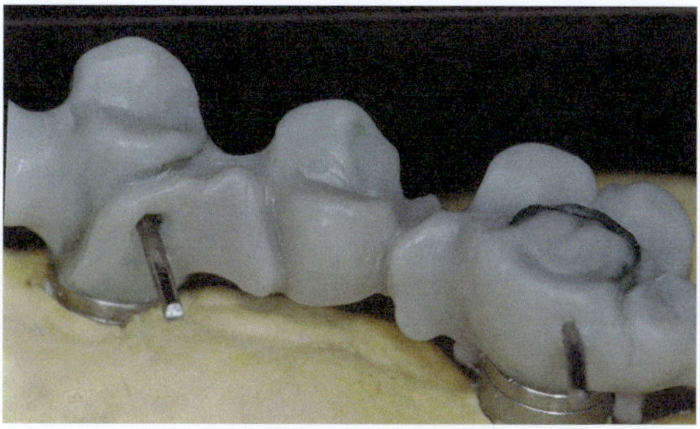

Fig. 9.44 Wax-up showing the palatal escape channel for the cement

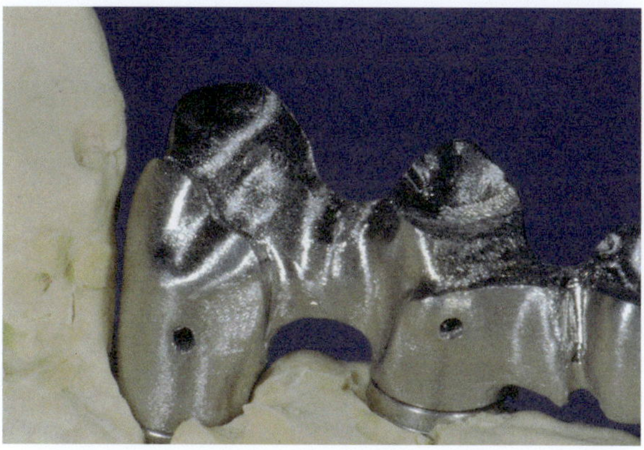

Fig. 9.45 Metal frame with a palatal cement escape channel

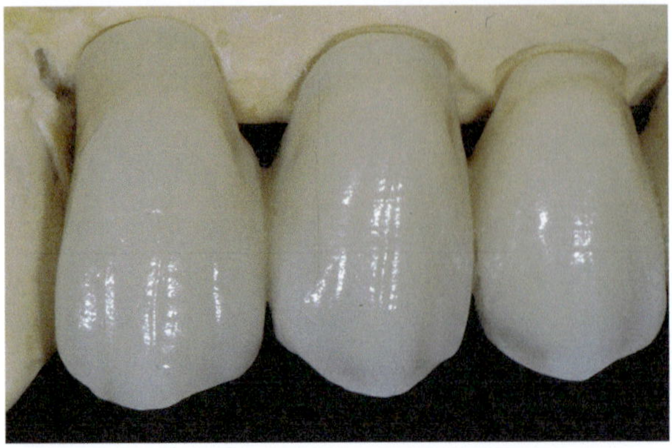

Fig. 9.46 Ceramic baked on gold alloy frame

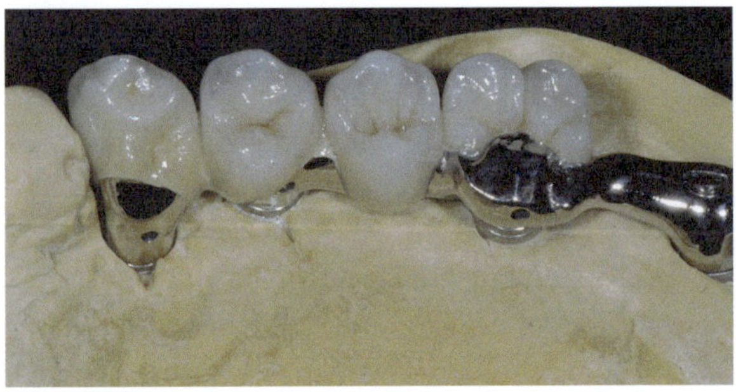

Fig. 9.47 Occlusal view of the pontic. Gold surfaces were necessary due to the occlusal conditions. The tubero-pterygoid implant was placed solely to secure the restoration; no prosthetic tooth was placed at this site. Immediate functional loading protocol

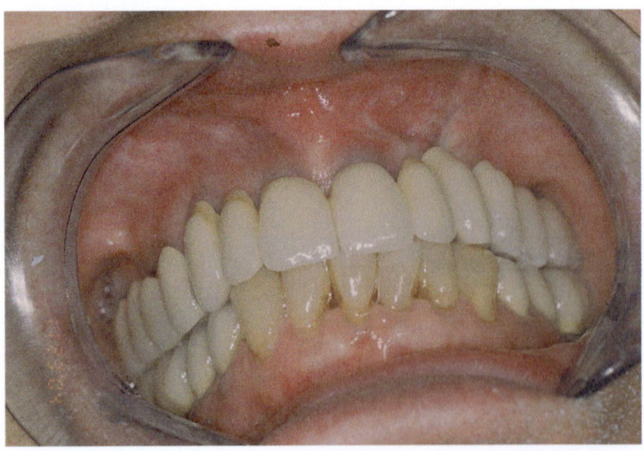

Fig. 9.48 Intraoral cosmetic aspect

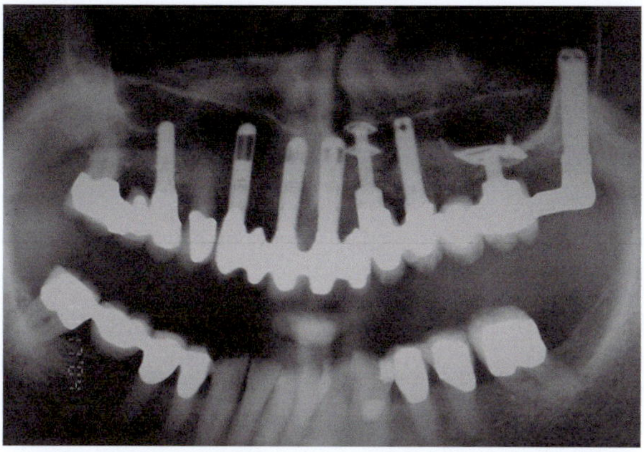

Fig. 9.49 Panoramic view of the final cemented and screw-retained bridge

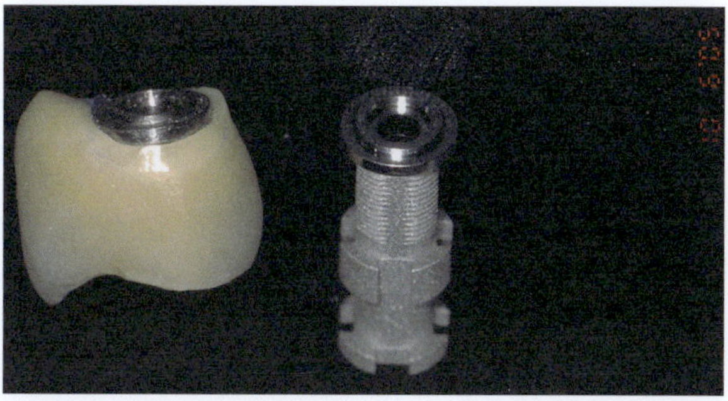

Fig. 9.50 Screw-retained zirconia-on-titanium single-tooth restoration

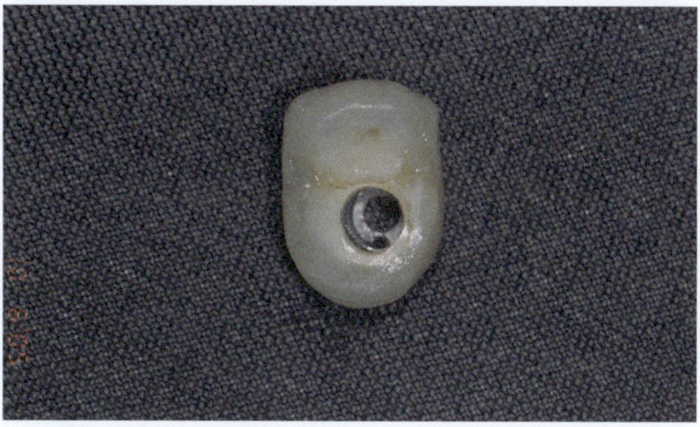

Fig. 9.51 Occlusal aspect

Cement-Retained Restorations (Figs. 9.52, 9.53, 9.54, 9.55, 9.56, 9.57 and 9.58)

Titanium hex abutment posts screwed onto the flat Monobloc emergence profile can be used when implants are parallel and for suitably located single implants.

- A pick-up impression is taken using titanium impression copings.
- The interarch relationship is recorded with a silicone bite or Beauty Pink® wax, depending on the clinical situation.
- If the implants are not perfectly parallel, the dental lab must prepare a customized angulated abutment with a positioning stent and a rigid plastic bite for a new occlusal record.
- A classic impression of the customized abutment is taken and sent to the dental lab, along with an occlusal record, for fabrication of the final cement-retained fixed bridge. During this time, the patient wears a transitional cemented acrylic fixed bridge.
- Use of specific intraoral and in-lab scan bodies allows virtual prosthodontics on basal implants. The scan body is placed on the implant directly in the patient's mouth; the scan data and an occlusal record are sent to the dental lab for preparation of a customized abutment (this applies to single-tooth replacements and small bridges only).

Digital Flow Prosthodontics

Increasing numbers of dental offices and laboratories are equipped for CAD-CAM and scan technologies. A trial wax-up and mock-up of the final restoration should always be checked in the patient's mouth for approval before fabricating the definitive basal implant-supported prosthesis.

Digital milling machines require accurate transfer of implant position before starting to make any prosthetic rehabilitation with an absolute passive fit. All

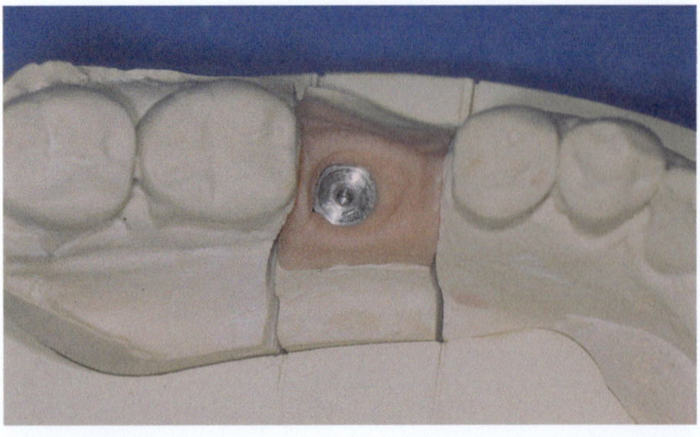

Fig. 9.52 The flat emergence profile is visible on the master model

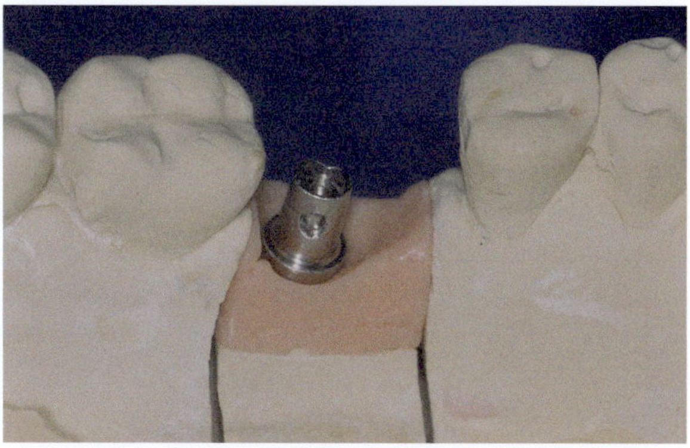

Fig. 9.53 Screw-secured straight abutment on the flat emergence. A lingual escape channel was prepared

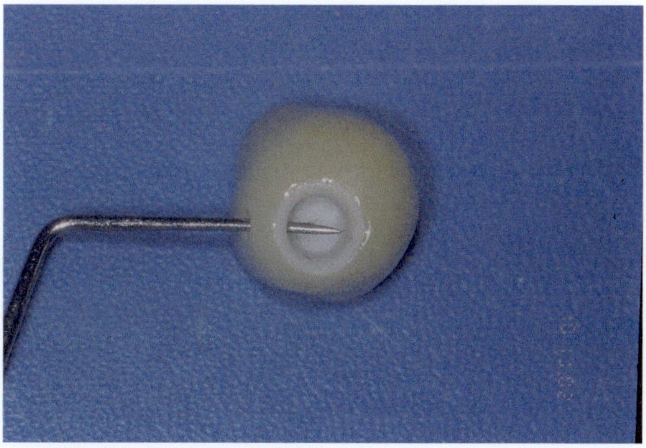

Fig. 9.54 Same escape channel in the zirconia tooth

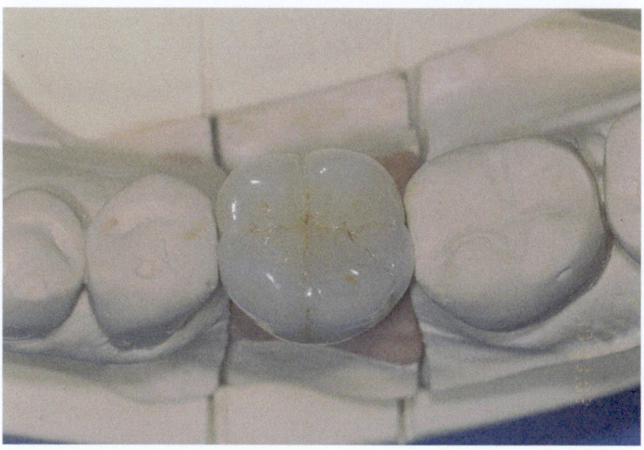

Fig. 9.55 Occlusal view of the cemented tooth

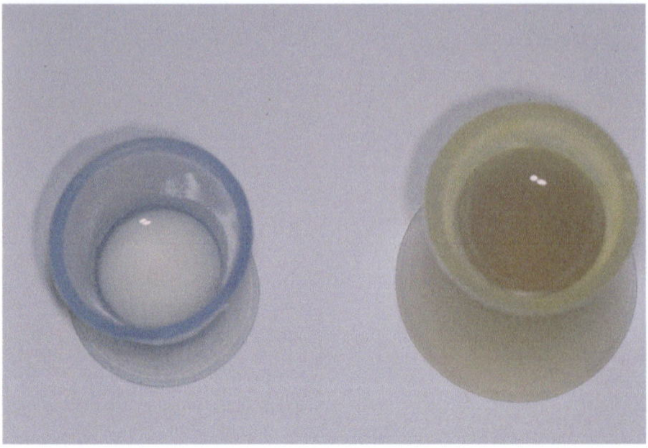

Fig. 9.56 Resin cement and monomer (liquid)

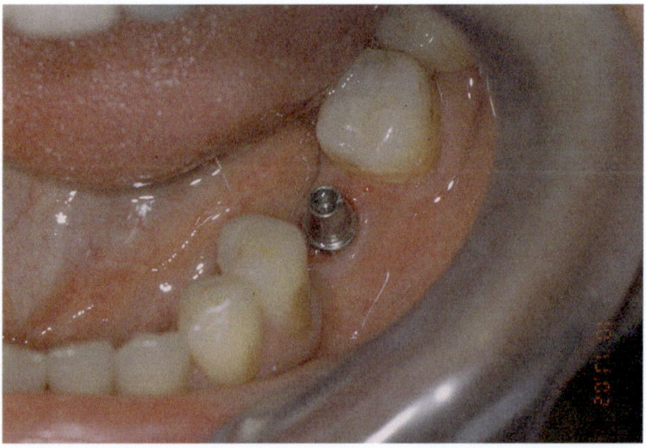

Fig. 9.57 Abutment in place

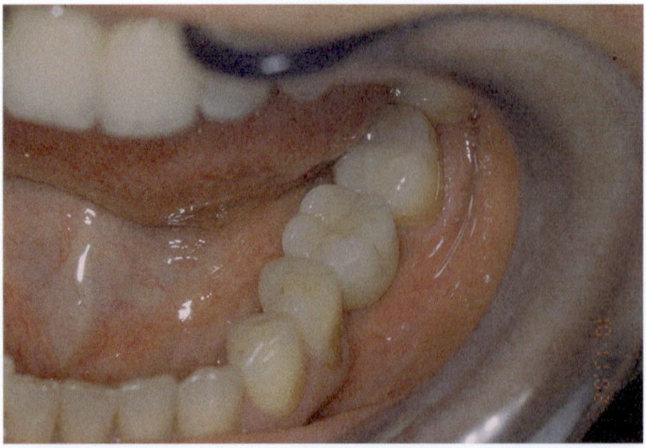

Fig. 9.58 Intraoral cosmetic aspect after cementing

transfer impression copings must be connected with plaster on the master model in the dental lab; they must then be checked in the patient's mouth by screwing them onto all of the implants. This allows easy detection and correction of any cracks in the connecting plaster before the final restoration is fabricated.

9.6 Prosthetic Materials for Transitional and Final Prostheses (Figs. 9.59, 9.60, 9.61, 9.62, 9.63, 9.64, 9.65, 9.66, 9.67, 9.68, 9.69, 9.70, 9.71, 9.72, 9.73, 9.74, 9.75, 9.76, 9.77, 9.78 and 9.79)

Immediate, screw-secured transitional restorations generally consist of a CrCo framework with machined titanium copings and conventional resin teeth (Phonares® denture teeth [Ivoclar Vivadent] for the anterior teeth, Premium® denture teeth [Heraeus Kulzer] for the premolars). Preparation of a transitional resin restoration on pick-up-type titanium impression copings cut to size is possible for single-tooth replacements. Esthetics, speech, mastication, and maintenance can all be evaluated

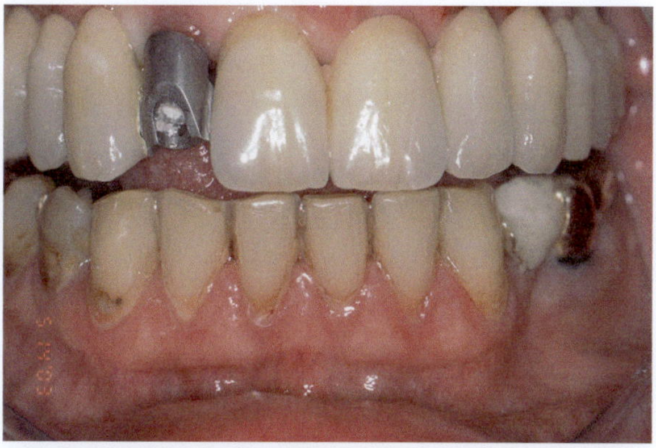

Fig. 9.59 Telescope screwed onto an implant with a flat emergence profile that was angled too far buccally

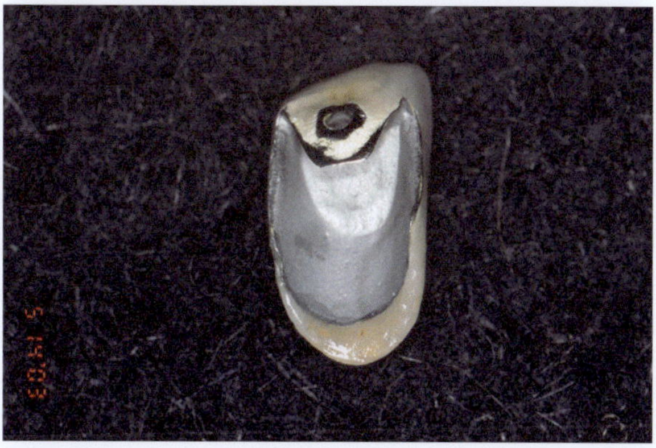

Fig. 9.60 Ceramic-baked-to-gold tooth to be cemented with resin cement

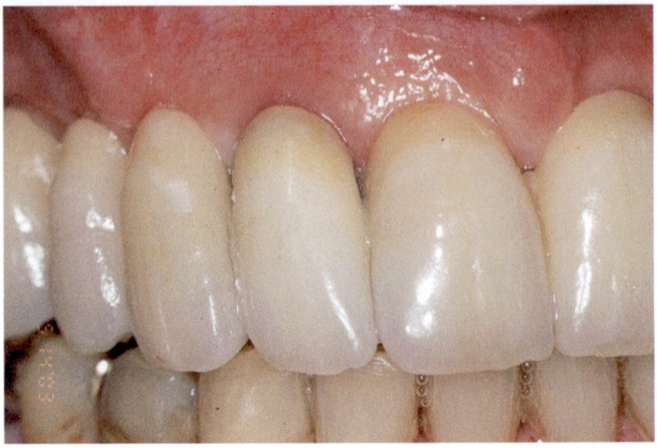

Fig. 9.61 Cosmetic outcome

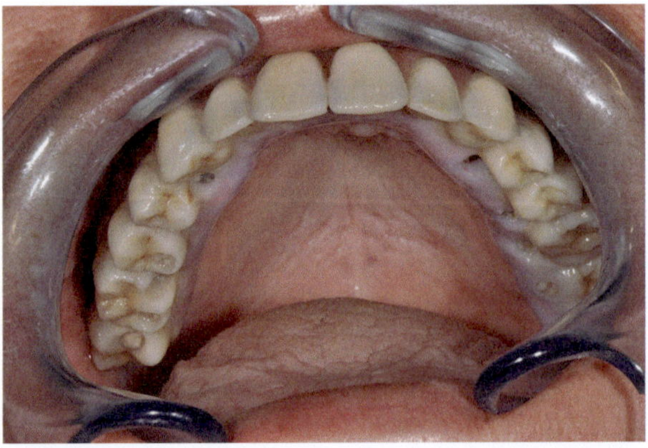

Fig. 9.62 Occlusal view of a full zirconia bridge (different patient)

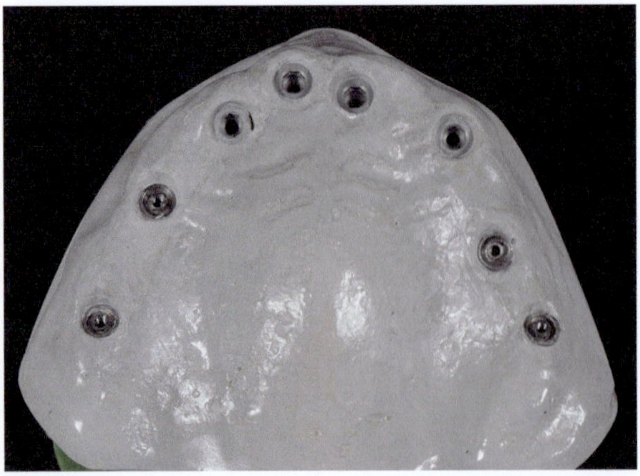

Fig. 9.63 Master model with Monobloc flat emergence profile analogs (screw-secured bridge)

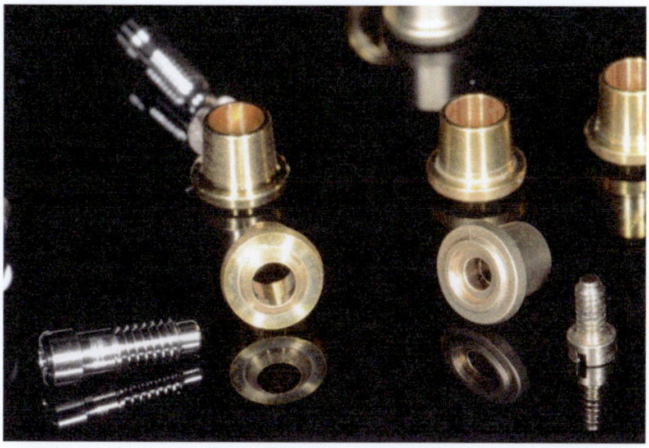

Fig. 9.64 Prosthetic components for a bridge screw-secured onto implants with a flat emergence profile

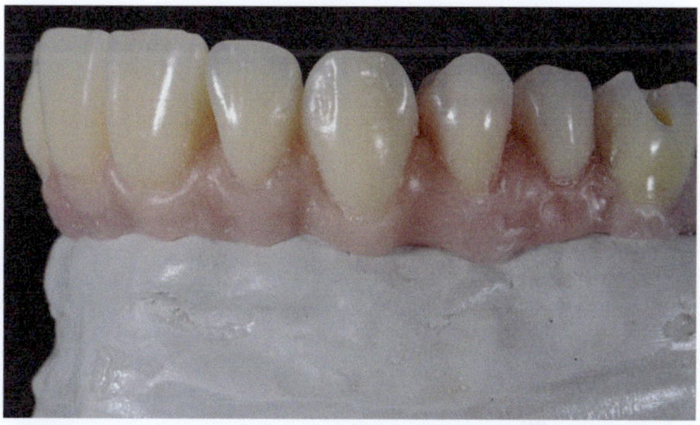

Fig. 9.65 Pink zirconia gingiva and full zirconia Zirkonzahn teeth

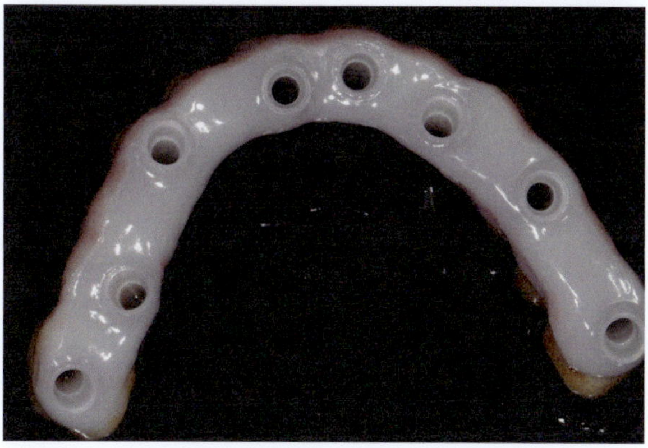

Fig. 9.66 Internal aspect of the full zirconia bridge

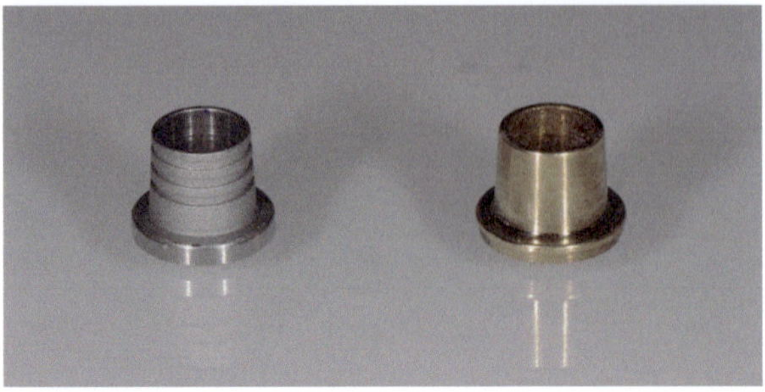

Fig. 9.67 Titanium bonding cylinder to be glued into the Zirkonzahn tooth; the brass centering cylinder on the right is only used on the master model in the dental laboratory

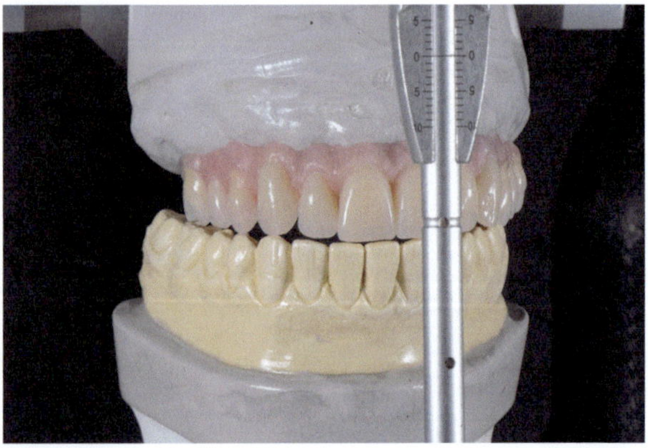

Fig. 9.68 Equilibration on an articulator

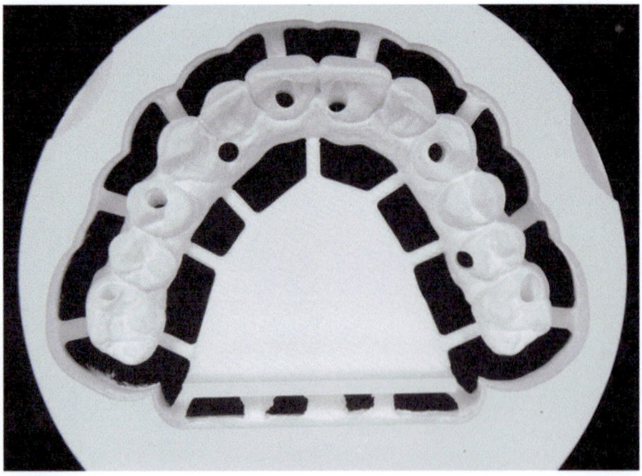

Fig. 9.69 Full zirconia prosthesis prepared with special milling burs

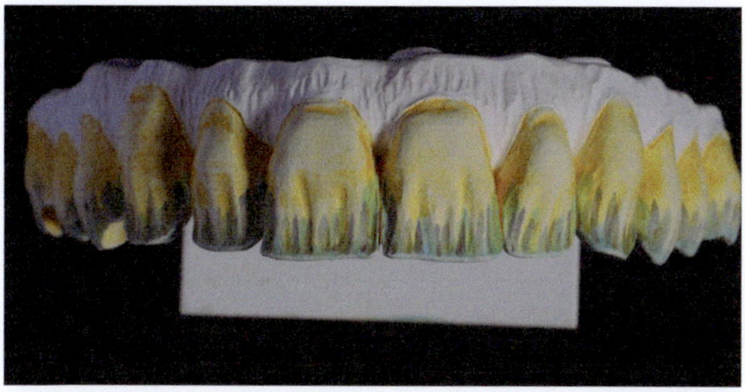

Fig. 9.70 Coloration prior to sintering

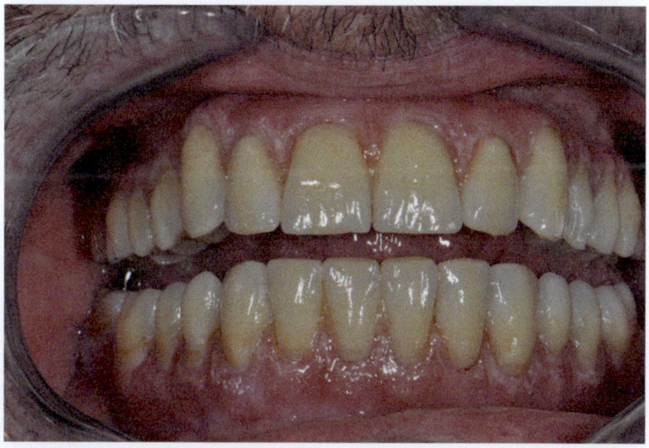

Fig. 9.71 Final cosmetic aspect of the upper and lower restorations (Zirkonzahn) screw-secured to basal implants

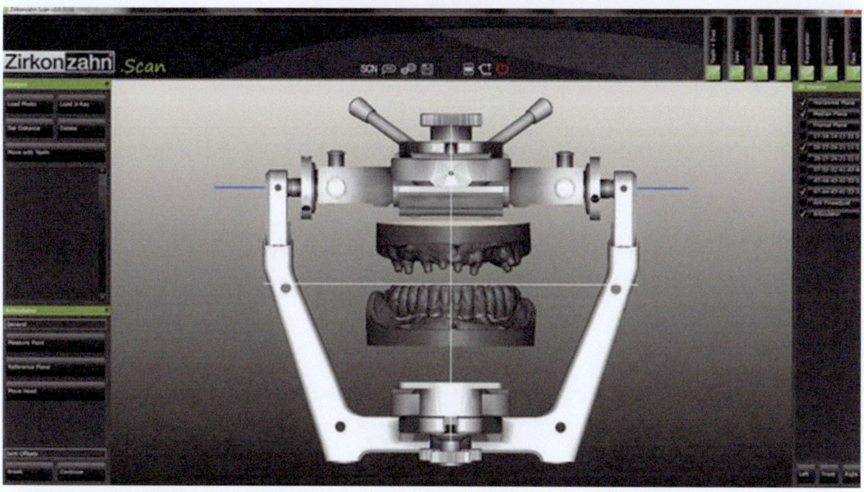

Fig. 9.72 Computerized view of the rehabilitation mounted on an articulator

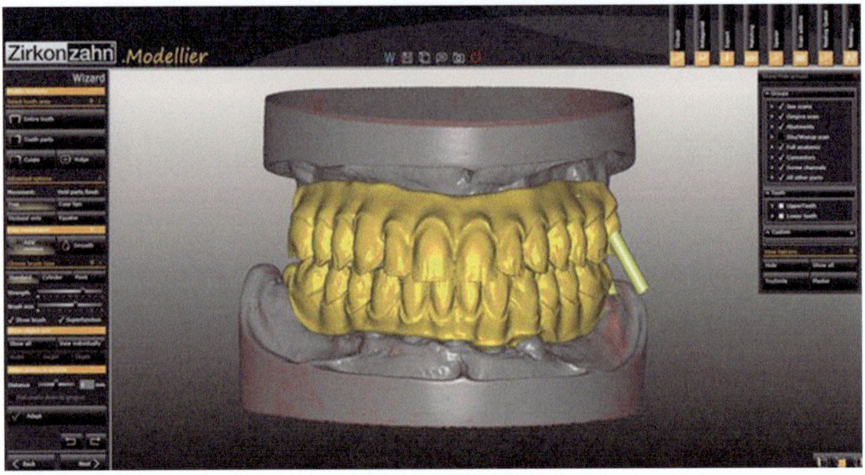

Fig. 9.73 Digital reconstruction of the future Zirkonzahn rehabilitation

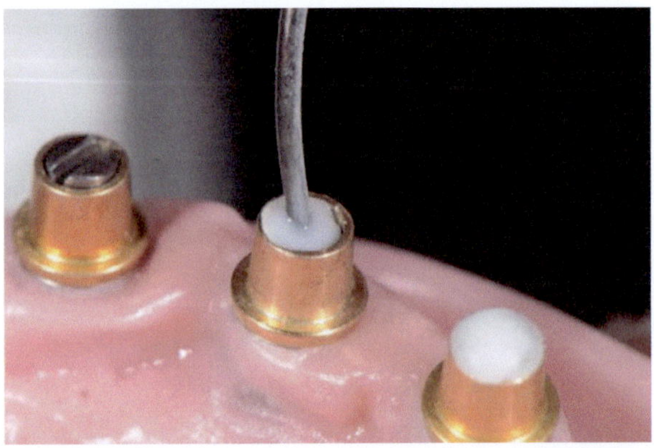

Fig. 9.74 Brass centering cylinders in place

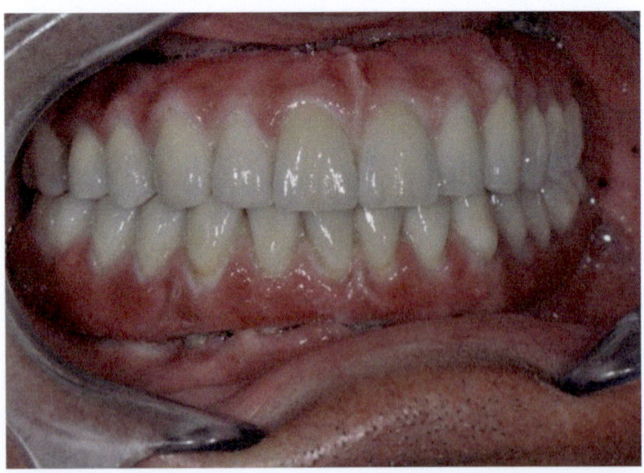

Fig. 9.75 Intraoral esthetic aspect

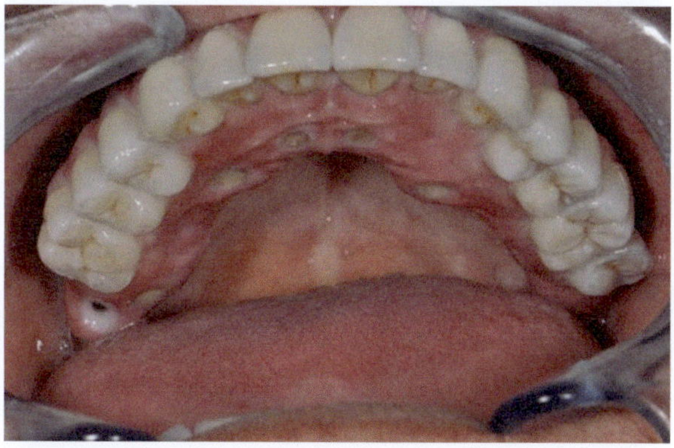

Fig. 9.76 Occlusal view of the Zirkonzahn rehabilitation

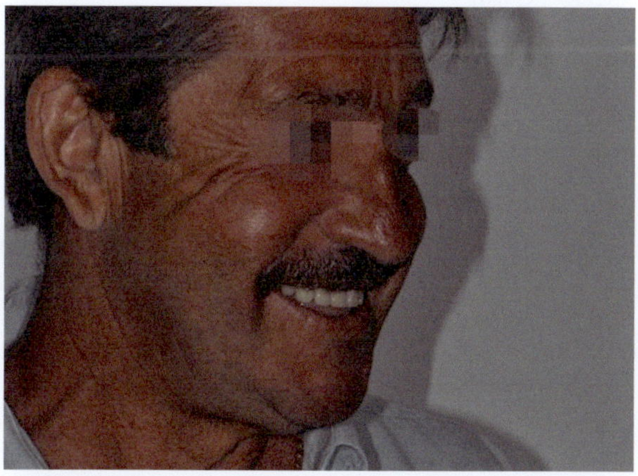

Fig. 9.77 Final esthetic outcome

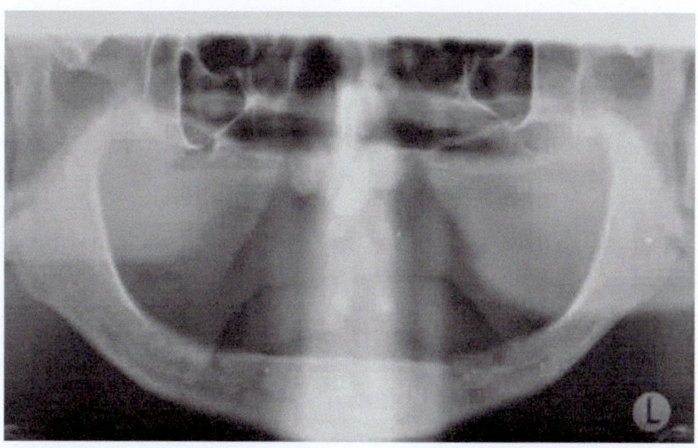

Fig. 9.78 Panoramic view of the initial intraoral status (2009)

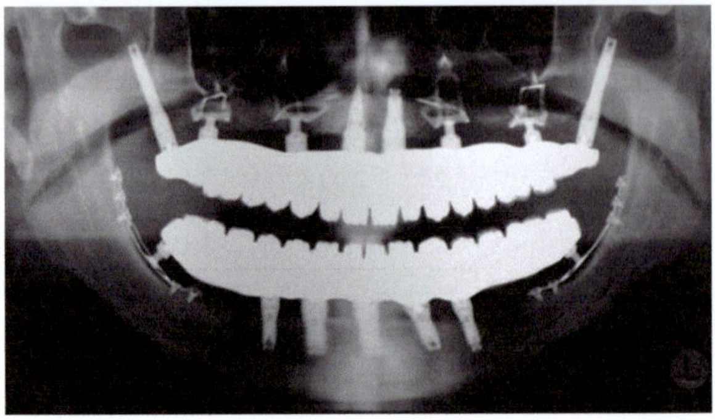

Fig. 9.79 Panoramic view of the restoration in 2017 (immediate functional loading protocol)

during the minimum 6-month period that the transitional appliance is in function. Use of machined abutments is generally preferable, but castable plastic copings can also be used.

6–12 months after validation of the transitional implant-supported tooth or prosthesis, the final restoration can be prepared by the laboratory with a minimum of modifications. The transitional prosthesis can be used as a transfer for the final restoration. In certain cases, it can even be maintained as the final restoration for clinical, mechanical, and economic reasons. Several options exist if the patient desires a more sophisticated final prosthesis: fabrication of a new framework, ceramic-fused-to-metal (precious metal, non-precious alloy or titanium), or prototyping technology (titanium on cobalt-chromium, which avoids the need to glue titanium cylinders into the framework).

Another possibility is full zirconia with titanium connecting components (titanium coping coupled to zirconia with Attachment Bond®) (Heraeus Kulzer, Germany) or a similar adhesive developed for cementing to zirconia. More recently, TRINIA® and PEEK abutments and frameworks have emerged as other options for implant-supported restorations.

Conflict of interest statement Gérard M. Scortecci is the inventor of the Diskimplant and holder of several associated patents that are exploited by the Victory company. He is an unpaid consultant to this firm and a minority shareholder in the company. No money was received from any of the companies mentioned in the book or from any of the companies whose products are mentioned.

Recommended Reading

1. Chen YW, Moussi J, Drury JL, Wataja JC. Zirconia in biomedical applications. Expert Rev Med Devices. 2016;16:1–19.
2. Cutts R. Implant digital workflow opportunities. Implants. 2018;2:34–7.
3. Gracis S, Michalakis K, Vigolo P, Vult von Steyern P, Zwahlen M, Sailer I. Internal vs. external connections for abutments/reconstructions: a systematic review. Clin Oral Implants Res. 2012;23(suppl 6):202–16.
4. Gapski R, Wang HL, Mascarenhes P, Lang NP. Critical review of immediate implant loading. Clinical Oral Implant Res. 2003;14:515–27.
5. Misch CE. Dental implant prosthetics. St. Louis, MO: Mosby; 2014.

6. Mohl ND, Zarb GA, Carlsson GE, Rugh JD. A textbook of occlusion. Chicago: Quintessence; 1988. p. 79–118.
7. Resnik R, Misch CE. Misch's avoiding complications in oral implantology. St. Louis, MO: Elsevier; 2017.
8. Schwitalla AD, Abou-Emara M, Zimmermann T, Spintig T, Beuer F, Lackmann J, Müller WD. The applicability of PEEK-based abutment screws. J Mech Behav Biomed Mater. 2016;63:244–51.
9. Scortecci GM, Misch CE, Benner KU, editors. Implants and restorative dentistry. London: Martin Dunitz; 2001.
10. Vigolo P, Givani A, Majzoub Z, Cordioli G. Cemented versus screw-retained implant-supported single-tooth crowns: a 4-year prospective clinical study. Int J Oral Maxillofac Implants. 2004;19(2):260–5.
11. Vigolo P, Mutinelli S, Givani A, Stellini E. Cemented versus screw-retained implant-supported single-tooth crowns: a 10-year randomized controlled trial. Eur J Oral Implantol. 2012;5(4):355–64.

Part III

Clinical Applications and Complications

Single-Tooth Replacement: The Esthetic Zone and Posterior Sectors

10

Gérard M. Scortecci, Charles Savoldelli, and Franck Afota

10.1 Single-Tooth Replacement with a Basal Implant

Epidemiology

In the anterior region, absence of a tooth is generally related to trauma or agenesis (lateral incisors); maxillary canines are sometimes impacted. Fracture, infection, and periodontal disease are the main causes of tooth loss in the molar and premolar sectors.

Agenesis

Agenesis can be managed in several ways. In some cases, a double Diskimplant® can be installed directly, without initial hard- or soft-tissue management. In other instances, a soft-tissue graft or a bone graft is required before an implant can be placed. If the mesiodistal space is too narrow crestally and/or apically, prior orthodontic movement and space maintainers are needed in order to obtain sufficient space for implant placement without injury of adjacent natural teeth. A minimum of 4 mm mesiodistally is required for narrow root-form implants versus 5.5 mm mesiodistally for Diskimplants®.

G. M. Scortecci (✉)
University of Nice-Sophia Antipolis Medical School, Nice, France

New York University, New York, NY, USA

University of Southern California, Los Angeles, CA, USA

Private Practice, Nice, France
e-mail: scortecci@wanadoo.fr

C. Savoldelli · F. Afota
Institut Universitaire de la Face et du Cou, Nice, France
e-mail: savoldelli.c@chu-nice.fr

© Springer Nature Switzerland AG 2019

G. M. Scortecci (ed.), *Basal Implantology*, https://doi.org/10.1007/978-3-319-44873-2_10

Immediate Basal Implant Placement Following Extraction

Basal implants are indicated when there is extensive loss of the buccal alveolar plate and not enough bone is available for direct placement of a root-form implant. If clinically possible, immediate implant placement is the recommended option. Removal of the tooth should be performed carefully so as to preserve the initial alveolar bone volume. The apical portion of the Diskimplant® (i.e., the basal disk) must be anchored firmly in the maxillary or mandibular bone and be wider than the extracted root. The remainder of the implant body must be solidly fixed in the dense palatal or lingual aspect of the remaining alveolar bone and fill in the crestal alveolar gap as closely as possible.

Delayed Implant Placement After Extraction

When immediate implant installation is not possible because of insufficient bone quality and/or quantity or because there is a high risk of infection, it is advisable to wait 3 months for alveolar bone reconstruction to take place, and all sources of infection have been eliminated. Repeat radiographic analysis is required before implant placement. Direct evaluation of bone density with a manual osseotensor is mandatory 45 days before installation of a basal implant.

Bone Grafting After Extraction

If a bone graft is necessary, the soft tissue at the extraction site must first be allowed to heal for 1 month in order to obtain a sufficient amount of mucosa to protect the future free bone graft. The best intraoral donor sites are the ramus and the mental area. Usually, implants are not installed at the time of bone grafting. It is preferable to let the free bone graft become incorporated (waiting period 3 months) with establishment of a new blood supply. This process of neo-angiogenesis is essential for successful implant integration. If there is enough remaining bone, root-form implants can be installed. If not, basal implants (double Diskimplants®) can be laterally inserted and left submerged for 6 months before loading. Immediate loading is possible in certain favorable clinical situations. Use of a night guard is advisable.

10.2 Loading Modalities for Single-Tooth Basal Implants

Immediate Functional Loading

Immediate loading of single-tooth and partial arch replacements remains controversial because this approach involves numerous hard-to-control parameters. In particular, patient compliance is mandatory. If clinical evaluation is favorable, a single-tooth restoration can be placed 24 hours after implant installation. Alternately, a fixed transitional titanium-resin unit can be fabricated immediately using a titanium pick-up impression coping to create a screw-retained Maryland bridge-type restoration. Indirect click-in type impression copings can be used with a regular impression tray and light and hard silicone impression materials. A full-arch night guard including the basal implant-supported tooth is advisable during the first 6 months post-op in order to guarantee initial and long-term stability.

Inclusion criteria for immediate functional loading (modified from [1]) are as follows:

- Non-smoking patient
- Physical and psychological health status compatible with the procedure
- Good oral conditions, including hygiene
- Amount and quality of available dense bone compatible with reliable and stable initial anchorage of a Diskimplant®
- Dental arch relationship allowing bilateral occlusal stability
- A minimum distance of 4 mm between the implant emergence (crestal level) and the occlusal surface of the opposite tooth

Exclusion criteria include:

- The canine, premolar, and molar areas: a submerged technique is recommended in these sectors.
- Patients with bruxism or tongue thrust habits.

Risk/Benefit Analysis

Delayed loading is the recommended procedure for 98% of single-tooth restorations on Diskimplants® and for 100% in posterior edentulous sectors. The waiting period is 6 months or more, depending on patient age (> 50 years) and initial bone volume and quality. However, whenever possible, it is always better to place a Diskimplant® immediately after an extraction in order to preserve the remaining alveolar bone. As the lateral osteotomy procedure provides a natural pathway for drainage, the risk of "trapping" a source of infection is very low.

10.3 Single-Tooth Impressions

Pick-Up Impression with an Anti-rotational Impression Coping

Before taking the impression, make sure that the titanium hex impression coping for single-tooth replacements (ref. TPMU) is positioned correctly on the Diskimplant® or PLM-3.5 abutment (check this radiographically). The TPMU coping is held in place with an M1.4 titanium laboratory screw (Diskimplant® carrier screw). A transparent plastic open impression tray is used with heavy silicone. Secure the impression coping to the tray with Duralay® or Luxabite® to prevent rotation during the connection of the implant analog (ref. APL) in the dental laboratory. This titanium pick-up-type impression coping can be reused to fabricate a transitional restoration with a denture tooth prior to fabrication of the final prosthetic element.

"Click-In" Impression Technique

The "click-in" or "pop in" impression coping (ref. TP) is compatible with standard commercial trays and silicone or hydrocolloid impression materials. The laboratory phase is the same as with pick-up-type impression copings. This technique can be used for all types of single-tooth restorations on a Monobloc abutment. Make sure that the impression coping "clicks" back into the impression, and then secure the impression coping/analog assembly before pouring the plaster into the impression tray.

10.4 Single-Tooth Prosthodontics

There are two techniques for single-tooth restorations, each with its advantages and drawbacks:

1. Screw-retained restoration directly on the Diskimplant®, when gingival thickness is less than 4 mm, or on a cylindrical transgingival titanium Monobloc abutment (ref. PLM-3.5)
2. Cement-retained restoration on a two-piece hex abutment post that is screw-secured directly onto the Diskimplant® or to a transgingival cylindrical Monobloc abutment.

In cosmetically demanding areas where the gingival thickness is less than 4 mm, the restoration can be prepared directly on the implant. If the implant emergence is buccal or incisal, cement-retained technology is indicated. The final decision depends on implant position, occlusion, gingival thickness, esthetics, and cost.

Screw-Retained, Single-Tooth Restorations (UCLA Concept)

When the gingival thickness is less than 3.5 mm, the UCLA concept can be used if the implant emergence is occlusal or lingual/palatal. If the gingival thickness is $\geq$3.5 mm, a screw-secured single-tooth restoration can be prepared on a titanium Monobloc abutment (PLM-3.5) placed on top of the implant. The emergence of the basal implant must be located in the middle of the cingulum for incisors and canines. Although occlusal screws may be visible and recurrent screw loosening may occur if the screw is not retightened 24 hours after installation, this type of restoration is easy to retrieve and repair. Anti-rotation is provided by the design of the Monobloc emergence profile (external hex plus conical seal) and use of appropriate prosthetic components for single units.

Impression

The impression is taken using a machined titanium, pick-up-type hex impression coping (ref. TPMU) held in place by an M1.4 laboratory screw. Hex impression copings provide maximum precision and anti-rotation effect due to friction grip (cylindrical impression copings are intended solely for bridges). A "click-in" impression coping (ref. TP) may also be used provided the implant is not excessively angulated. A Monobloc analog (ref. APL) is then screwed onto the assembly which is given to the dental laboratory.

Laboratory Procedure

The laboratory phase for screw-retained, single-tooth restorations directly on Diskimplants® and on Monobloc abutments is the same for both "click-in" and "pick-up"-type impression techniques.

A single-tooth unit can be fabricated using a castable plastic single-unit coping (PCMU) or by modifying a hex impression coping (ref. TPMU). These components are held onto the Monobloc analog with the M1.4 laboratory screw.

- The plastic castable coping for single units features a hex for anti-rotation. It must be waxed and overcast in order to prepare a suitable emergence profile for the corresponding prosthetic tooth.
- A machined titanium hex impression coping can be shortened to prepare a relatively inexpensive composite crown directly.

The single-tooth prosthetic element is secured using an M1.4 retaining screw tightened manually to 10–15 Ncm.

M1.4 Screws

Gold M1.4 retaining screws (ref. VFO-M1.4) are recommended for fixation of single crowns as they are easy to retrieve if they fracture. Titanium retaining screws (ref. VFT-M1.4) should be used with caution owing to the risk of formation of a cold solder. The long titanium M1.4 carrier screws supplied with Diskimplants® can be cut down in the dental laboratory (1.5 mm from the occlusal level) and used for temporary single crowns on implants or Monobloc abutments. All retaining screws should be retightened after 24 hours to prevent screw loosening.

Cement-Retained Single-Tooth Restorations

If the implant emergence is buccal, a cement-retained restoration on a customized, screw-secured UCLA abutment is indicated. Depending on implant position and gingival thickness, a machined titanium hex abutment post (ref. FMT-5, FMT-6, or FMT-7) can be screw-secured directly into the basal implant or into a transgingival

PLM-3.5 abutment placed on top of the implant. Cementation to a hex abutment post screw-secured directly into the implant is indicated if the implant emergence requires angle correction and gingival thickness is less than 4 mm.

Impression

- The hex abutment post can be left in the mouth and an impression taken directly, just as for a natural tooth.
- Alternately, a hex impression coping for single-tooth units (ref. TPMU) can be used to take the impression.

Laboratory Procedure

If a hex abutment post is not left in the mouth, the dental laboratory can either use a machined hex post or fabricate a post using a castable plastic single-unit coping. This coping must be re-shaped, waxed, and overcast; the final unit must be trimmed and highly polished in order to obtain a suitable emergence profile for the final tooth. The dental technician then prepares the single-unit ceramic crown to be cemented directly onto the screw-secured hex abutment post or custom post. Three or four layers of die spacer should be used to allow room for the resin cement that absorbs shocks during function and parafunction.

Cementing

Duralay® or a resin cement is recommended to hold the single crown to the post. The slot of the abutment post retaining screw should be protected with eugenol-free temporary cement or a Teflon™ pellet. In order to eliminate any air trapped during cementation, the technician should prepare an escape channel for the resin cement (approx. 1 or 2 mm in diameter) on the lingual side of the crown and another escape channel on the corresponding screw-secured abutment post. The two channel openings are aligned to create a continuous resin pin through the cingulum of the single crown and through the screw-secured hex abutment post.

Retrieval of a Cemented Crown

If retrieval of the cemented crown proves necessary, the resin pin can be eliminated easily using a carbide bur mounted on a high-speed handpiece. Drilling without spray causes the resin cement to expand. A drop of eugenol is then placed in the "now open" channel to dissolve the resin. A new drilling sequence is then performed at high speed with a small diamond bur, again without spray. Another drop of eugenol is next introduced in the small access channel. The patient must wait 20 minutes in the waiting room for the product to soften the resin cement (or they can return the next day, if necessary). A crown removal appliance is then inserted in the access channel on the lingual side of the crown to be retrieved. A gentle tap is sufficient to separate the resin-cemented crown from the screw-secured abutment post. This is a simple means to safely retrieve a definitive cement-retained single-tooth restoration on an implant.

10.5 Cleft Palate and Agenesis: Surgical Management with Iliac Bone Grafting of the Palate (Figs. 10.1, 10.2, 10.3, 10.4, 10.5, 10.6, 10.7, 10.8, 10.9, 10.10, 10.11, 10.12, 10.13, 10.14, 10.15, 10.16, and 10.17)

This patient was followed up since the age of 7. The cleft was successfully closed with an iliac crest bone graft, but the height of the bone available under the nasal floor was insufficient for installation of even a short root-form implant. Both disks of a 7-mm-diameter double Diskimplant® advantageously engaged the remaining nasal bone in addition to the autologous grafted bone. The delayed loading protocol included a 6-month waiting period before functional loading. At follow-up in January 2018, after 2 years of service, the implant was fully osseointegrated.

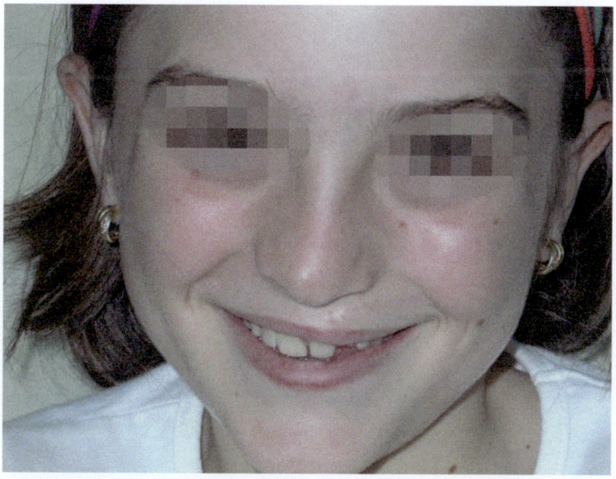

Fig. 10.1 Patient aged 7 years: extraoral view (cleft palate)

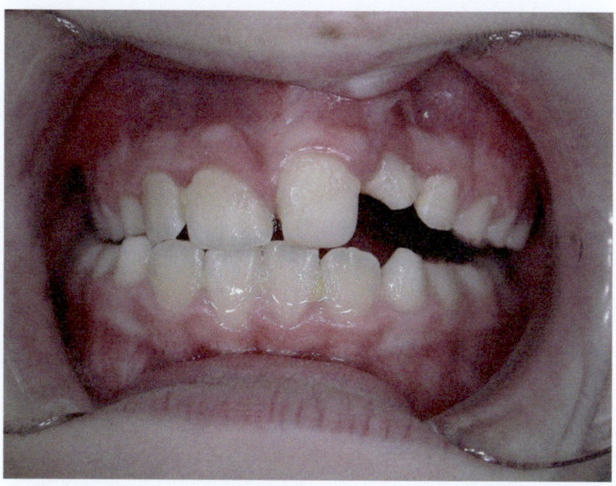

Fig. 10.2 Same patient as Fig. 10.1: intraoral view

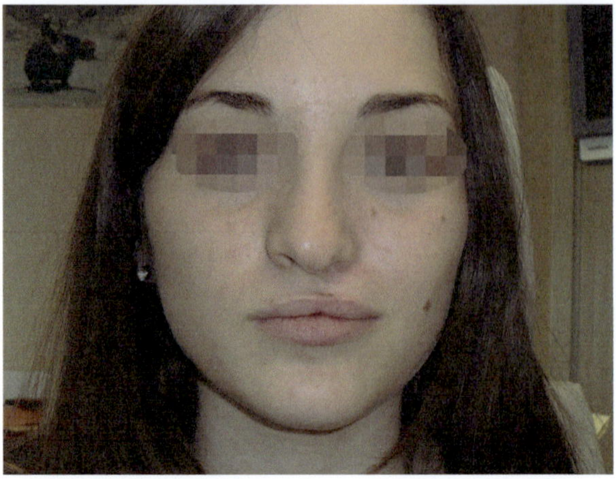

Fig. 10.3 Extraoral view at age 18 years

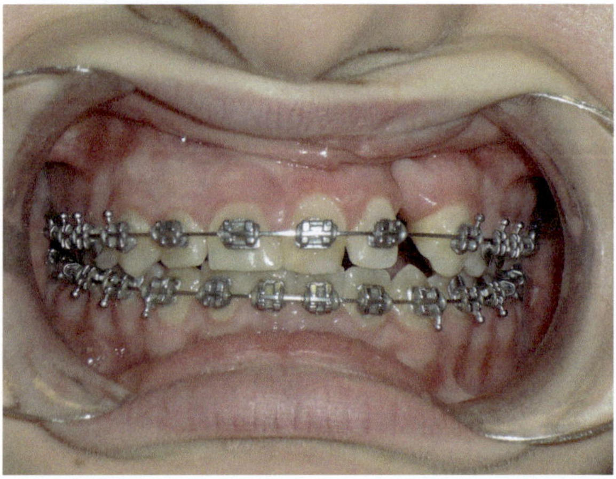

Fig. 10.4 Intraoral view before surgery

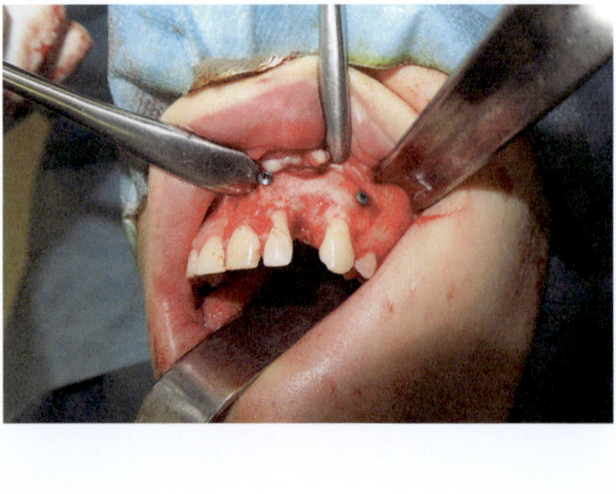

Fig. 10.5 The braces were removed and replaced by an Invisalign®-like space maintainer. Intraoral view of the bone exposure due to elevation of an extensive full-thickness flap. The base of the nasal floor is visible

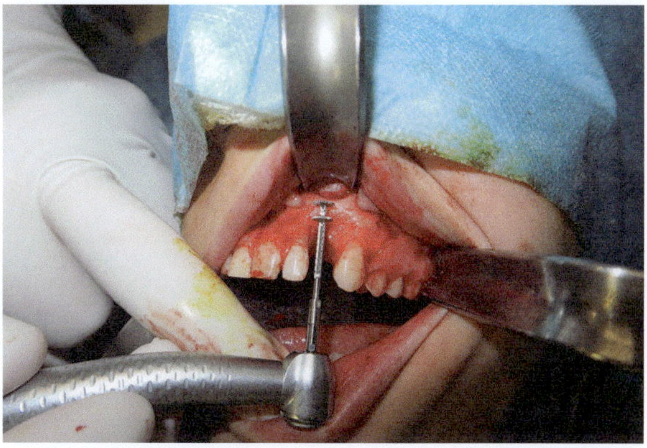

Fig. 10.6 A 5-mm-diameter double cutter is used to determine the osteotomy site. The position can easily be checked at this step by taking an intraoral radiograph. If necessary, the osteotomy site can be moved

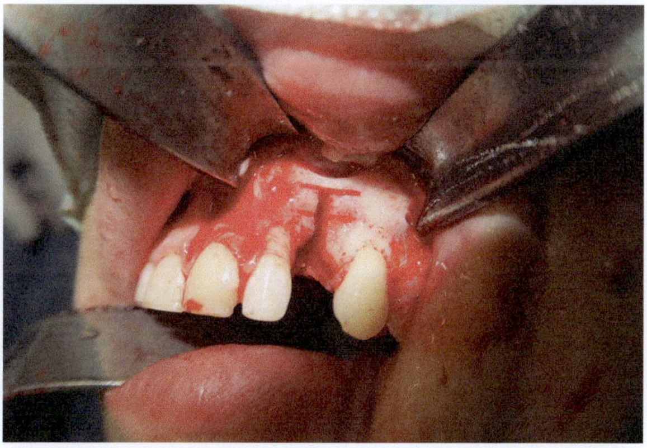

Fig. 10.7 A 7-mm-diameter cutter is used to finalize the "cut" in the bone-grafted area

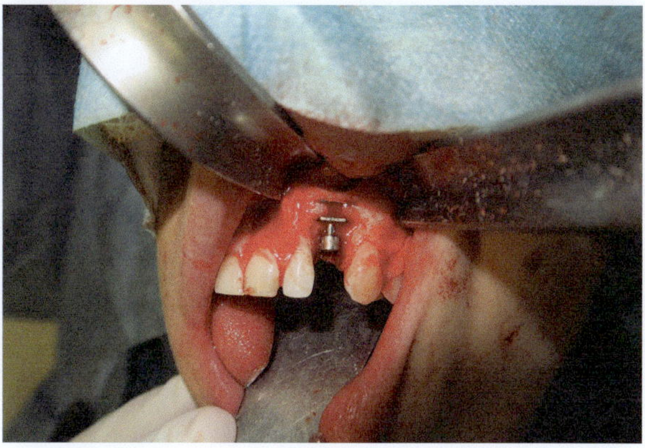

Fig. 10.8 The double Diskimplant® is gently impacted and immediate absolute stability is checked

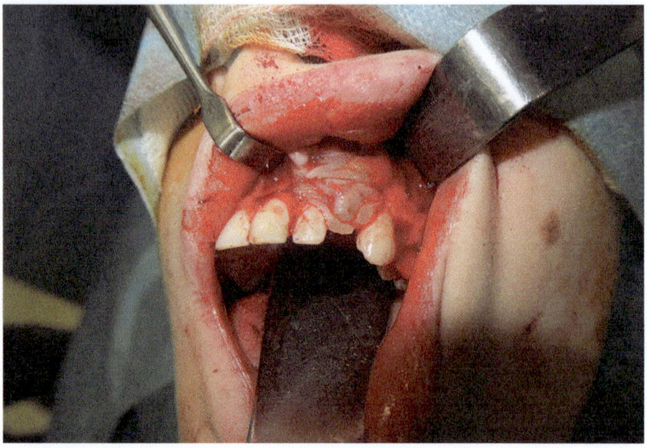

Fig. 10.9 Bone substitute material is used to completely cover the Diskimplant® buccally, crestally, and palatally

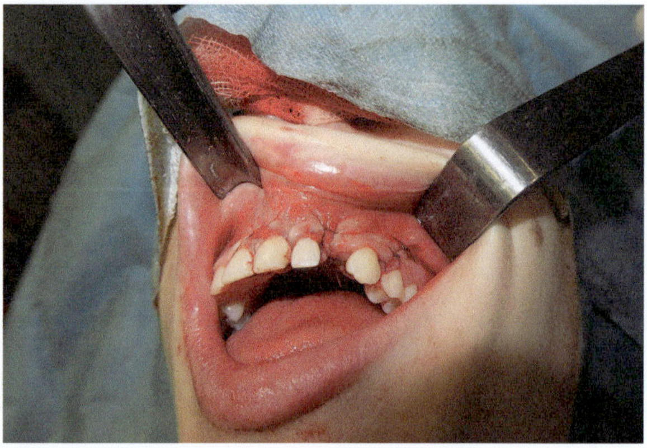

Fig. 10.10 PRF membranes are placed, and a passive, full-thickness flap is repositioned and meticulously sutured with 4/0 sutures (Glycolon®)

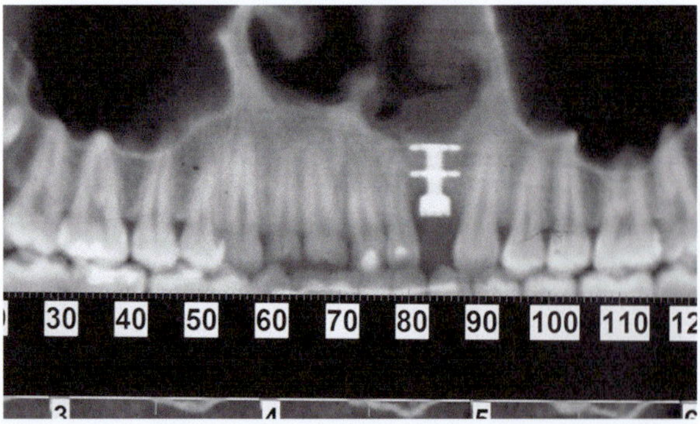

Fig. 10.11 Panoramic radiograph at 9 months. The 7-mm-diameter Diskimplant® is mesially and distally anchored in native living bone; the rest of the implant is in the remaining iliac crest graft. The distance between the two disks is 3 mm. The apical disk lies 1 mm under the nasal floor

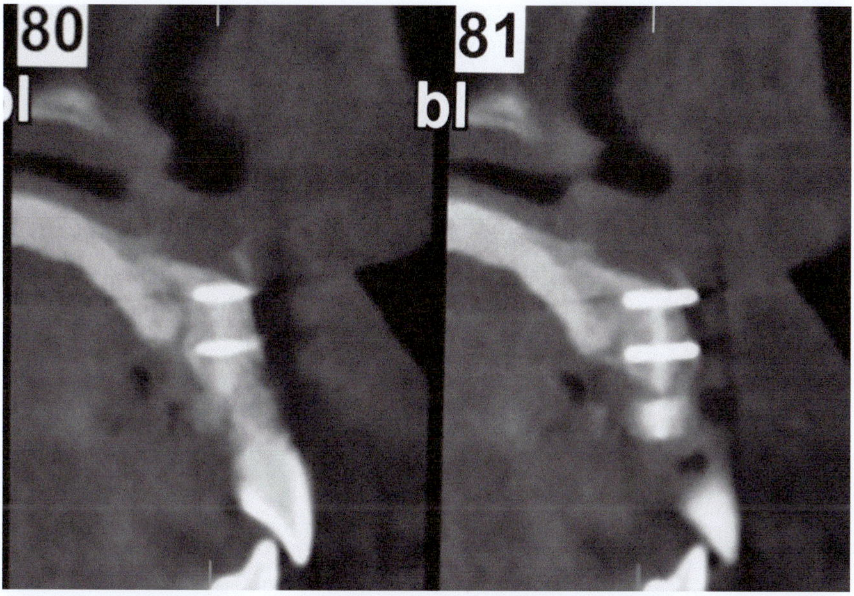

Fig. 10.12 Cone beam CT: sagittal view showing the difficulty of the situation. The crestal emergence of the implant remains in the prosthetic corridor for a screw-secured single tooth

Fig. 10.13 Removable Invisalign® appliance with an incorporated resin tooth

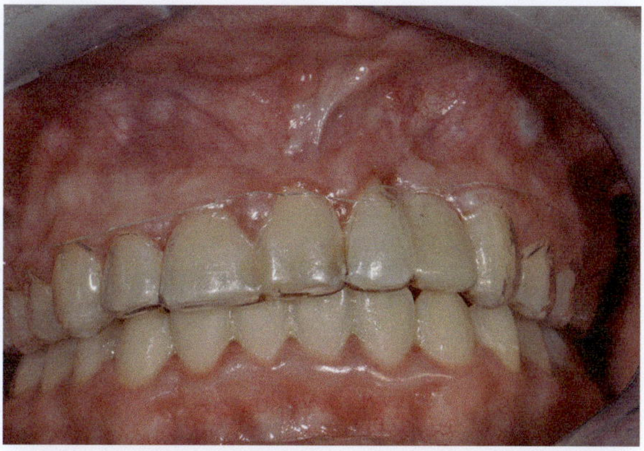

Fig. 10.14 After a 9-month waiting period, the double Diskimplant® appears osseointegrated clinically and radiologically (no pain, mobility, sign of infection, or radiolucency)

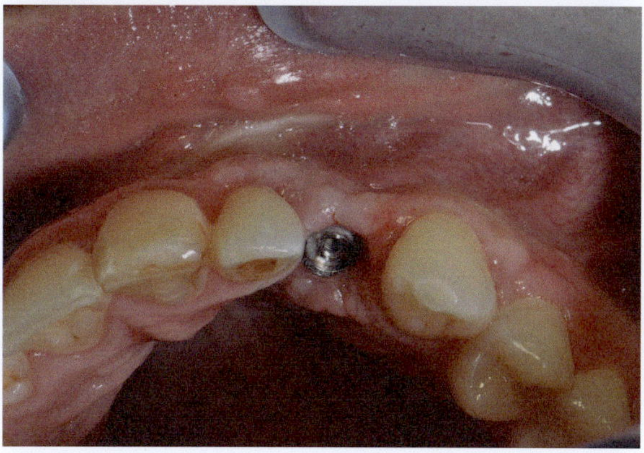

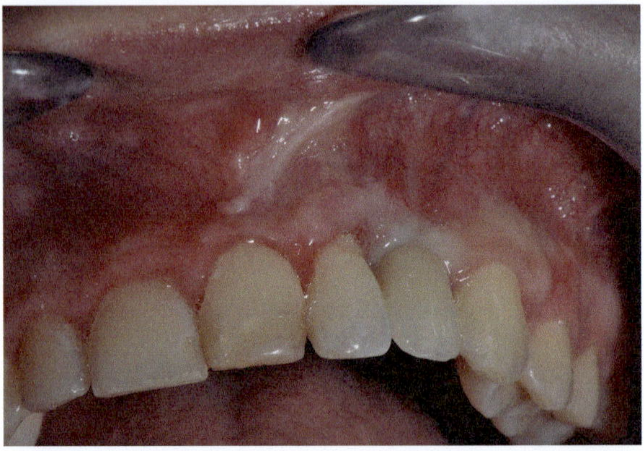

Fig. 10.15 A transitional titanium/composite resin tooth was screw-secured on the double Diskimplant® and placed in function for 1 year (a night guard was worn)

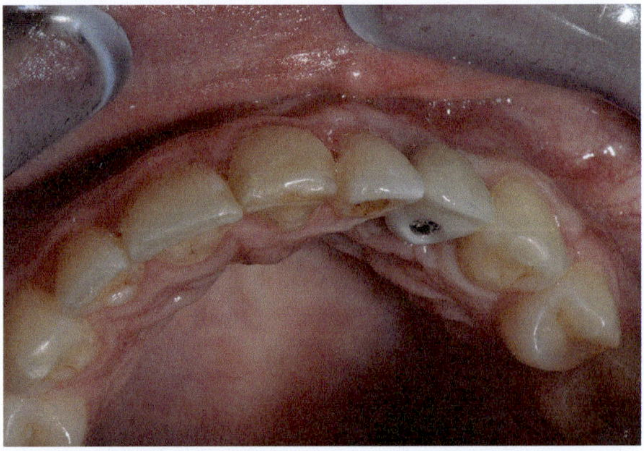

Fig. 10.16 Placement of a zirconia-to-titanium, screw-secured final tooth

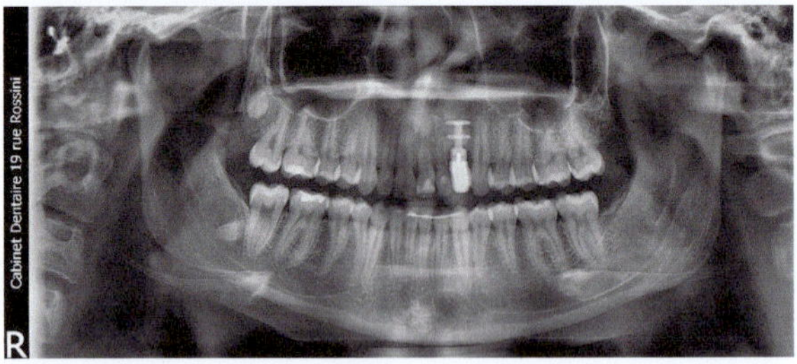

Fig. 10.17 Panoramic radiograph 2.5 years post-op

10.6 Management of the Anterior Region

Single-Tooth Basal Implant (Maxilla) After Traumatic Loss of the Buccal Plate (Delayed Loading) (Figs. 10.18, 10.19, 10.20, 10.21, 10.22, 10.23, 10.24, 10.25, 10.26, 10.27, 10.28, 10.29, 10.30, 10.31, and 10.32)

The buccal plate and tooth 11 were lost during a fall from a bicycle. An initial autologous ramus graft failed, and the patient refused a second bone grafting procedure. After obtaining her informed consent and esthetico-functional analysis including a

3D cone beam exam and the Diskimplant® software library, it was decided to place an asymmetrical double Diskimplant® (base diameter 7 × 5 mm, distance between the two disks 3 mm). As the most apical disk was located 13.5 mm from the bone level emergence, a cutter extender (Orthoroad, France) was required.

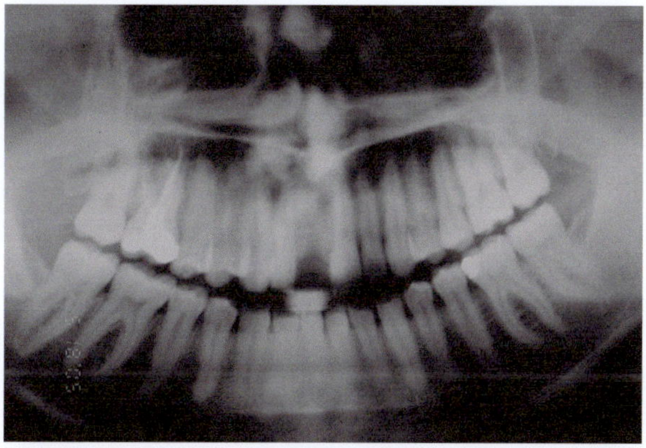

Fig. 10.18 Panoramic view showing post-traumatic loss of the upper right central incisor

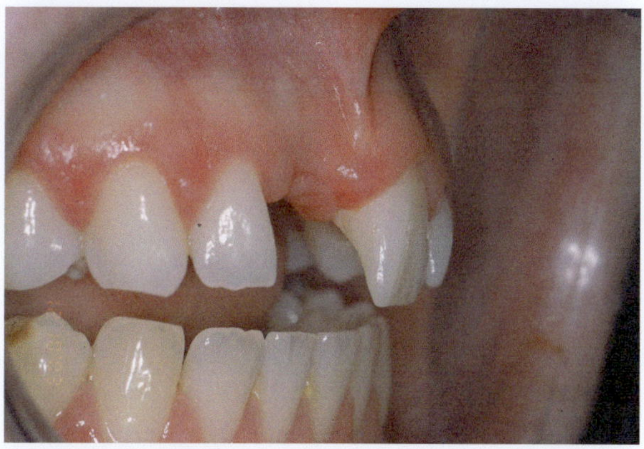

Fig. 10.19 Intraoral view of the knife ridge 6 months post-trauma

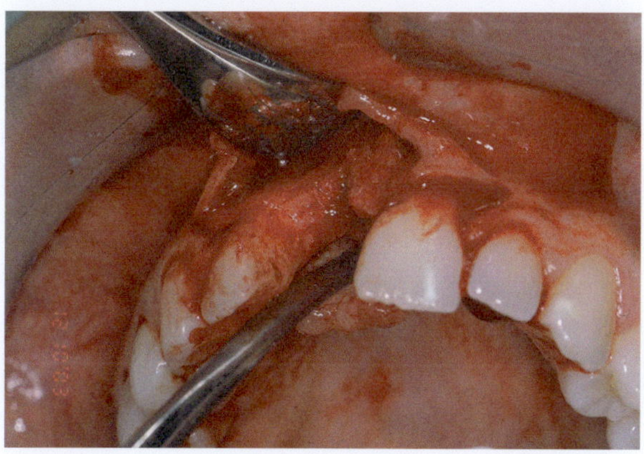

Fig. 10.20 An initial free autologous bone graft failed due to the iatrogenic effect of the temporary removable single-tooth prosthesis

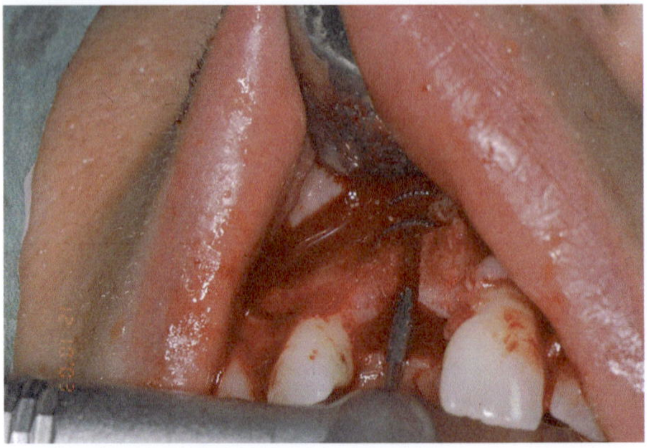

Fig. 10.21 Lateral osteotomy with a 7-mm-diameter double disk titanium cutter

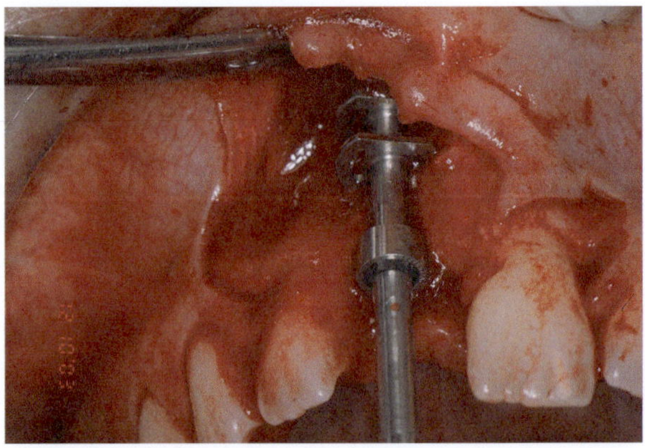

Fig. 10.22 A 7-mm-diameter double Diskimplant® with a long shaft was used to create a crestal notch in order to place the Diskimplant® emergence at bone level

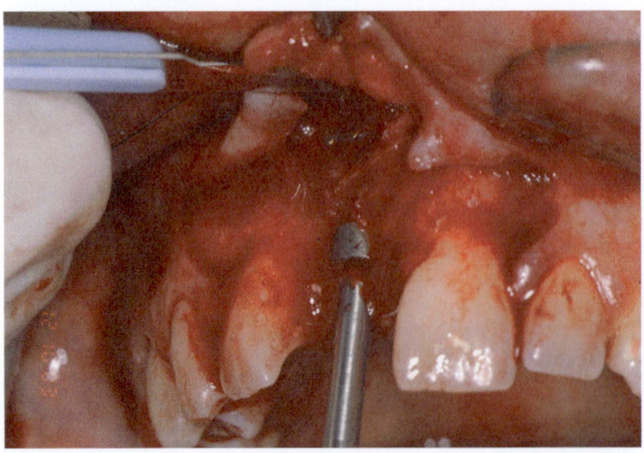

Fig. 10.23 Autologous bone chips collected from the vertical buccal plate were used to cover the lateral bone cut

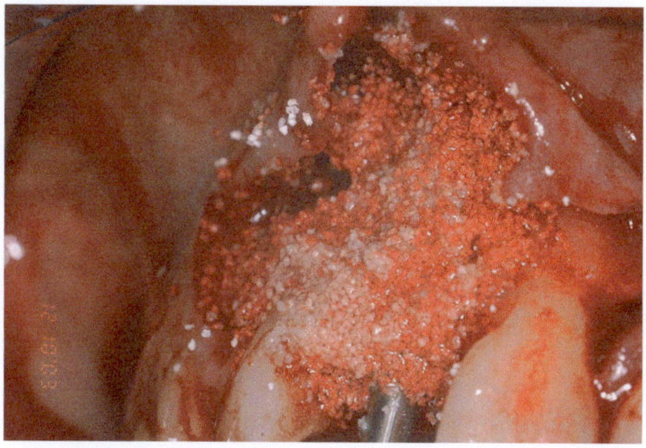

Fig. 10.24 Bone substitute material and PRF were used to fill in the defect and the crestal portion of the Diskimplant® emergence

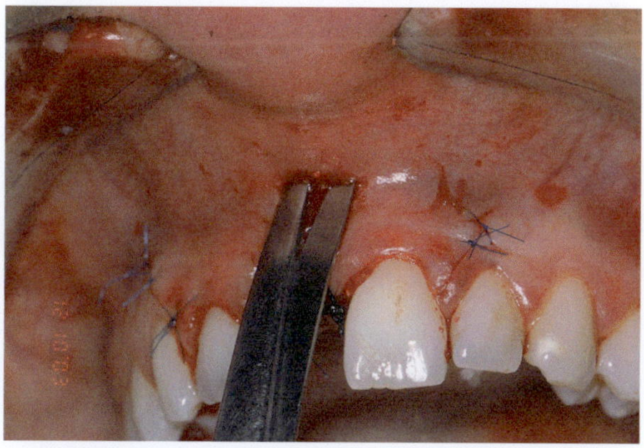

Fig. 10.25 The full-thickness flap was repositioned passively and sutured with 6/0 sutures

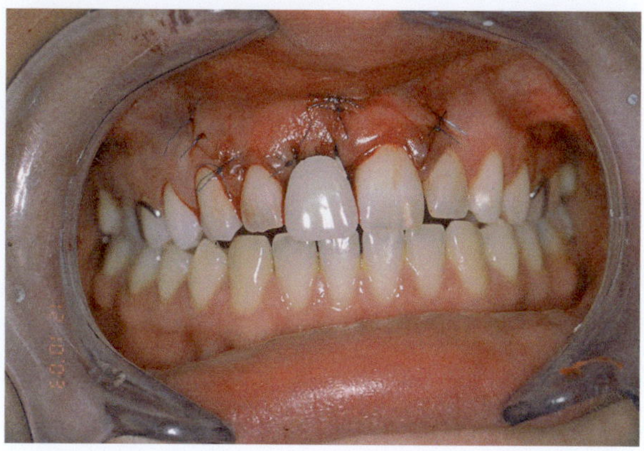

Fig. 10.26 Temporary, removable single-tooth appliance without any occlusal contact to avoid placing pressure on the soft tissues

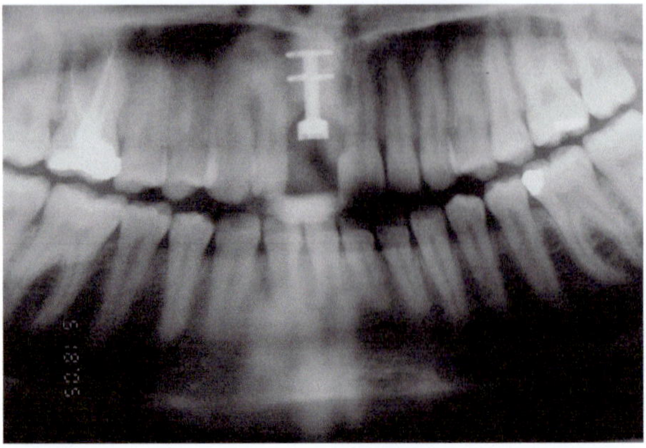

Fig. 10.27 Panoramic view at 6 months

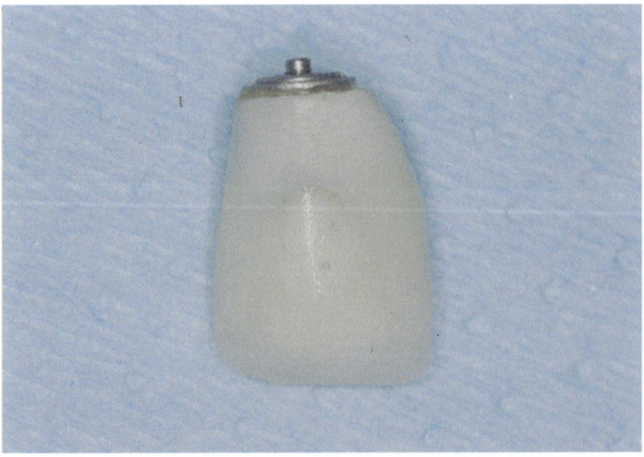

Fig. 10.28 Final screw-secured, zirconia-glued-to-titanium restoration fabricated after the patient had used a fixed transitional resin tooth for 1 year

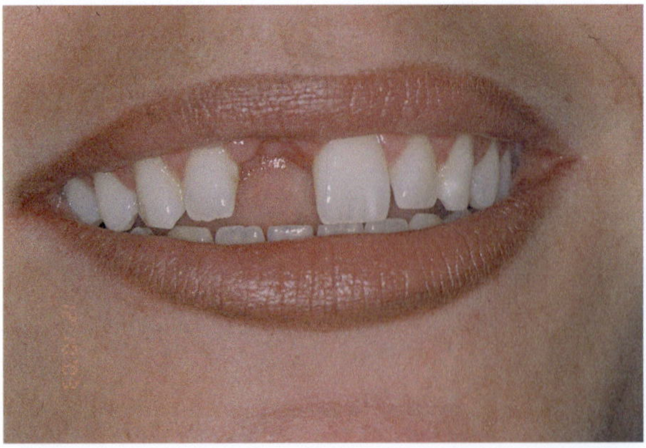

Fig. 10.29 Final gingivo-alveolar aspect of the initial defect site 2 years post-op

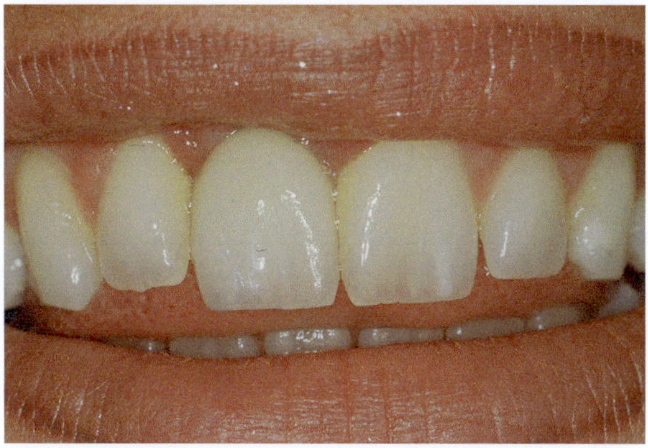

Fig. 10.30 Intraoral cosmetic aspect 4 years post-op (same patient as Fig. 10.29)

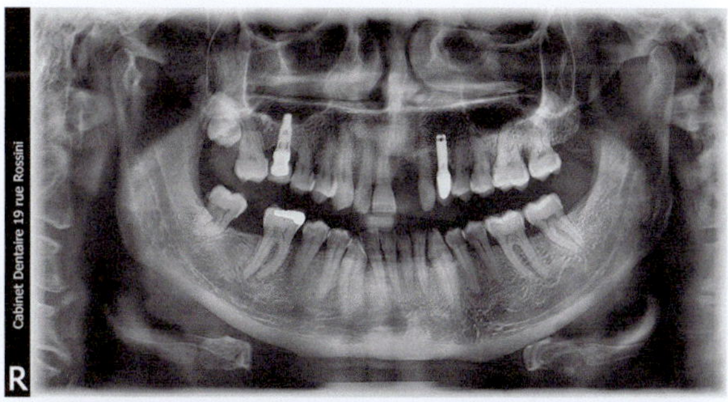

Fig. 10.31 Loss of the upper left central incisor in 2001

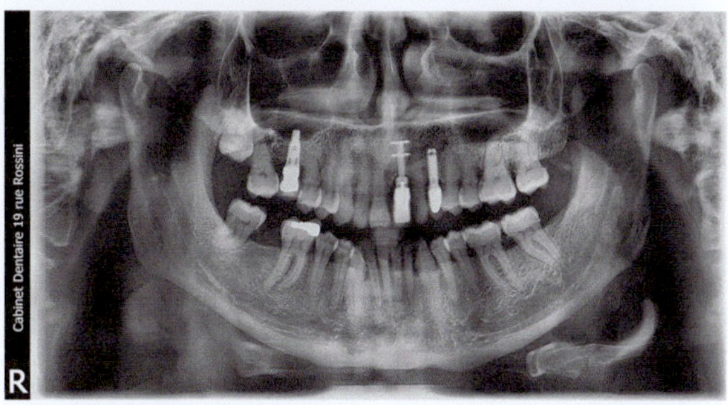

Fig. 10.32 Panoramic radiograph 16 years post-op (2017)

Following a flash of 3 g of amoxicillin 30 minutes before surgery, the protocol was as follows:

- Local-regional anesthesia.
- Crestal incision with distal and mesial releasing incisions.
- Elevation of a full-thickness mucoperiosteal flap.
- Osteotomy with a cutter under copious irrigation.

- Implant impacted from one cortical plate to the other.
- The buccal cut was filled in with small autologous bone chips and a bone substitute material and covered by PRF membranes.
- Flap sutured without tension (4/0 or 5/0 Glycolon® sutures).
- 6-month waiting period (delayed loading).

Single-Tooth Basal Implant After Traumatic Tooth Loss: Immediate Loading (Figs. 10.33, 10.34, 10.35, 10.36, 10.37, 10.38, 10.39, 10.40, 10.41, 10.42, 10.43, 10.44, and 10.45)

Two months after this patient broke his central incisor, the fractured tooth was removed and replaced by a double Diskimplant®. An immediately loaded Maryland appliance was screw-secured to the basal implant.

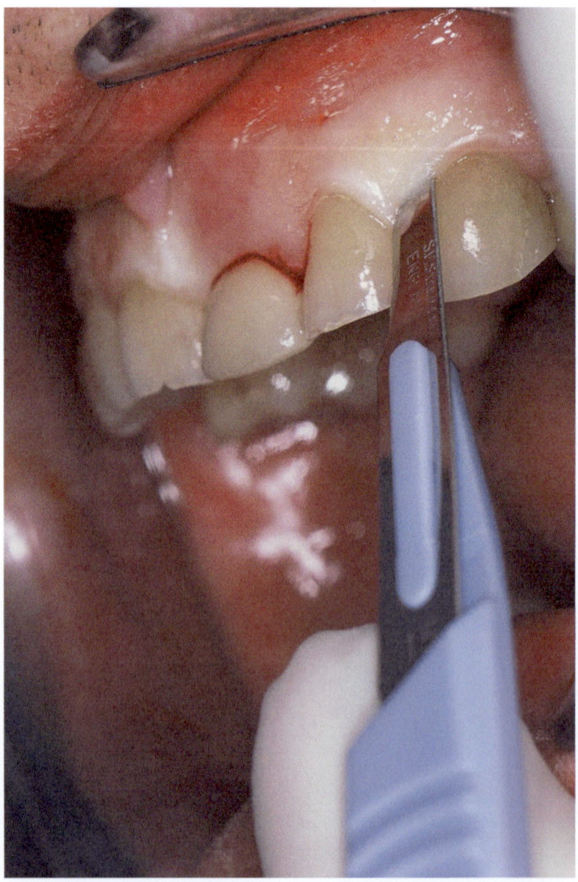

Fig. 10.33 Intraoral view of an upper left central incisor that had fractured 1 year earlier. The patient had no pain, but a chronic fistula was periodically treated with antibiotics and mouthwash. A long full-thickness flap including both adjacent teeth was elevated

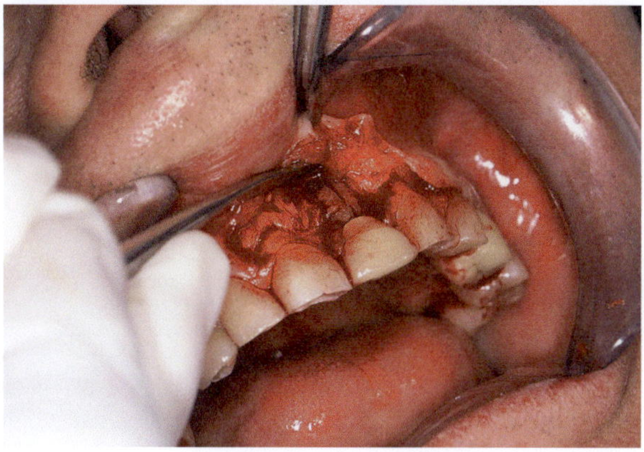

Fig. 10.34 Extensive vestibular defect. The entire alveolar buccal wall has been lost

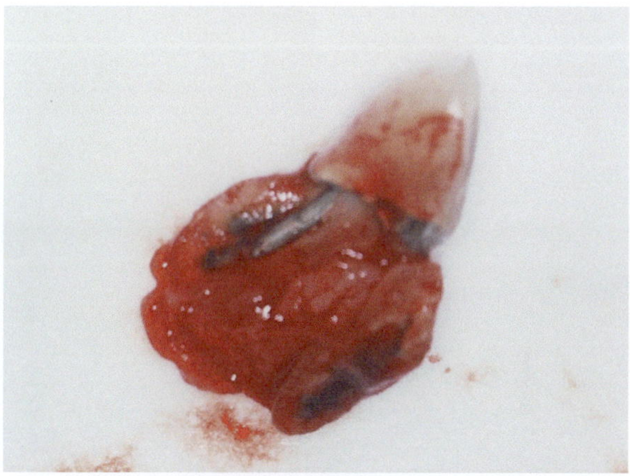

Fig. 10.35 The fractured tooth was removed with a large segment of inflammatory soft tissue (12 × 8 mm)

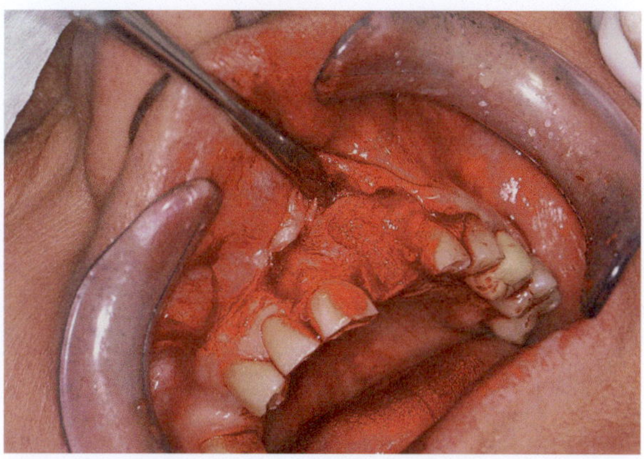

Fig. 10.36 Meticulous cleaning with 10% Betadine® and 3% peroxide plus saline solution

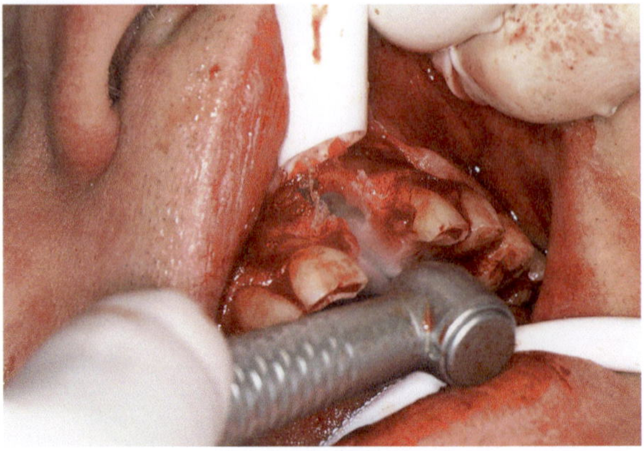

Fig. 10.37 Lateral osteotomy with a 5-mm-diameter triple-disk cutter and then a 7-mm-diameter cutter

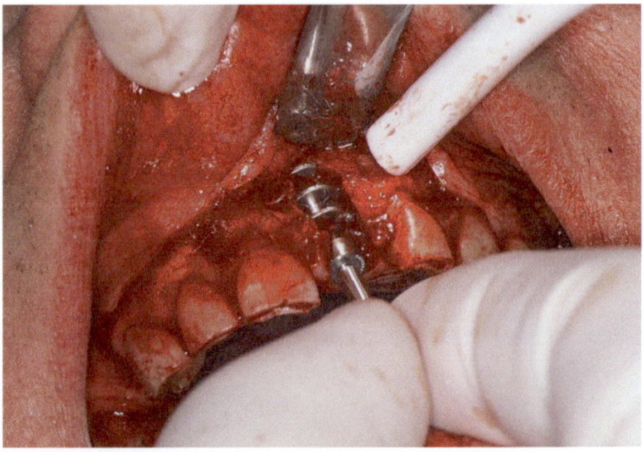

Fig. 10.38 Placement of a 7-mm-diameter triple-disk Diskimplant®

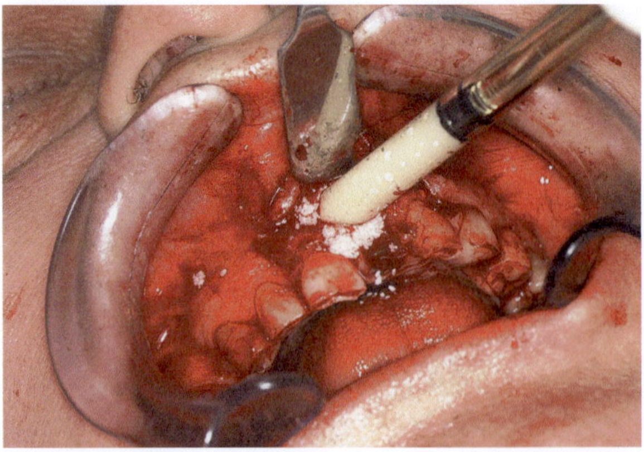

Fig. 10.39 Placement of bone substitute material (ProOsteon®)

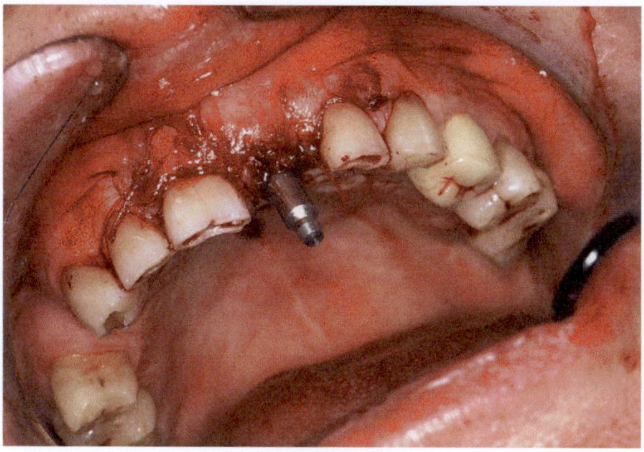

Fig. 10.40 Flap sutured passively with 5/0 sutures. A click-in impression coping was used

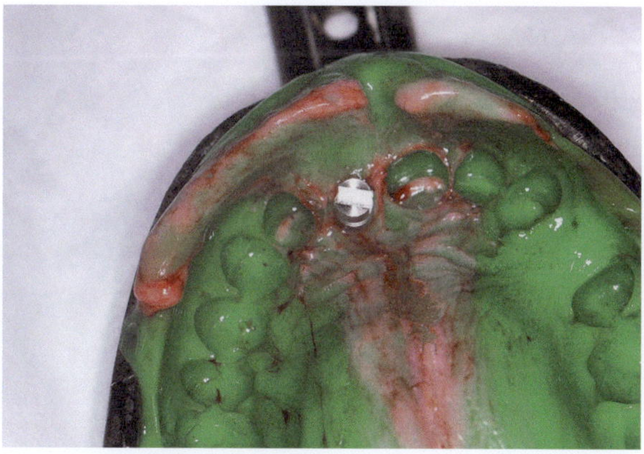

Fig. 10.41 Hydrocolloid impression; impression coping and implant replica (analog) in place

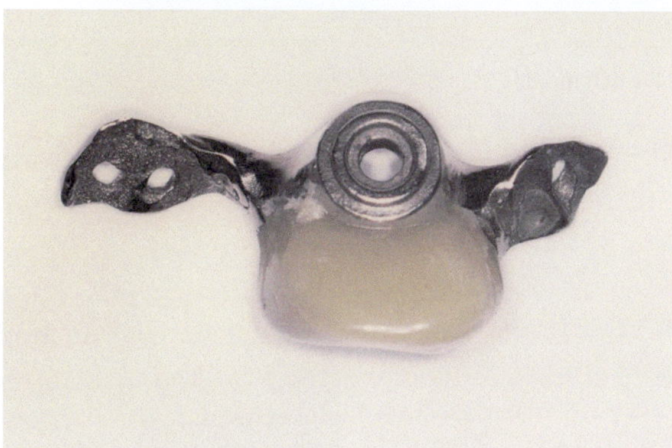

Fig. 10.42 Immediate, transitional single-tooth Maryland bridge-type restoration (screw-secured resin-to-metal)

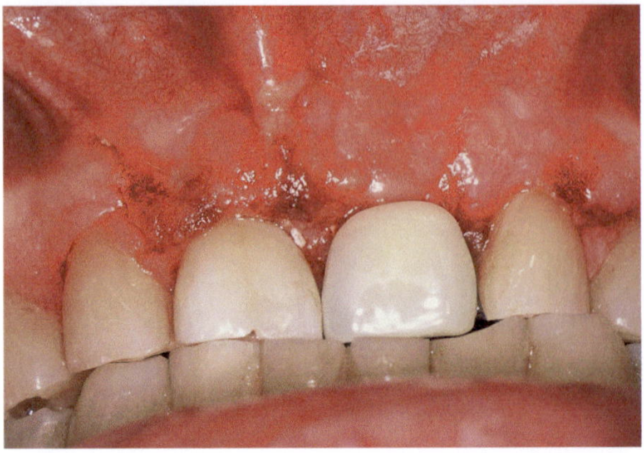

Fig. 10.43 Cosmetic aspect: intraoral buccal view

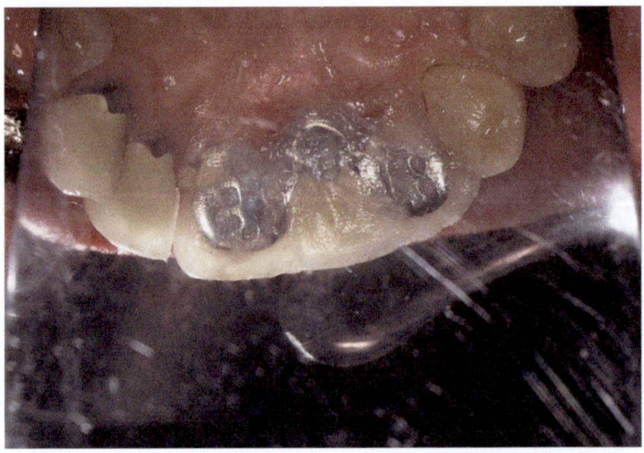

Fig. 10.44 Palatal view of the screw-secured Maryland bridge glued to the adjacent teeth

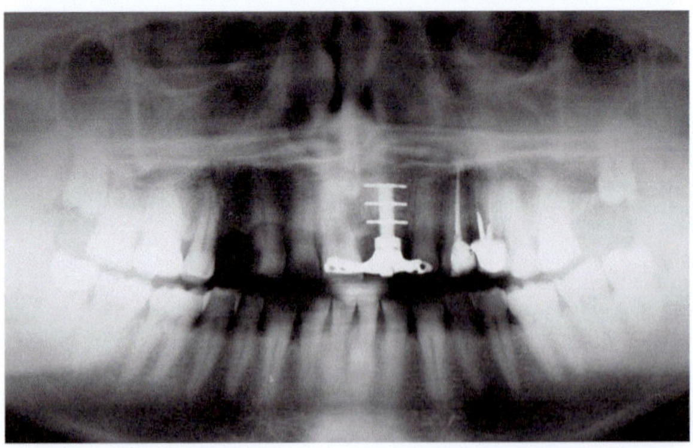

Fig. 10.45 Panoramic view at 6 months

10.7 Management of the Posterior Region (Figs. 10.46, 10.47, 10.48, 10.49, 10.50, 10.51, 10.52, and 10.53)

This patient aged 66 years was rehabilitated by installing Diskimplants® in the posterior maxilla and three root-form implants in the mandible. After a 1-year course of chemotherapy for breast cancer, she lost two of the root-form implants (one in the left posterior region and one on the right side). Following discussion with her oncologist, it was decided to place new implants. As the spongiosa did not appear sufficiently dense, two 9-mm-diameter Diskimplants® were installed between the cortical plates on each side. Individual ceramic prosthetic teeth were fabricated 6 months later. Nine years post-op, the patient was in complete remission, and all implants appeared clinically and radiologically integrated.

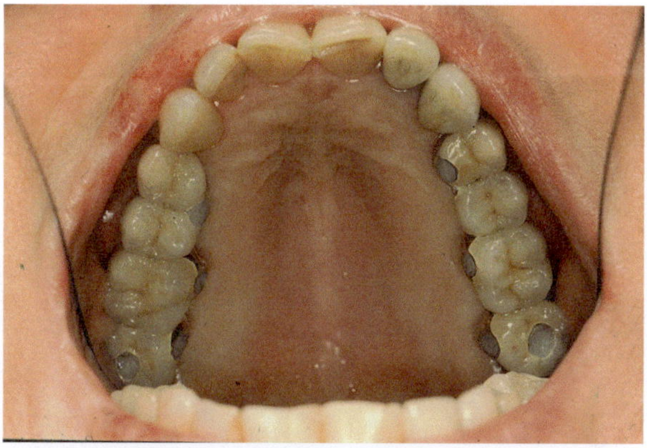

Fig. 10.46 Intraoral view in 2008 of an upper jaw that had been rehabilitated in 1998 (Diskimplants® and tubero-pterygoid implants)

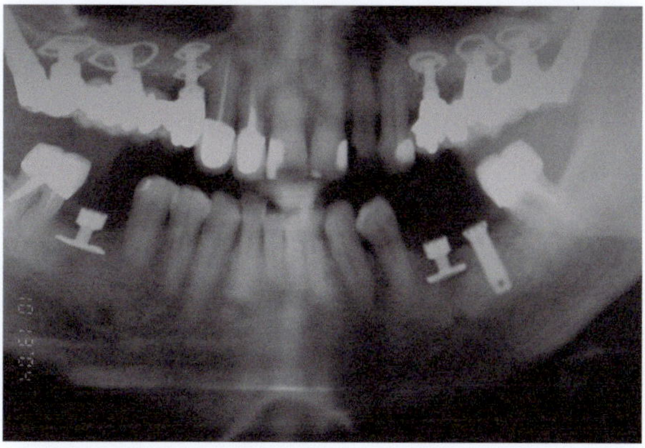

Fig. 10.47 Panoramic view 6 months post-op: these two Diskimplants® were installed in the posterior mandible in 2008 (submerged technique), 2 months after two root-form implants had been lost in the same sector

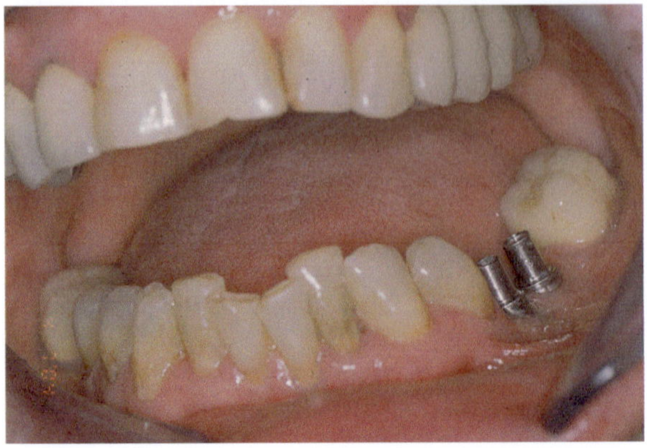

Fig. 10.48 An abutment was screw-secured onto each implant

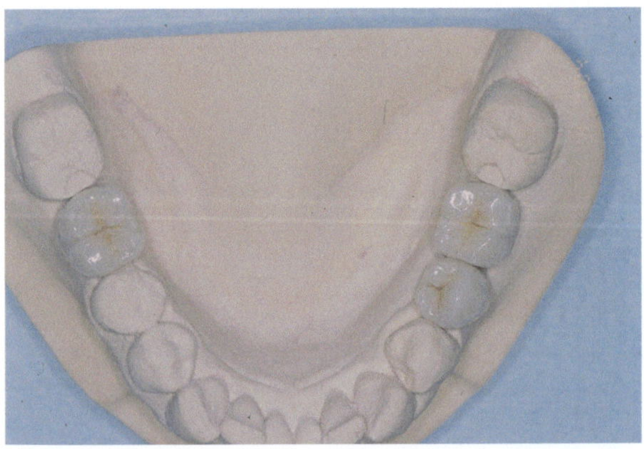

Fig. 10.49 Master model for three individual crowns (Empress® ceramic)

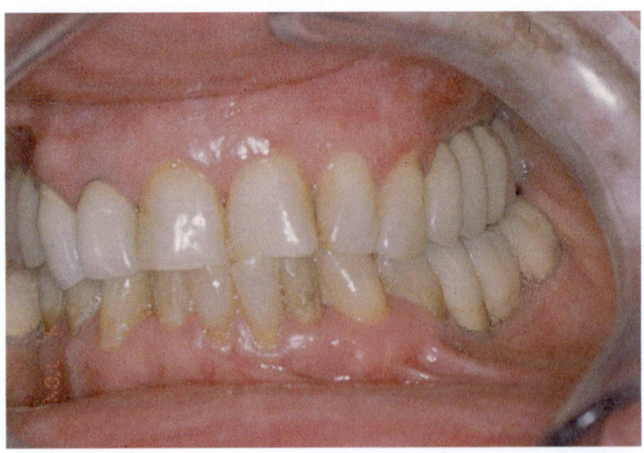

Fig. 10.50 Intraoral view of the crowns screw-secured to the implants in the upper jaw; cemented single implant-supported tooth in the mandible

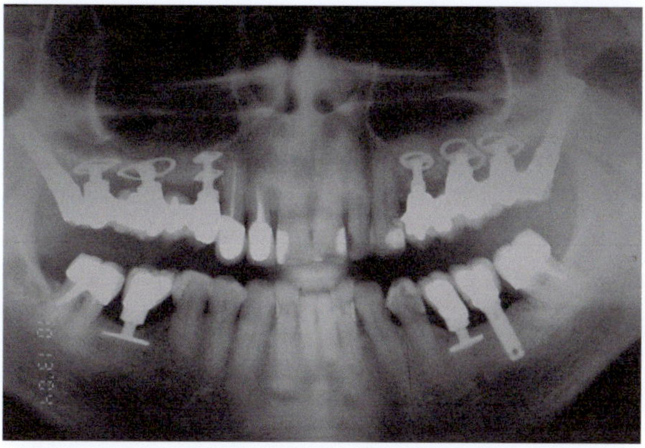

Fig. 10.51 Panoramic view in 2016

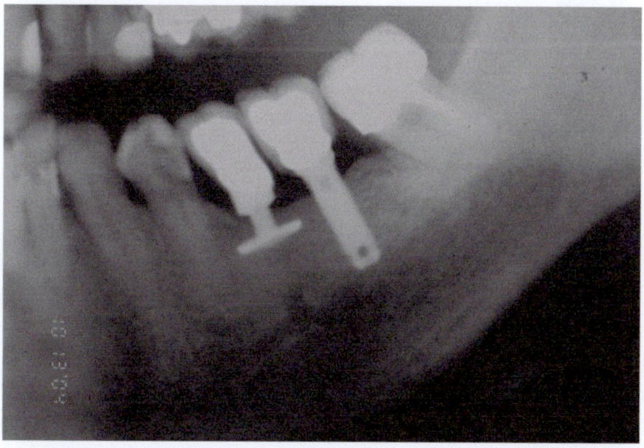

Fig. 10.52 Periapical radiograph of the left posterior mandible: no bone loss or peri-implantitis

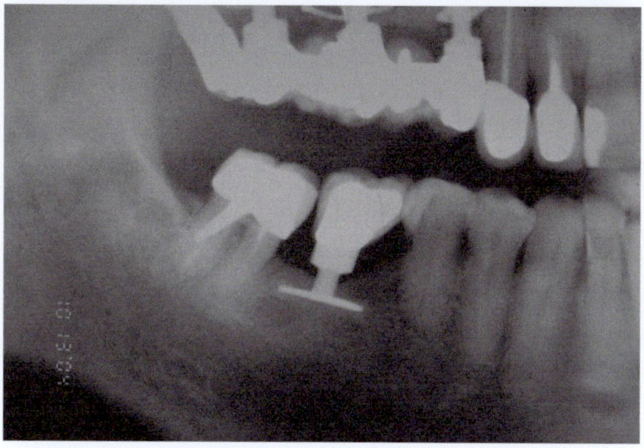

Fig. 10.53 Same situation on the right side

Conflict of interest statement Gérard M. Scortecci is the inventor of the Diskimplant and holder of several associated patents that are exploited by the Victory company. He is an unpaid consultant to this firm and a minority shareholder in the company. No money was received from any of the companies mentioned in the book or from any of the companies whose products are mentioned.

Recommended Reading

1. Ericsson I, Nilson H, Lindh T, Nilner K, Randow J. Immediate functional loading of Brånemark single-tooth implants. An 18 months' clinical pilot follow-up study. Clin Oral Implants Res. 2000;11:26–33.
2. Afota F. Stratégies chirurgicales pré-implantaires et implantaires des séquelles de fentes labio-maxillo-palatines: Etat de l'art et analyse de cas. Thèse de Docteur en Chirurgie Dentaire, n° 42-57-16-22, Université de Nice-Sophia Antipolis (DDS thesis); 2016.
3. Andersson B. Implants for single-tooth replacement. A clinical and experimental study on the Brånemark CeraOne system. Swed Dent J suppl. 1995;108:1–41.
4. Andersson B, Odman P, Lindvall AM, Brånemark PI. Cemented single crowns on osseointegrated implants after 5 years. Results from a prospective study on CeraOne. Int J Prosthodont. 1998;11:212–8.
5. Ekfeldt A, Carlsson GE, Borjesson G. Clinical evaluation of single-tooth restorations supported by osseointegrated implants: a retrospective study. Int J Oral Maxillofac Implants. 1994;9:179–83.
6. Ekfeldt A, Fürst B, Carlsson GE. Zirconia abutments for single-tooth implant restorations; a 10- to 11-year follow-up study. Clin Oral Implants Res. 2017;28:1303–8. https://doi.org/10.1111/clr.12975.
7. Engquist B, Nilson H, Astrand P. Single-tooth replacement by osseointegrated Brånemark implants. Clin Oral Implants Res. 1995;6:238–45.
8. Ericsson I, Randow K, Glantz PO, Lindhe J, Nilner K. Some clinical and radiographical features of submerged and non-submerged titanium implants. Clin Oral Implants Res. 1994;5:185–9.
9. Ericsson I, Randow K, Nilner K, Petersson A. Some clinical and radiographical features of submerged and non-submerged titanium implants. A 5-year follow-up study. Clin Oral Implants Res. 1997;8:422–6.
10. Ganeles J, Wesmeijer D. Early and immediately restored and loaded dental implants for single-tooth and partial-arch applications. Int J Oral Maxillofac Implants. 2004;19 suppl:92–102.
11. Jemt T, Petersson P. A 3-year follow-up study on single implant treatment. J Dent. 1993;21:203–8.
12. Misch CE. Contemporary implant dentistry. 2nd ed. St Louis: Mosby; 1999. p. 397–428.
13. Ohrnell LO, Palmquist J, Brånemark PI. Single tooth replacement. In: Worthington P, Brånemark PI, editors. Advanced Osseointegration Surgery: Applications in the Maxillofacial region. Chicago: Quintessence; 1992. p. 211–32.
14. Palacci P. Peri-implant soft-tissue management: papilla regeneration technique. In: Palacci P, Ericsson I, Engstrand P, Rangert B, editors. Optimal implant positioning and soft-tissue management for the Brånemark system. Berlin: Quintessence; 1995. p. 59–70.
15. Palmer RM, Smith BJ, Palmer PJ, Floyd PD. A prospective study on Astra single tooth implants. Clin Oral Implants Res. 1997;8:173–9.
16. Parel SM, Sullivan DY. Esthetics and osseointegration. Dallas: Osseointegration Seminars; 1989.
17. Scheller H, Urgell JP, Kultje C, Klineberg I, Goldberg PV, Stevenson-Moore P, et al. A 5-year multicenter study on implant-supported single crown restorations. Int J Oral Maxillofac Implants. 1998;13:212–8.
18. Schmitt A, Zarb GA. The longitudinal effectiveness of osseointegrated dental implants for single tooth replacement. J Prosthodont. 1993;6:197–202.

Further Reading

Piattelli A, Paolantonio M, Scarano A. Immediate loading of titanium plasma-sprayed screw-shaped implants in man: a clinical and histological report of two cases. J Periodontol. 1997; 68:591–7.

Randow K, Ericsson I, Nilner K, Petersson A, Glantz PO. Immediate functional loading of Brånemark implants. An 18-month clinical follow-up study. Clin Oral Implants Res. 1999;10:8–15.

Resnik RR, Misch CE. Misch's avoiding complications in oral implantology. St. Louis: Elsevier; 2017.

Schnitman PA, Wöhrle PS, Rubenstein JE. Immediate fixed interim prostheses supported by two-stage threaded implants: methodology and results. J Oral Implantol. 1990;16:96–105.

Schnitman PA, Wöhrle PS, Rubenstein JE, Da Silva JD, Wang NH. Ten-year results for Brånemark implants immediately loaded with fixed prostheses at implant placement. Int J Oral Maxillofac Implants. 1997;12:495–503.

Scortecci G, Bourbon B. Prothèse sur Diskimplant®: la dent unitaire. RFPD Actual. 1991;31:21–9.

Scortecci G. Immediate function of cortically anchored disk-design implants without bone augmentation in moderately to severely resorbed completely edentulous maxillae. Oral Implantol. 1999;25(2):70–9.

Tarnow DP, Emitiag S, Classi A. Immediate loading of threaded implants at stage one surgery in edentulous arches. Ten consecutive case reports with 1- to 5-year data. Int J Oral Maxillofac Implants. 1997;12(3):319–24.

Partial Edentulism

11

Gérard M. Scortecci and Carl E. Misch

11.1 The Complexity of Partial Edentulism

Epidemiology of Partial Edentulism

Millions of individuals worldwide over the age of 18 years are partially edentulous. Such clinical situations are often more complex to handle than total edentulism and interdental single-tooth replacement. Patterns of partial tooth loss can be classified into three categories: (i) single interdental, (ii) multiple interdental, and (iii) free-end loss. Accepted treatments include fixed restorations on natural abutments, removable partial dentures, and implant-supported fixed partial dentures.

Patient Selection and Treatment Planning

Treatment planning for basal implant placement in partially edentulous patients must be designed mechanically for long-term success. This requires a thorough evaluation of the status of the remaining teeth and oral hygiene. All tooth-related pathologies must be treated or brought under control before surgery. The extent of the planned restoration and the related cost must be clearly explained to the patient before implant surgery is performed. In particular, individuals who have lost teeth in different quadrants and periodontally compromised, partially edentulous patients with limited

C. E. Misch (Deceased)

G. M. Scortecci (✉)
University of Nice-Sophia Antipolis Medical School, Nice, France

New York University, New York, NY, USA

University of Southern California, Los Angeles, CA, USA

Private Practice, Nice, France
e-mail: scortecci@wanadoo.fr

© Springer Nature Switzerland AG 2019

G. M. Scortecci (ed.), *Basal Implantology*, https://doi.org/10.1007/978-3-319-44873-2_11

finances are often best managed with a conventional removable appliance until a state of total edentulism is reached, at which time implants may be reconsidered. This approach can sometimes actually prove less expensive in the long run.

Selection criteria for implant placement in partially edentulous patients include:

- Psychological and physical health (general and local) compatible with implant surgery. Only individuals who are able to maintain an acceptable level of oral hygiene should be considered acceptable candidates. Heavy smokers must be fully informed of the potential risk of implant loss.
- Bone quality and quantity at the surgical site capable of providing reliable support for the selected endosseous implants.
- Favorable occlusion (at least 4 mm of available prosthetic space between the gingival level and the opposite occlusal surface).

Periodontal Conditions

Although dental implants can be used safely for selected, partially edentulous patients with periodontal disease, conventional prostheses are often more predictable and less expensive, especially if the disease process is ongoing. Patients with advanced periodontitis must be fully informed of the long-term clinical and financial aspects of implant treatment because repeated implant surgery and related costs must be expected during subsequent years as additional teeth are lost.

Occlusal Conditions: Parafunctions

The type of edentulism and the presence or absence of the canine teeth correspond to completely different clinical situations. Bruxism and clenching habits in particular must be detected at this point. Preparation of models mounted in occlusion on semi-adjustable or fully adjustable articulators permits anticipation of problems, evaluation of the prosthetic space and the required number of implants, and fabrication of a surgical template for implant placement. An increase in the vertical dimension may prove necessary, but such cases require a major full-mouth rehabilitation.

- *Kennedy class II patients*: if the cross side is compromised, rehabilitation must be included in the treatment plan and carried out first.
- *Kennedy class I patients*: both sides must receive dental implants. Surgery can be performed simultaneously or consecutively, but the fixed implant-supported partial denture must be installed simultaneously on both edentulous sides in order to restore normal function and avoid TMJ disorders.

Cantilevers on implants should be avoided for partially edentulous patients, especially when opposite natural dentition is present, because they are a major source of fatigue problems, screw loosening, and fracture of components and/or implants [1, 2].

Temporomandibular Joint (TMJ) Disorders

Acute pain and/or reduced mouth opening must be treated prior to implant installation. Occlusion can then be re-evaluated using a conventional removable denture and bite plane.

Infra-sinus Area

When implants are planned for the posterior maxilla, the patient should always be asked two questions: "have you ever been treated for sinusitis or rhinitis?" and "do you suffer from allergies involving the sinuses?". If the patient answers yes to one or both of these questions, he or she should first be referred to an ENT specialist, even if the CT scan or cone-beam CT does not reveal any radiologically evident pathology. A resorbed posterior maxilla is an indication for a sinus lift or installation of a zygomatic and/or pterygoid basal implant.

Delayed Versus Immediate Loading Protocol

The number and location of implants, bone quality and quality, and dental, occlusal, and periodontal conditions must all be evaluated carefully prior to making a decision. A delayed loading protocol is usually preferable for treatment of partial edentulism (one to three implants). However, immediate functional loading provides predictable results in selected cases when three or more basal implants are planned and occlusal conditions are favorable [3].

Connection with Natural Teeth

It is technically possible to include natural teeth in an implant-supported denture [4]. This approach can be used in certain cases with a fair long-term prognosis. However, as teeth and implants react differently, connection with natural teeth should generally be avoided for mechanical and biological reasons:

- Mechanically speaking, implants are rigid, whereas teeth are slightly mobile because of the periodontal ligament.
- Biologically, including natural teeth in a highly rigid system eliminates functional stimulation. Periodontal problems and tooth intrusion can occur. Teeth are sensitive to decay and may be lost. The entire fixed partial denture may then have to be redone and new implants installed in the extraction sites.

Such problems must be anticipated before connecting implants with teeth [4–13]. Moreover, for psychological reasons, patients generally prefer to keep their remaining teeth "as they are" rather than have them included in an implant-supported denture.

11.2 Case Studies

Case Study 1: Kennedy Class II (Immediate Functional Loading Protocol) (Figs. 11.1, 11.2 and 11.3)

These two patients were fully informed of their clinical situation and were given a choice between a sinus lift procedure and basal implants. Conventional root-form implants had been in service in the mandible before the upper jaw was finalized. The posterior maxillae were rehabilitated with Diskimplants® and a tubero-pterygoid root-form implant (panoramic checkup at 20 years: 1995–2015).

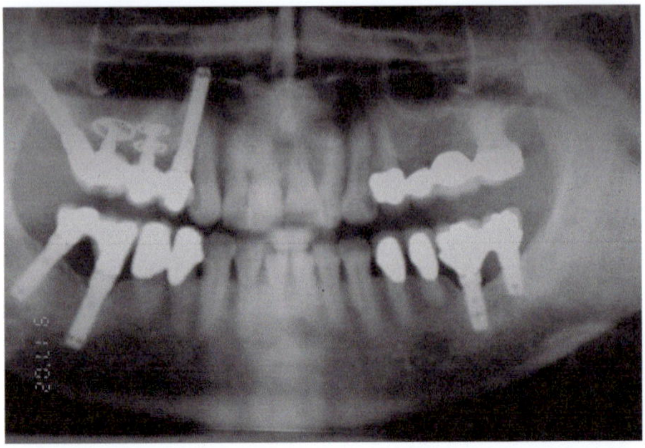

Fig. 11.1 Panoramic view of basal implants located under the right sinus after 20 years of service

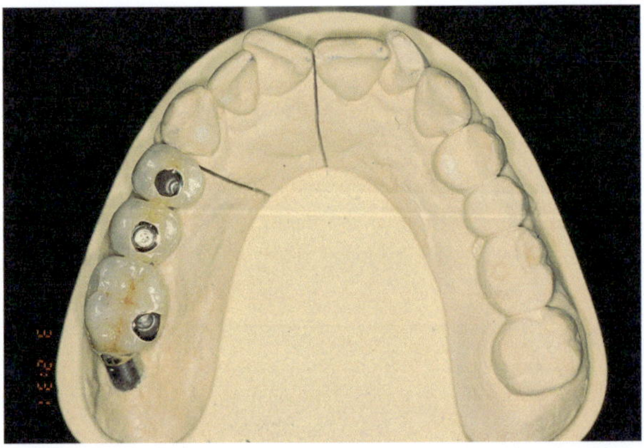

Fig. 11.2 Occlusal view of the ceramic-baked-to-gold final rehabilitation (same patient as Fig. 11.1)

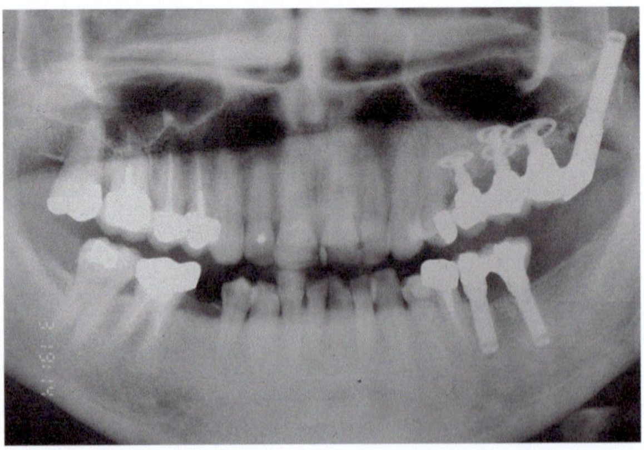

Fig. 11.3 Basal Diskimplants® under the left sinus and one pterygoid implant. Immediate loading protocol. Panograph after 24 years of function

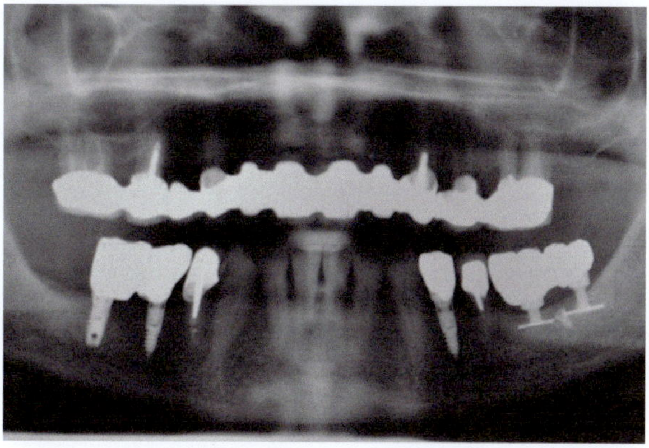

Fig. 11.4 Atrophic posterior left mandible: two mono-disk Diskimplants® were left submerged for 6 months before loading. Two short (6 mm) implants had been lost previously. Panoramic view 4 years post-op

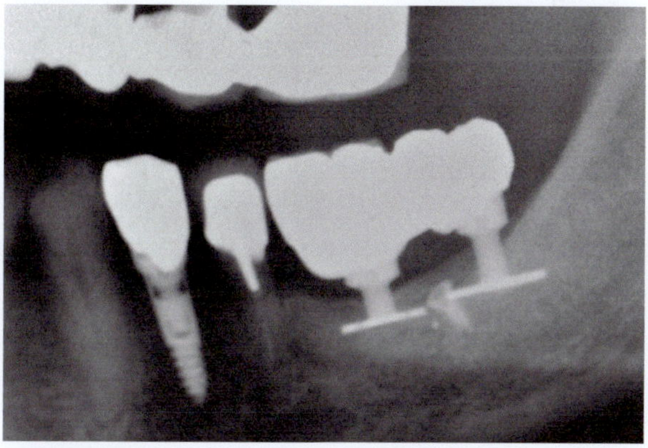

Fig. 11.5 Periapical view. An orthopedic bone screw was inserted against the distal Diskimplant® to improve primary stability

Case Study 2: Posterior Mandible (Figs. 11.4 and 11.5)
Following placement of short implants in the posterior left mandible in 2009, peri-implantitis developed over the next 3 years. In 2012 these implants were lost and replaced by two mono-disk Diskimplants® (dia. 9 mm) that were left submerged for 6 months. A panoramic radiograph and retro-alveolar films taken in 2017 revealed complete osseointegration (bone depth <3 mm).

Case Study 3: Partial Edentulism, Kennedy Class II with Two Impacted Canines (Figs. 11.6, 11.7, 11.8, 11.9, 11.10 and 11.11)
This patient wished to keep her three front teeth. Retrieval of the two impacted canines would have definitively compromised the entire premaxilla, with loss of the front teeth and extensive bone defects.

In 1991, both sides were equipped with root-form and basal implants using an immediate loading protocol (the prosthesis was placed after 48 h). The provisional rehabilitations were monitored for 1 year. After individual verification of all implants to check

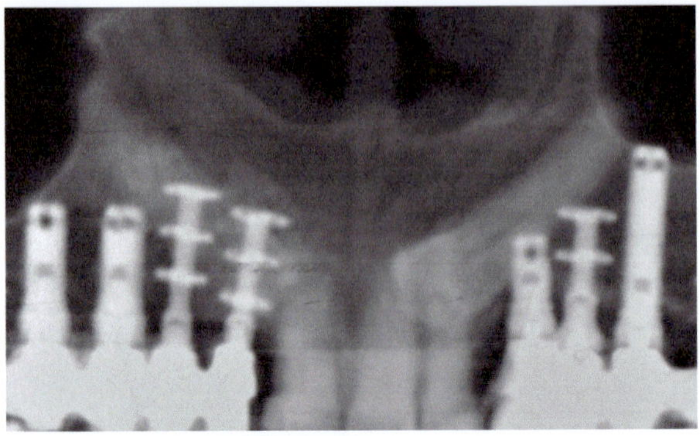

Fig. 11.6 Two impacted upper canines left in place. Basal and axial implants had been placed 23 years earlier.

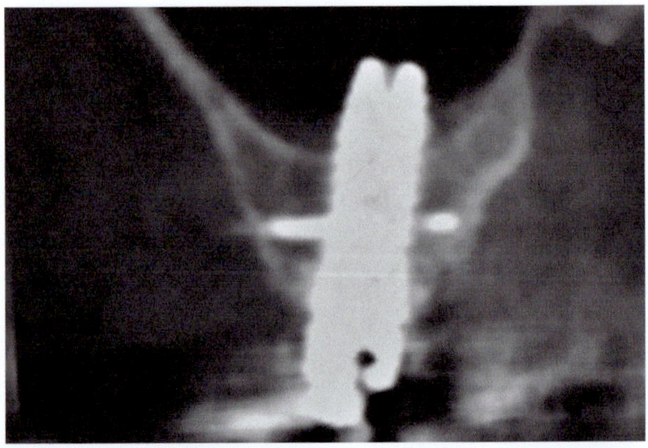

Fig. 11.7 Same patient as Fig. 11.6. This patient fractured the shaft of a mono-disk Diskimplant® under the right sinus when she bit down on a hard object. A Fractal® root-form implant (Victory, France) was placed through the fractured disk

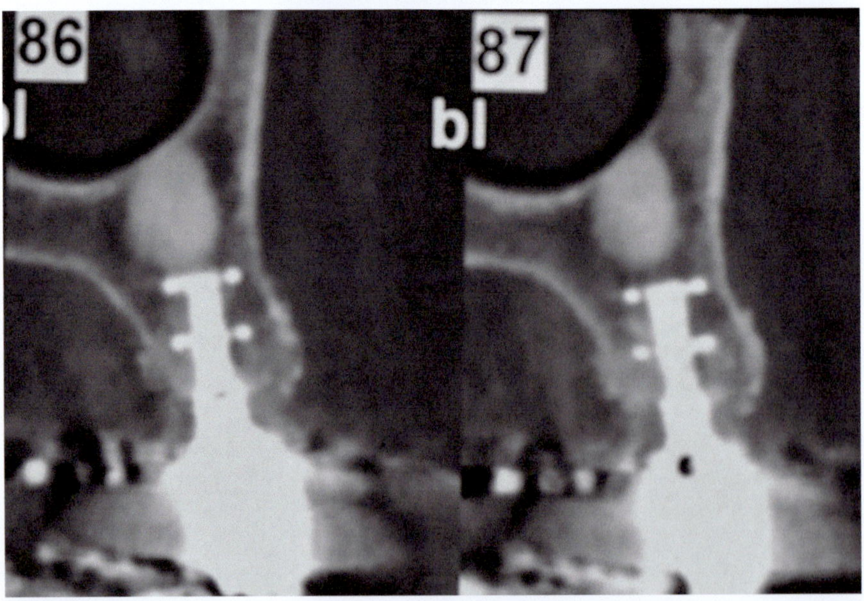

Fig. 11.8 CT scan of a double Diskimplant® under the impacted upper left canine

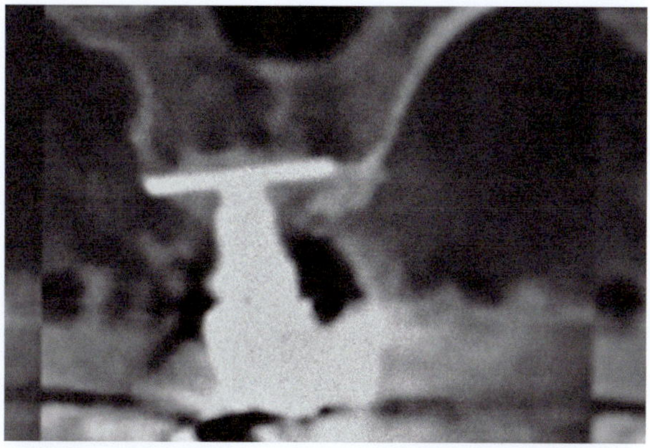

Fig. 11.9 Mono-disk Diskimplant® under the left sinus

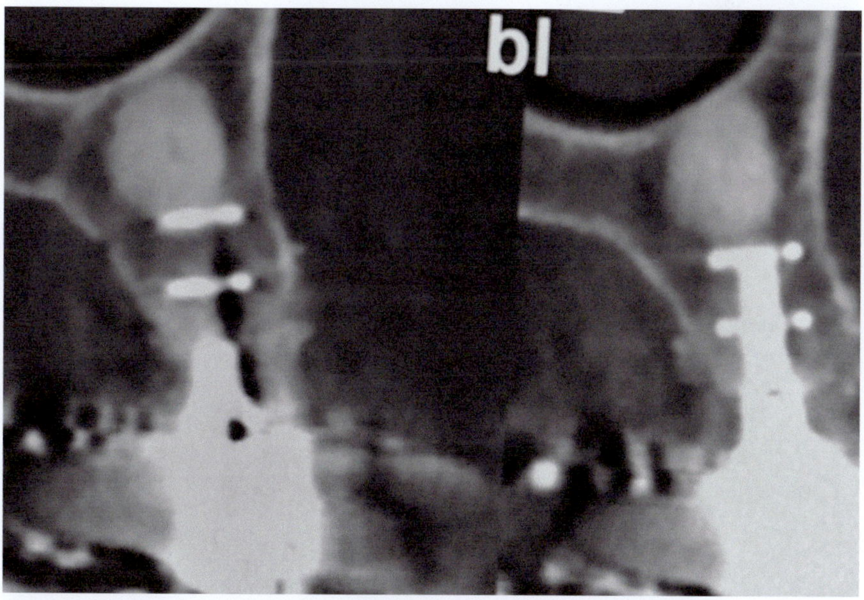

Fig. 11.10 Double Diskimplant® touching the canine without any untoward reaction after 23 years of service

osseointegration, the final prostheses were installed in 1993. In 2007, the patient bit on a hard object in a piece of food that loosened the right prosthesis and fractured the shaft of the Diskimplant® in the upper right second molar position. A root-form implant was inserted through the Diskimplant® with the fractured shaft and left submerged for 6 months. The upper bridge was cut at the level of the first molar and then screwed back into place. A new upper right bridge was fabricated in 2008. In 2017, the entire partial rehabilitation was still in service. A cone-beam CT scan revealed complete osseointegration with no bone loss or peri-implantitis, not even in the impacted canine area. In some areas, less than 1 or 2 mm of bone covered the disk.

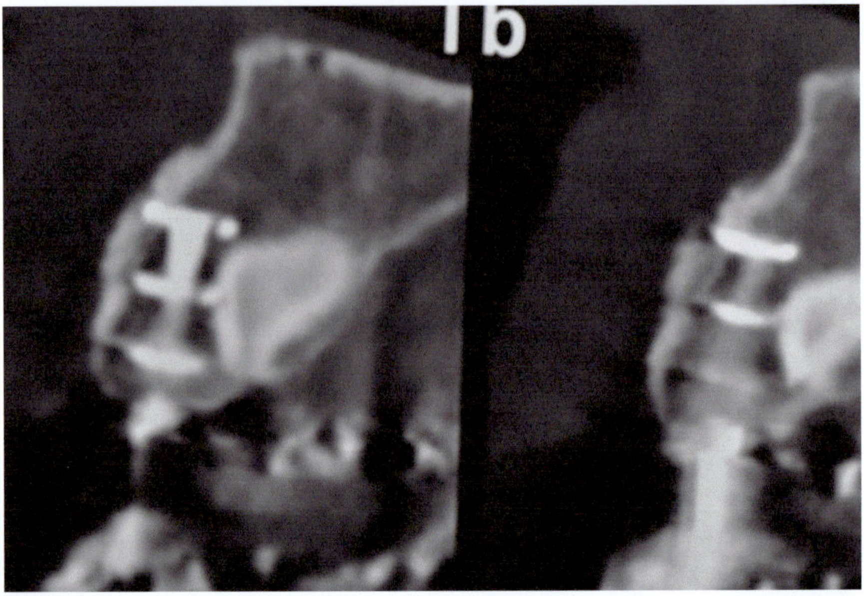

Fig. 11.11 CT scan showing a triple Diskimplant® in front of the upper right canine. Note the complete bony reconstruction of the triple-disk bone cuts

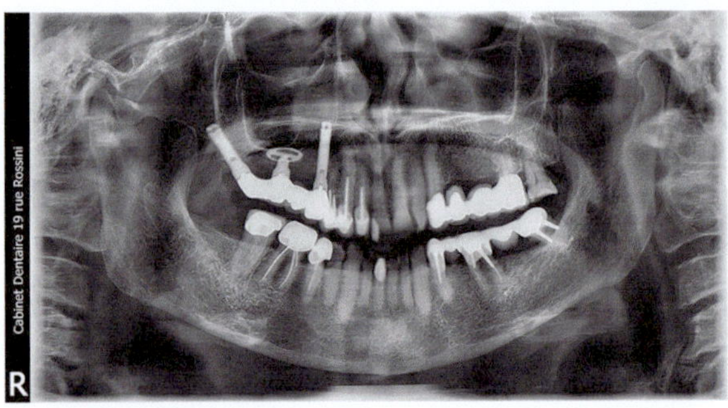

Fig. 11.12 Mono-disk Diskimplant® placed under the sinus and a root-form pterygoid implant after 17 years of service

Case Study 4: Complex Partial Edentulism (Figs. 11.12 and 11.13)

- Kennedy class II in the upper right: verification after 22 years of service (1996–2018).
- Kennedy class I maxilla and class II mandible: the upper right was rehabilitated in 1992 and the restoration was still in service in 2017. The upper left and lower left were rehabilitated 10 years later (2002). Checkup in 2017.

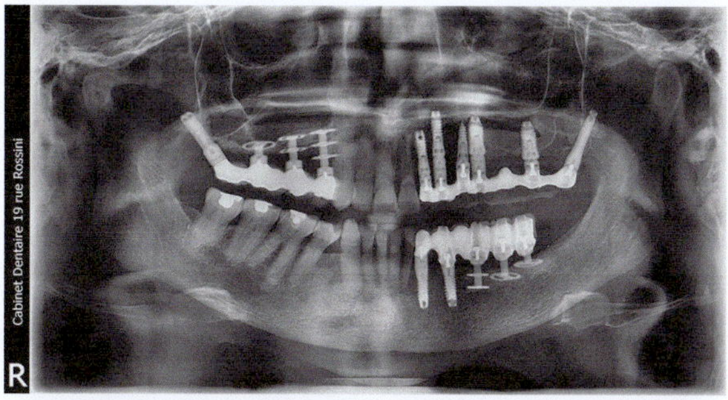

Fig. 11.13 Panoramic view showing the complexity of partial edentulism over a period of time: the upper right was equipped 24 years ago, the lower left 12 years ago, and the upper left 6 years ago

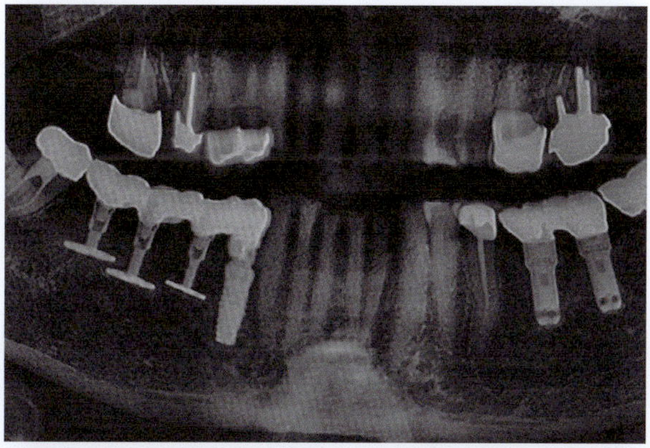

Fig. 11.14 Three Diskimplants® were installed in 1987 (*ad modum Brånemark* machined surface identical to that of the root-form implant placed in the lower left in 1995). The patient broke his first premolar in 2012. Panoramic view in 2017: no peri-implantitis

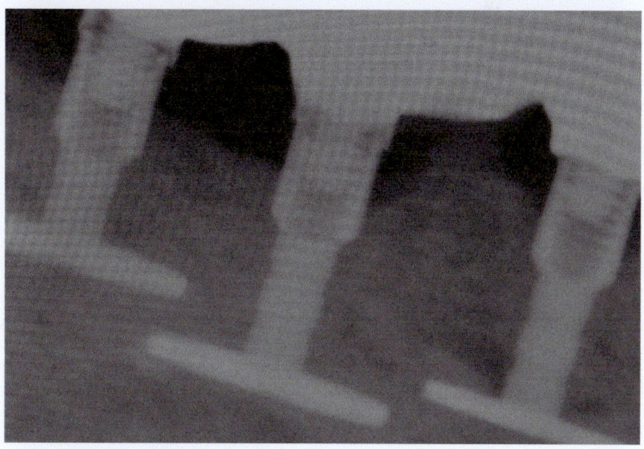

Fig. 11.15 Retro-alveolar view after 30 years of function revealing a bone gain without peri-implantitis (same patient as Fig. 11.14)

Case Study 5: Posterior Mandible (Figs. 11.14 and 11.15)
Three Diskimplants® were installed in 1988; the two left root-form implants were placed in 1992. After a checkup in 1994, the patient was lost to follow-up for 20 years. When seen again in 2014, she had just lost her lower right first molar. A root-form implant was placed and a new bridge was fabricated. Periapical radiographs in 2017 revealed a bone gain at the crestal level after the 29 years of service of the Diskimplants® that were still functional.

Case Study 6: Ameloblastoma (Figs. 11.16, 11.17, 11.18, 11.19, 11.20, 11.21, 11.22, 11.23 and 11.24)
The anterior portion of the lower jaw was completely removed, and a vascularized, pedicular bone graft was obtained from the fibula in a 12-hour surgery including micro-sutures with 9/0 sutures under a microscope to connect the vascularized bone

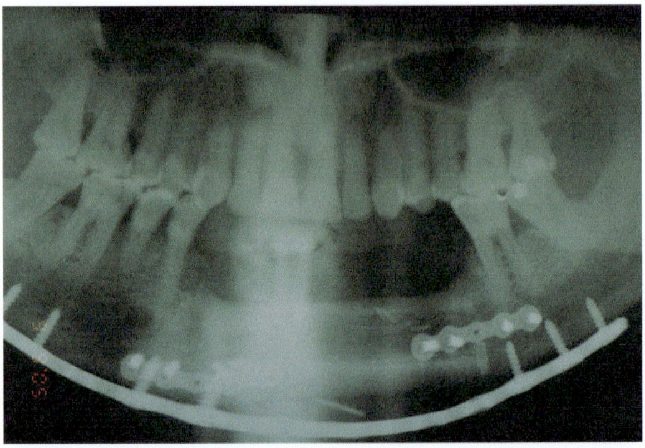

Fig. 11.16 Pedicular fibula graft after complete removal of the anterior mandible for treatment of an ameloblastoma

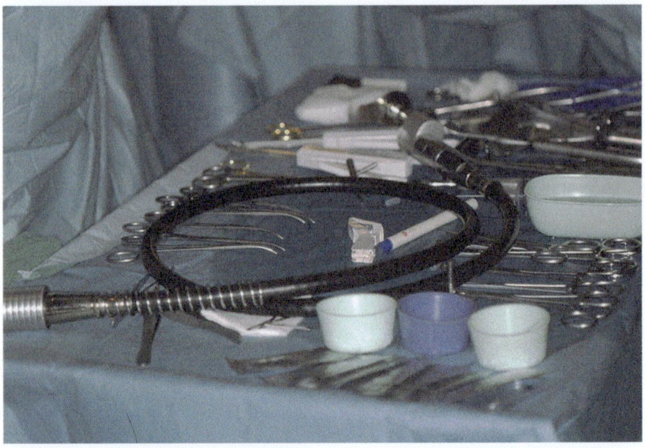

Fig. 11.17 Instruments for transplantation of the pedicular graft

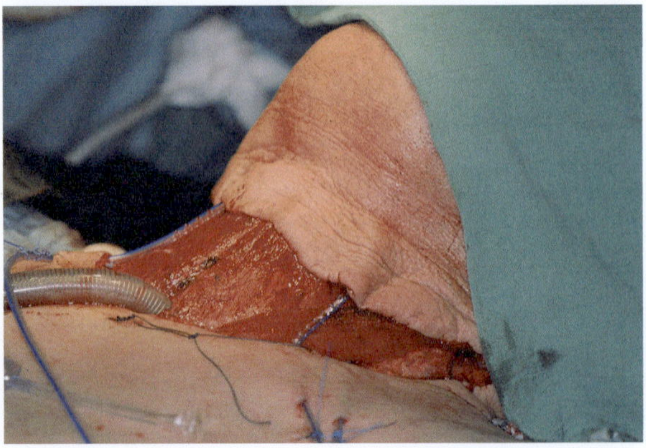

Fig. 11.18 Submandibular incision and tracheotomy for an extraoral surgical approach

transplant to the superior thyroid artery. Implant rehabilitation was decided on after the surgery had proved successful (1 year post-op). Three root-form implants (two Fractal® implants and one Diskimplant®) were installed just above the screw-retained plate that was left in place. Seven years later, the implants were still in service, with no signs of mobility or bone loss.

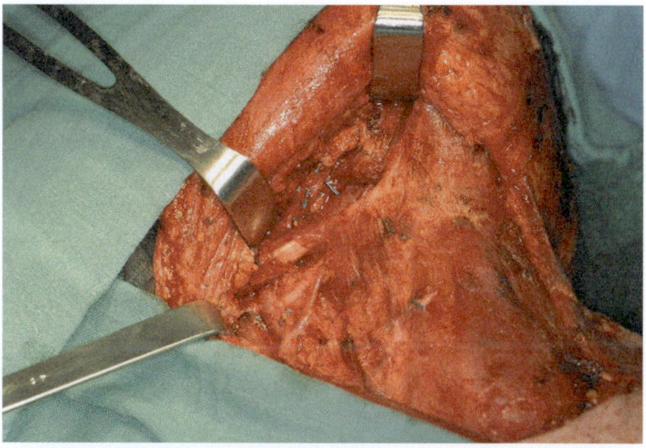

Fig. 11.19 Vascular recipient bed for the pedicular graft

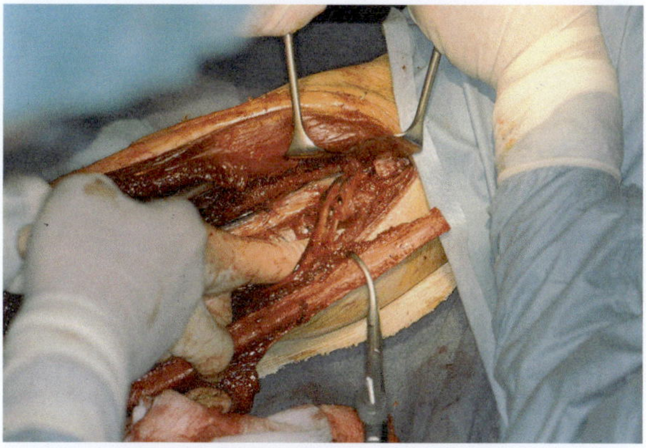

Fig. 11.20 Removal of the cutaneous pedicular fibula graft from the leg

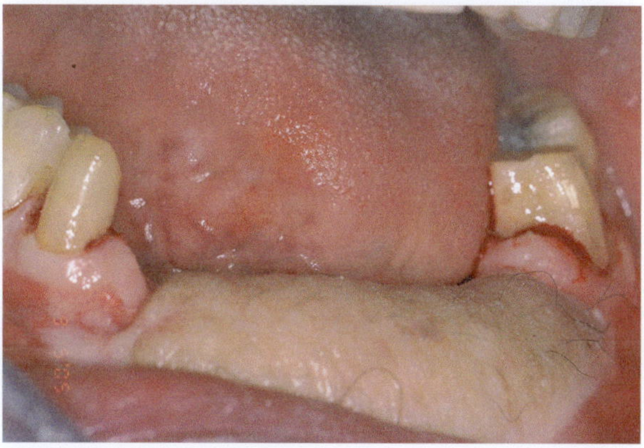

Fig. 11.21 Intraoral view at 6 months

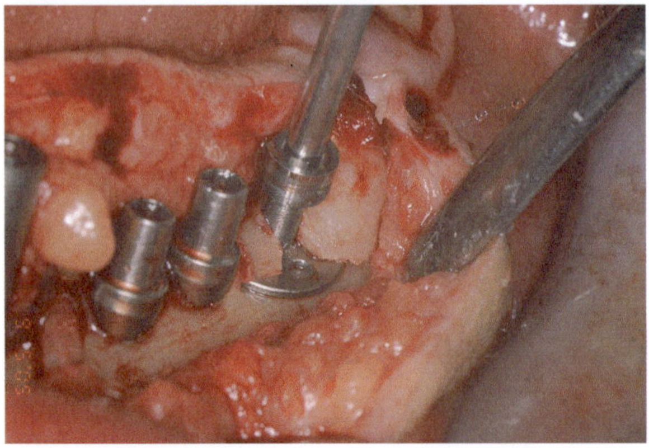

Fig. 11.22 Four Fractal® root-form implants and one mono-disk Diskimplant® installed above the orthopedic plate

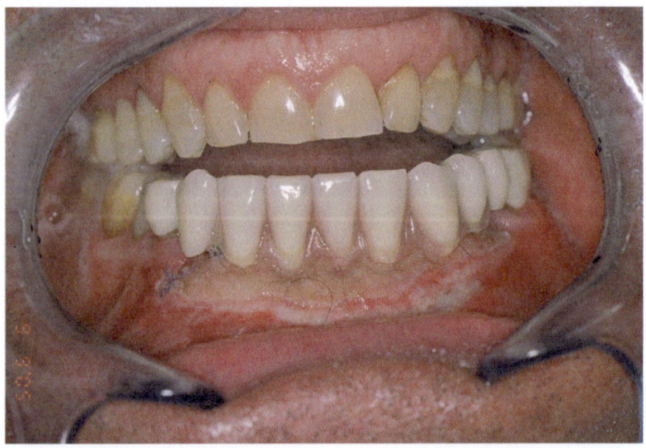

Fig. 11.23 Cosmetic aspect after 4 days (immediate loading protocol)

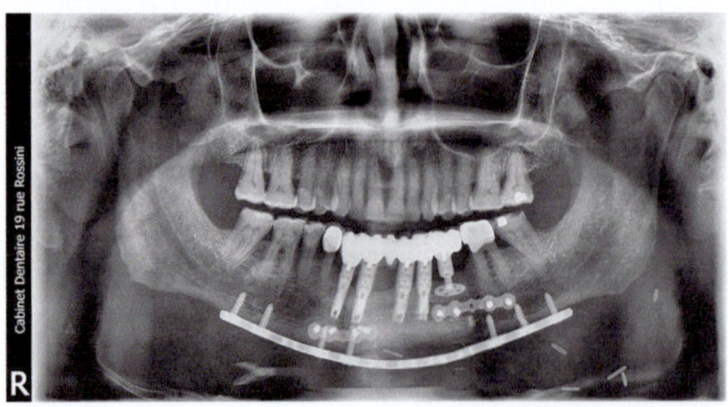

Fig. 11.24 Panoramic view of the screw-secured, full zirconia bridge after 12 years of function

Case Study 7: Posterior Mandible (Fig. 11.25)
Long-term follow-up after 15 years of function of a Kennedy class I posterior mandible with a knife ridge: a bone gain is visible on both sides. This case illustrates the advantage of dental implants compared to removable partial dentures that cause continuous bone loss over time.

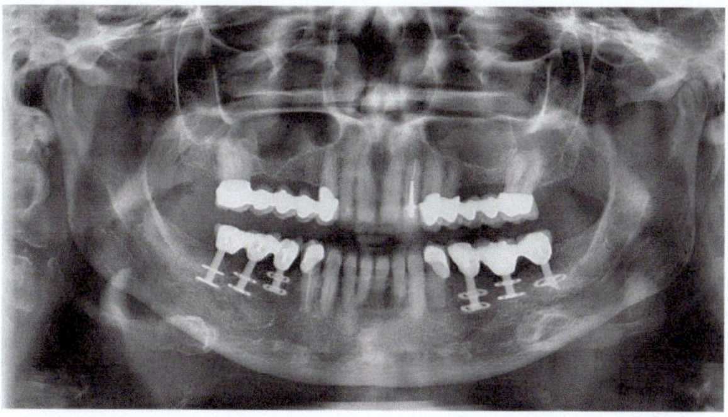

Fig. 11.25 Panoramic view after 15 years. The implants placed in this mandibular knife ridge using a delayed loading protocol feature a machined, *ad modum Brånemark* surface. A bone gain is visible at the crest level behind the last molar on each side. No peri-implantitis

Conflict of interest statement Gérard M. Scortecci is the inventor of the Diskimplant and holder of several associated patents that are exploited by the Victory company. He is an unpaid consultant to this firm and a minority shareholder in the company. No money was received from any of the companies mentioned in the book or from any of the companies whose products are mentioned.

Recommended Reading

1. Balshi TJ. An analysis and management of fractured implants: a clinical report. Int J Oral Maxillofac Impl. 1996;11:660–6.
2. Resnik RR, Misch CE. Misch's avoiding complications in oral implantology. Amsterdam: Elsevier; 2017.
3. Scortecci G. Immediate function of cortically anchored disk-design implants without bone augmentation in moderately to severely resorbed completely edentulous maxillae. Oral Implantol. 1999;XXV(2):70–9.
4. Lindhe J. Clinical periodontology and implant dentistry. 3rd ed. Copenhagen: Munksgaard; 1998.
5. Brånemark PI, Hansson BO, Adell R, et al. Osseointegrated implants in the treatment of the edentulous jaw. Experience from a 10-year period. Scan J Plast Reconstr Surg. 1977;2(suppl 10):1–132.
6. Odin G, Scortecci G, Levratto F, Morin L. Techniques avancées en implantologie basale chirurgico-prothétique. Stratégie Prothétique. 2011;11(3):1–10.
7. Odin G, Misch CE, Binderman I, Scortecci G. Fixed rehabilitation of severely atrophic jaws using immediately loaded basal disk implants after in situ bone activation. J Oral Implantol. 2012;XXXVIII(5):611–6.
8. Quine S, Morrell S. Hopelessness, depression and oral health concerns reported by community dwelling older Australians. Community Dent Health. 2009;26:177–82.
9. Rodrigues SM, Oliveira AC, Vargas AMD, Moreira AN, Ferreira E. Implications of edentulism on quality of life among elderly. Int J Environ Res Public Health. 2012;9:100–9.
10. Saman DM, Lemieux A, Arevalo O, Lutfiyya MN. A population-based study of edentulism in the US. BMC Public Health. 2014;14:65.
11. Schrott A, Riggi-Heiniger M, Maruo K, Gallucci GO. Implant loading protocols for partially edentulous patients with extended edentulous sites-a systematic review and meta-analysis. Int J Oral Maxillofac Implants. 2014;29(suppl):239–55.
12. Scortecci G, Misch CE, Benner KU. Implants and restorative dentistry. London: Martin Dunitz; 2001.
13. Weber HP, Sukotjo C. Does the type of implant prosthesis affect outcomes in the partially edentulous patient? Int J Oral Maxillofac Implants. 2007;22(suppl):140–72.

Completely Edentulous Atrophic Jaws and Extreme Clinical Situations

12

Jean-Marie Donsimoni, Gérard M. Scortecci, Carl E. Misch, Guillaume Odin, and Jean-Paul Meningaud

12.1 Basal Implant Therapy for the Completely Edentulous Atrophic Maxilla (Figs. 12.1, 12.2, 12.3, 12.4, 12.5, 12.6, 12.7, 12.8, 12.9, 12.10, 12.11, 12.12, 12.13, 12.14, 12.15, 12.16, 12.17, 12.18, 12.19, 12.20, 12.21, 12.22, 12.23, 12.24, 12.25, 12.26, 12.27, 12.28, 12.29, 12.30, 12.31, 12.32, 12.33, 12.34, and 12.35)

The upper dental arch is formed by a process of two paired bones that are fused together to form the anterior lower walls and floor of the nasal cavity. The maxillary complex sustains and protects the organs of sight, smell, and taste. Each hemi-maxilla contains an air-filled sinus that is connected by a continuous membrane with other sinuses in the upper face.

C. E. Misch (Deceased)

J.-M. Donsimoni
Centre Médical Europe, Paris, France
e-mail: jean-marie@donsimoni.com

G. M. Scortecci (✉)
University of Nice-Sophia Antipolis Medical School, Nice, France

New York University, New York, NY, USA

University of Southern California, Los Angeles, CA, USA

Private Practice, Nice, France
e-mail: scortecci@wanadoo.fr

G. Odin
ENT and Maxillo-facial Surgery Department, Institut Universitaire de la Face et du Cou, University of Nice-Sophia Antipolis Medical School, Nice, France
e-mail: odin.g@chu-nice.fr

J.-P. Meningaud
Hôpital Henri Mondor, Créteil, France

© Springer Nature Switzerland AG 2019

G. M. Scortecci (ed.), *Basal Implantology*, https://doi.org/10.1007/978-3-319-44873-2_12

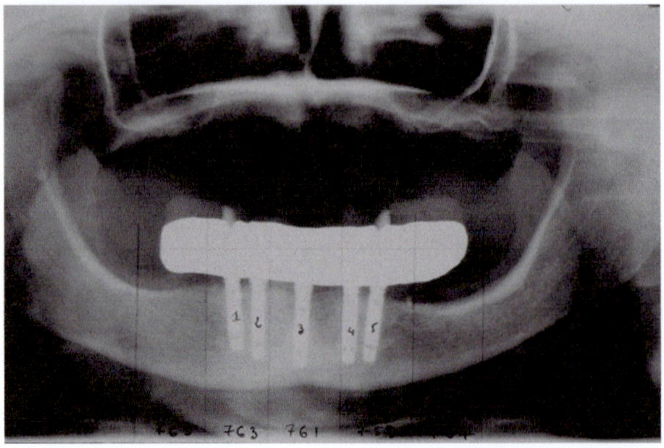

Fig. 12.1 Panoramic view in 2004. Extremely atrophic maxilla of a 78-year-old patient

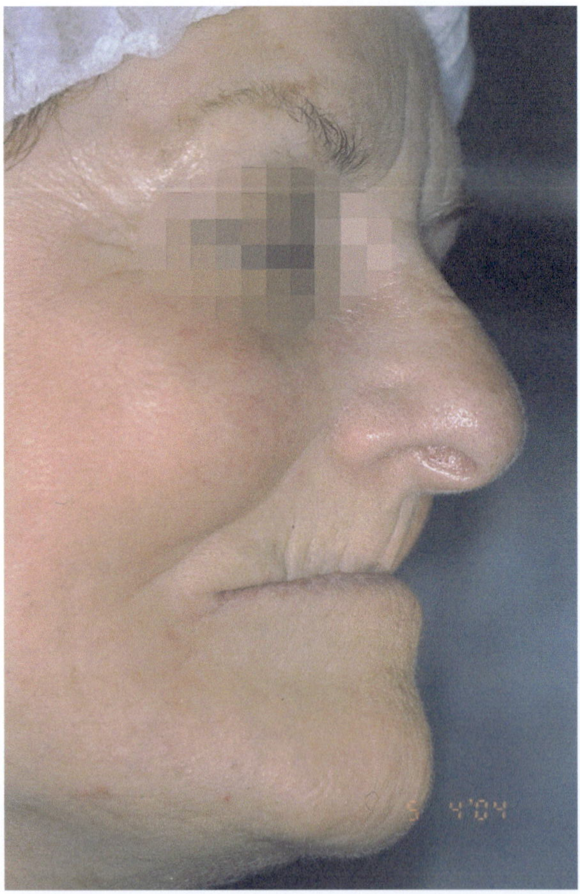

Fig. 12.2 Typical "bird-like" profile of an atrophic maxilla without the full denture (same patient as Fig. 12.1)

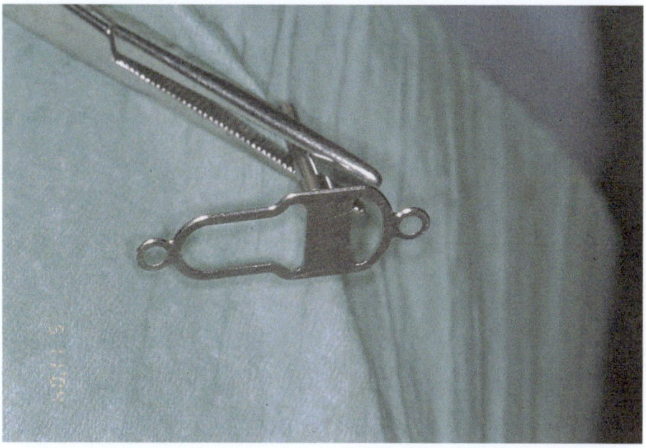

Fig. 12.3 Plate-form Diskimplant® (33 mm × 9 mm; Victory, France) that is installed laterally after osteotomy of the crestal bone with a cutter

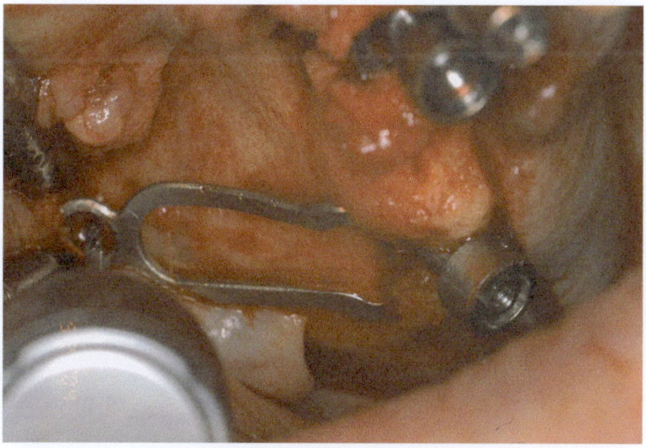

Fig. 12.4 Plate-form Diskimplant® screw-secured to the dense bone of the zygomatic arch (same patient as Fig. 12.1)

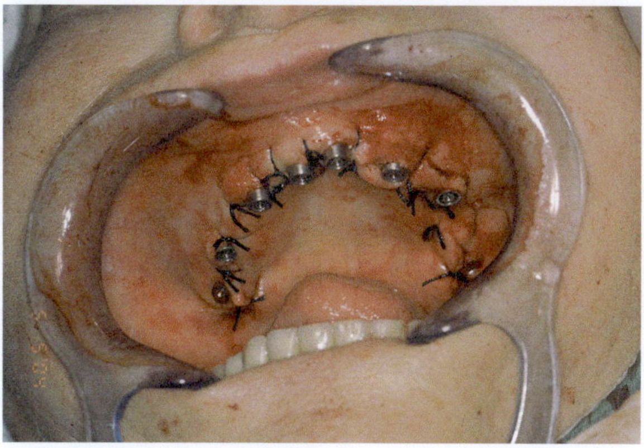

Fig. 12.5 After a horizontal, apical periosteal incision and six syringes of biomaterial (non-resorbable HA), the full-thickness flap is tightly sutured without tension

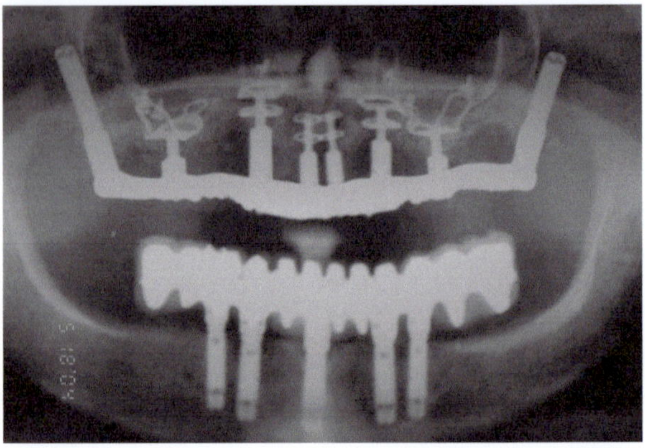

Fig. 12.6 Panoramic radiograph after 2 years showing full osseointegration of all of the implants placed (same patient as Fig. 12.1)

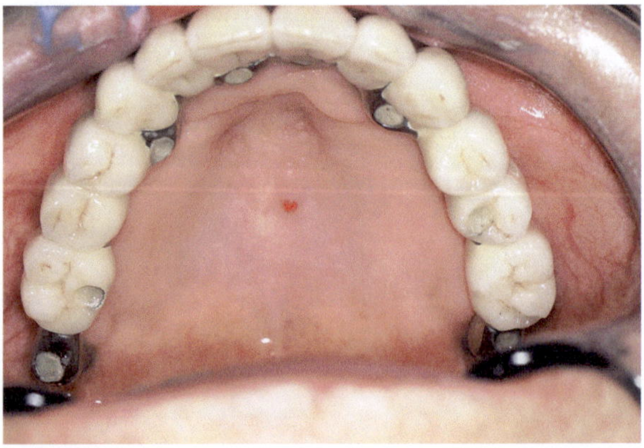

Fig. 12.7 After 2 years of service, the transitional bridge was retrieved, and the osseointegration of all implants was checked by imaging studies and clinical examination. The porcelain-fused-to-metal final restoration was then fabricated (same patient as Fig. 12.1)

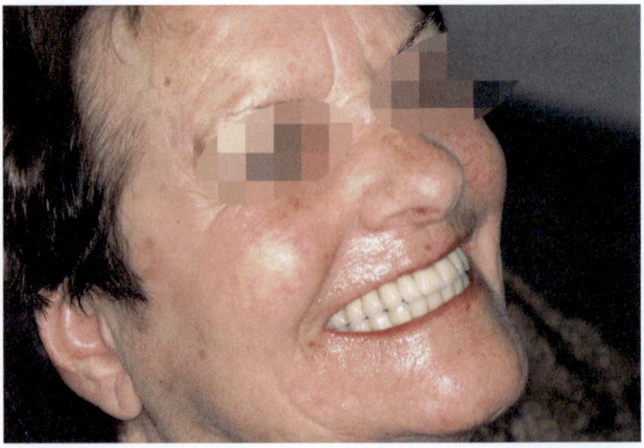

Fig. 12.8 Cosmetic outcome 2 years post-op (same patient as Fig. 12.1)

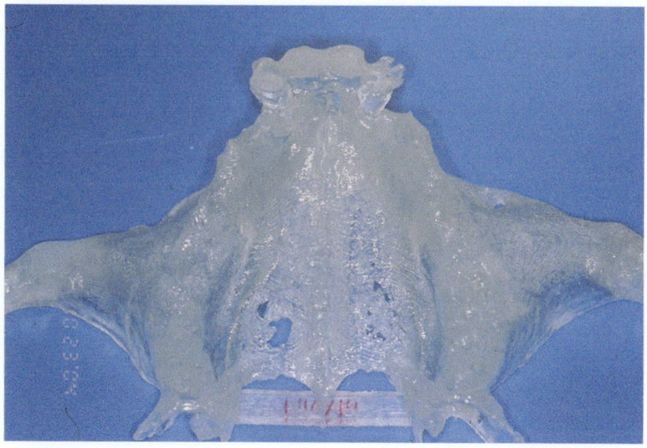

Fig. 12.9 Stereolithographic model of an extremely resorbed maxilla. The remaining teeth were affected by periodontal disease and had to be removed; basal implants were installed immediately

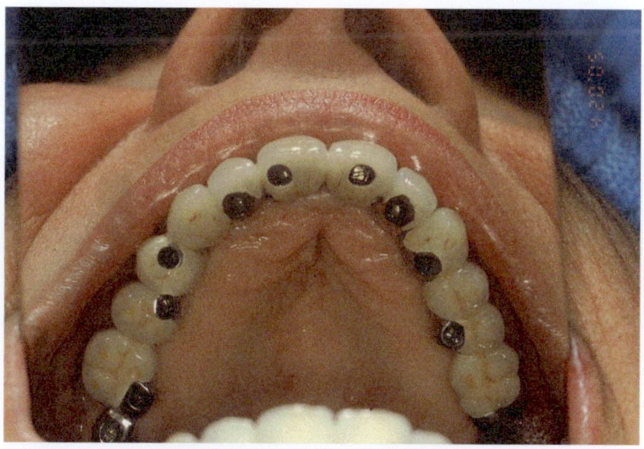

Fig. 12.10 Intraoral view of the screw-secured, ceramic-baked-to-metal final prosthesis in 2001 (2 years post-op) (same patient as Fig. 12.9)

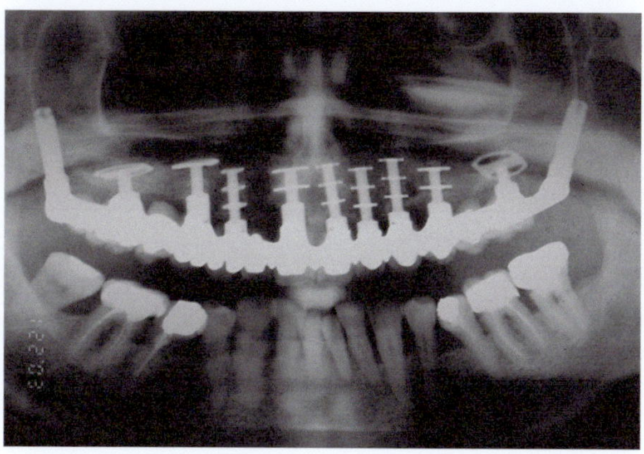

Fig. 12.11 Panoramic radiograph after 18 years of service (2017) (same patient as Figs. 12.9 and 12.10)

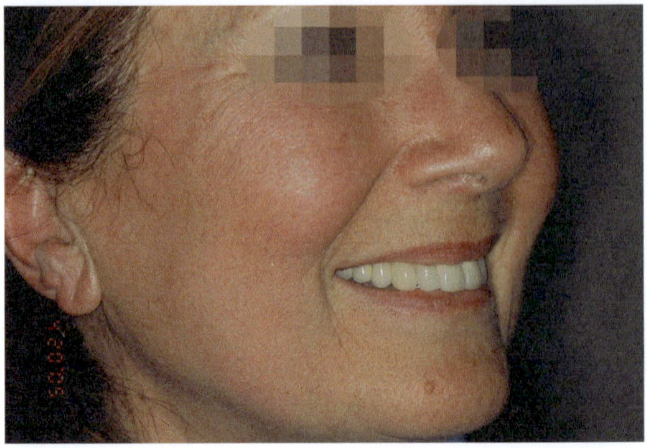

Fig. 12.12 Cosmetic aspect (same patient as Fig. 12.11)

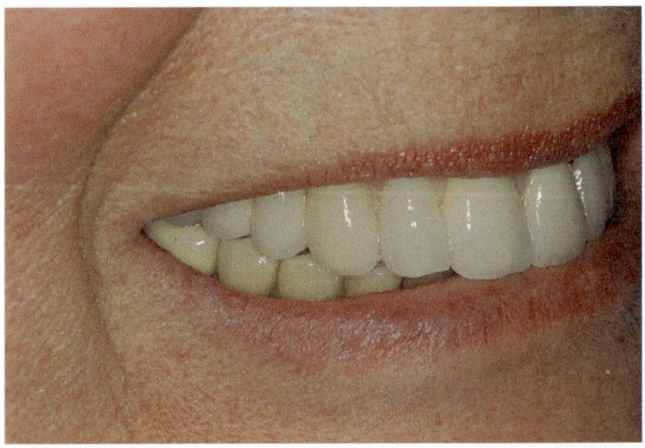

Fig. 12.13 Pink ceramic was used to improve the patient's "gummy smile" (same patient as Fig. 12.12)

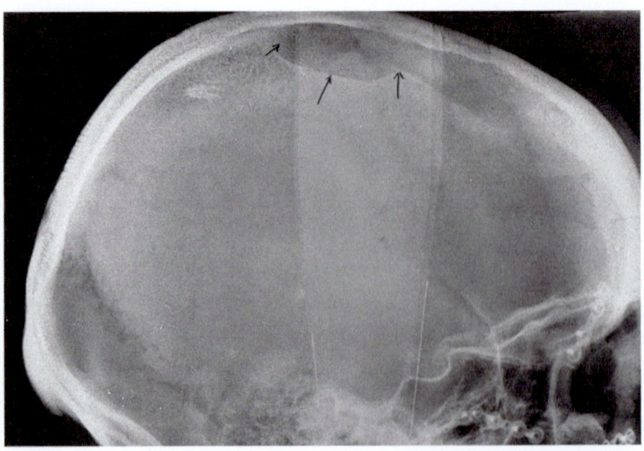

Fig. 12.14 Following traumatic injuries in a major car accident, autologous grafts were taken from the hip, and calvaria (arrows) was used to reconstruct the upper jaw, but there was not enough bone to install root-form implants. Basal implants were placed in 2003

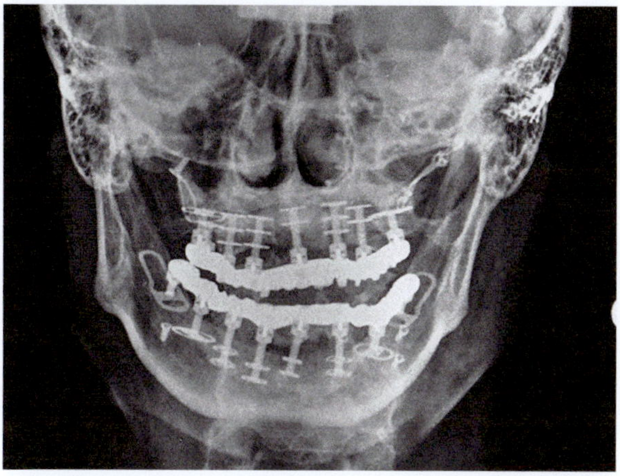

Fig. 12.15 Front view of the upper and lower jaws. Basal implant rehabilitation 14 years post-op (same patient as Fig. 12.14)

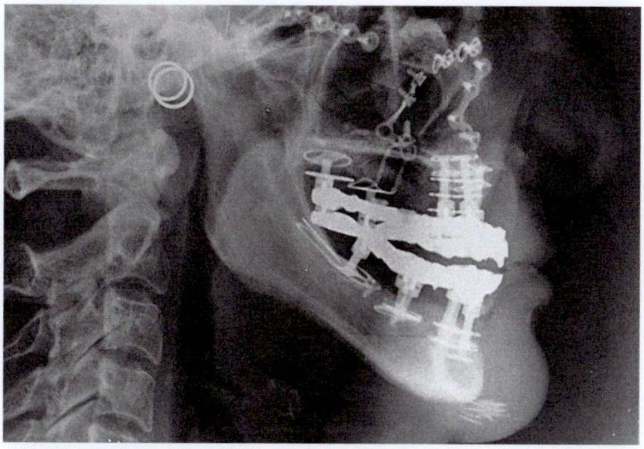

Fig. 12.16 Sagittal view of the jaws 14 years post-op (same patient as Fig. 12.14)

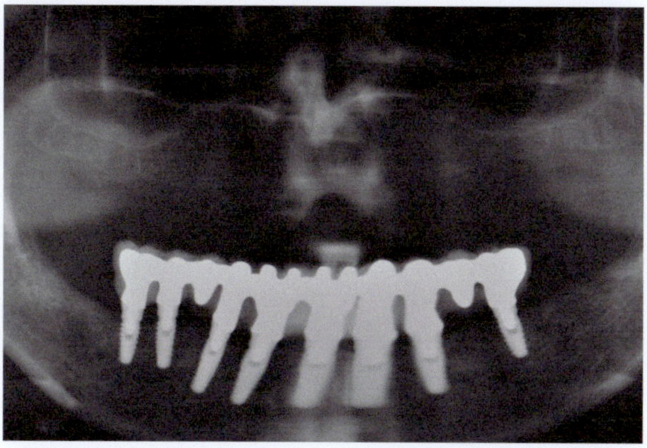

Fig. 12.17 Panoramic view of an atrophic maxilla in 2001

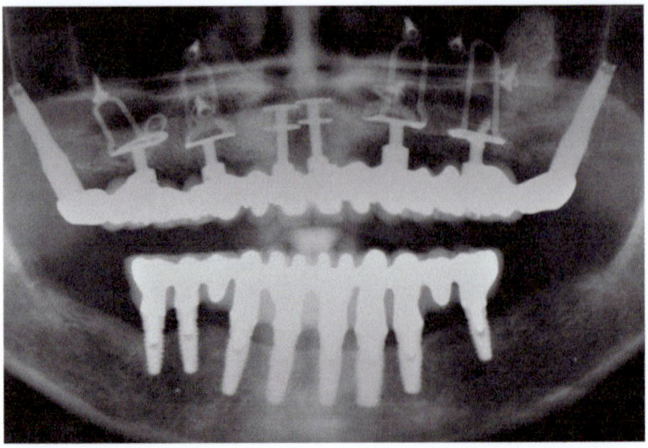

Fig. 12.18 Panoramic view in February 2014 showing the final, fixed screw-secured ceramic-baked-to-metal restoration (same patient as Fig. 12.17)

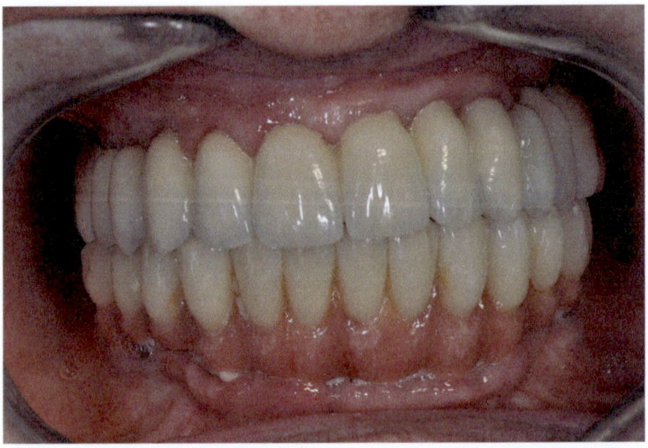

Fig. 12.19 Intraoral cosmetic aspect (same patient as Fig. 12.17)

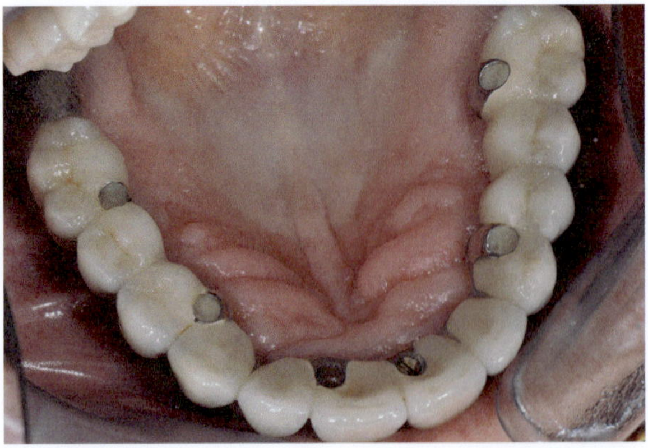

Fig. 12.20 Palatal view of the screw-secured ceramic bridge (same patient as Fig. 12.17)

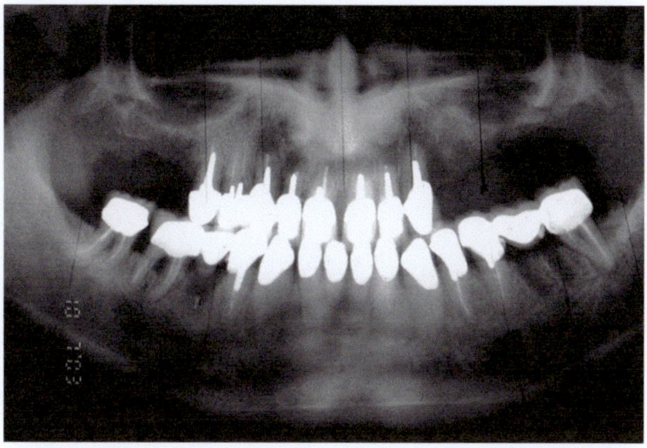

Fig. 12.21 Initial status prior to extraction/immediate implant placement

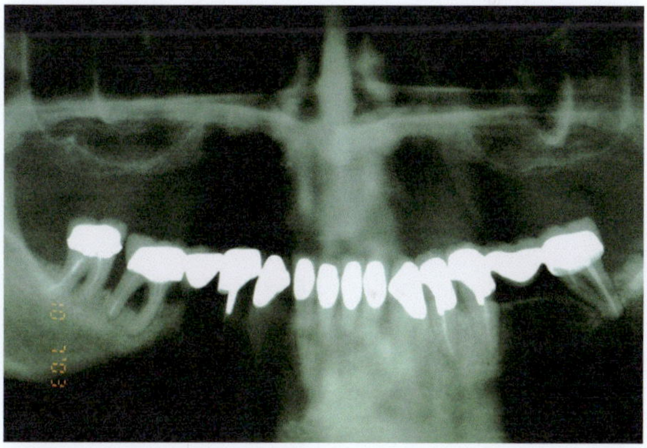

Fig. 12.22 An immediate function, ceramic-to-metal bridge was secured to root-form implants placed immediately in the extraction sites in 2002 (same patient as Fig. 12.21)

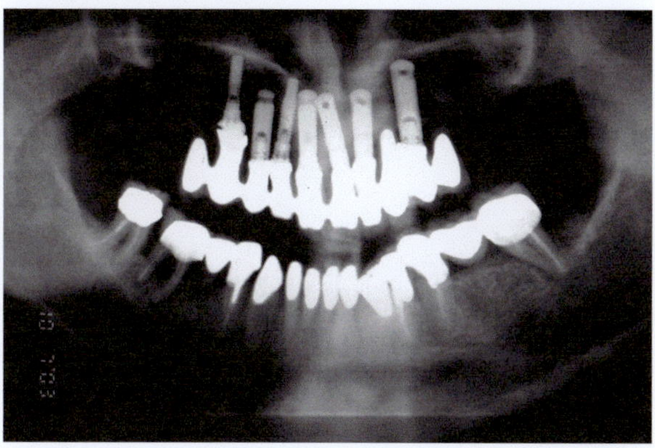

Fig. 12.23 After 6 months of function, all of the root-form implants were mobile and had to be removed. This panoramic radiograph taken in 2003 reveals the tremendous bone loss that had occurred. Alveolar bone preservation did not succeed after immediate implant placement (same patient as Fig. 12.21)

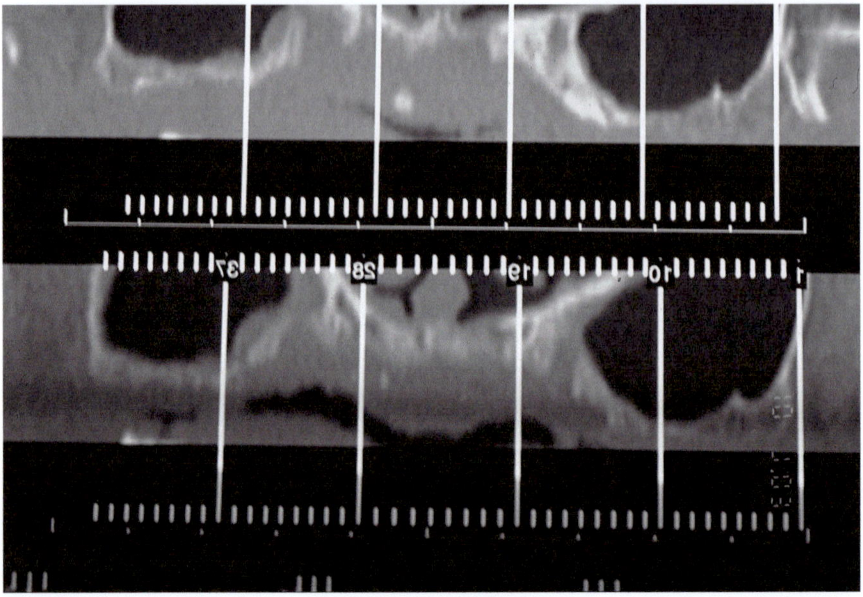

Fig. 12.24 CT scan illustrating the severe bone resorption after total implant loss (same patient as Fig. 12.21)

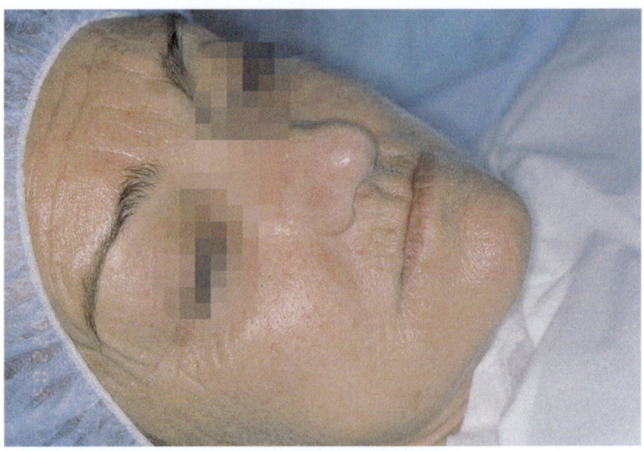

Fig. 12.25 Facial aspect after severe maxillary bone resorption (same patient as Fig. 12.21)

The maxillary alveolar bone is highly responsive to biochemical and physical stimuli. Excessive external stimuli of mechanical origin can destroy the alveolar bone in a continuous process. During a lifetime, the dental arch gradually resorbs, primarily as a result of loss of teeth and periodontal disease associated with systemic disorders. Alteration of the bone's internal architecture occurs first, with thinning of the trabeculae that become increasingly fragile. Up to 75% of bone mass may be lost before the external shape of the ridge is modified. Evaluation of potential implant sites by conventional radiographs alone can thus be misleading.

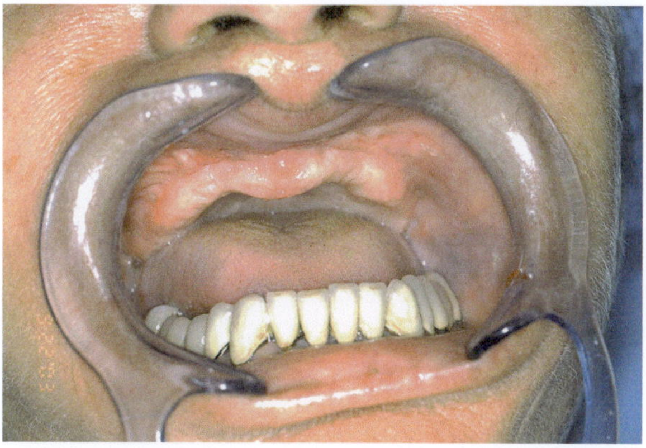

Fig. 12.26 Intraoral view of the hard and soft tissue loss

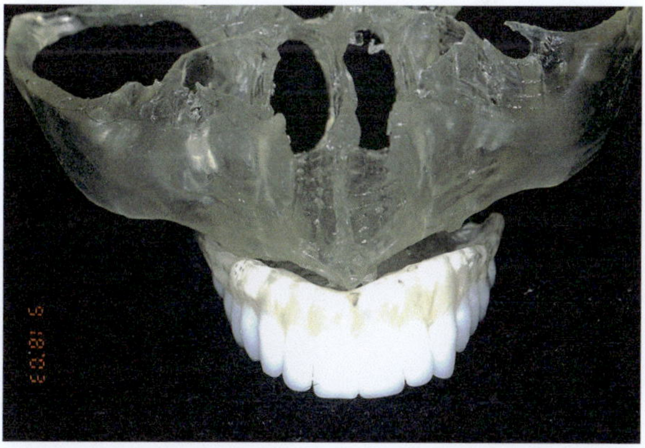

Fig. 12.27 Stereolithographic model and full upper denture (barium teeth) (same patient as Fig. 12.21)

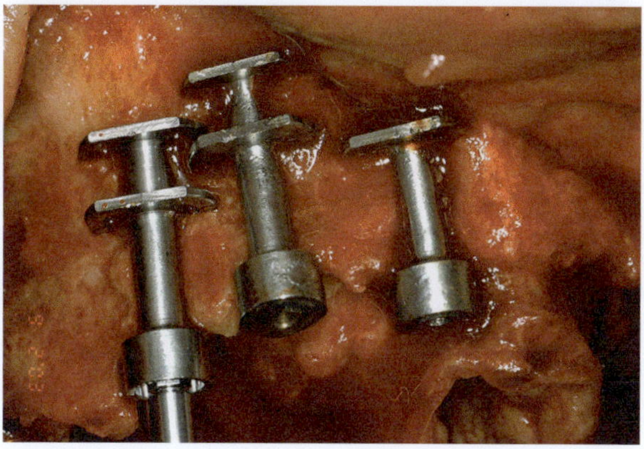

Fig. 12.28 A double Diskimplant® is particularly indicated in knife ridges of the premaxilla

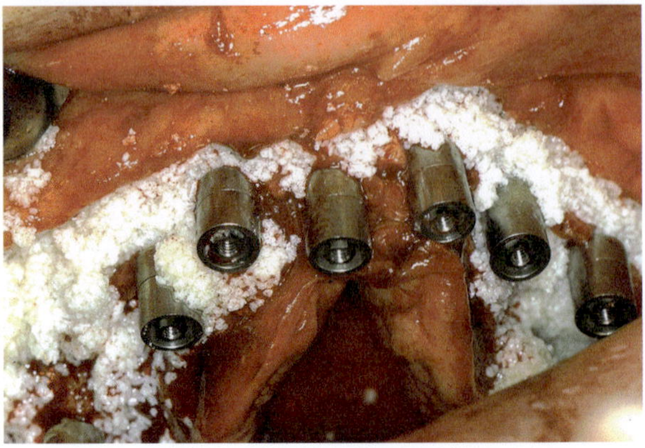

Fig. 12.29 Bone substitute material (non-resorbable HA) was used to cover the protruding portion of the basal implants (same patient as Fig. 12.21)

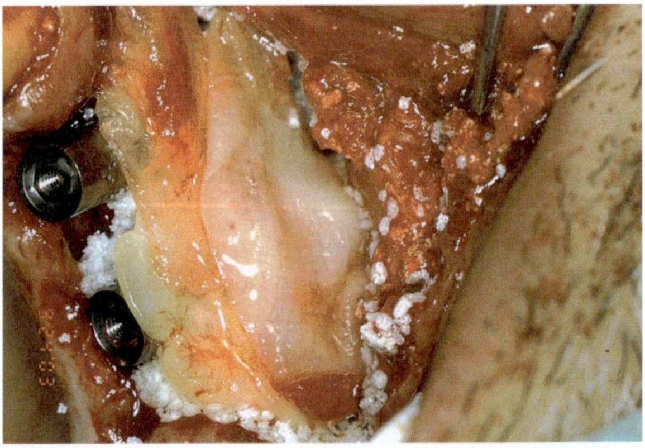

Fig. 12.30 A PRF membrane was added to maintain the bone substitute material and promote tissue repair and bone formation (same patient as Fig. 12.21)

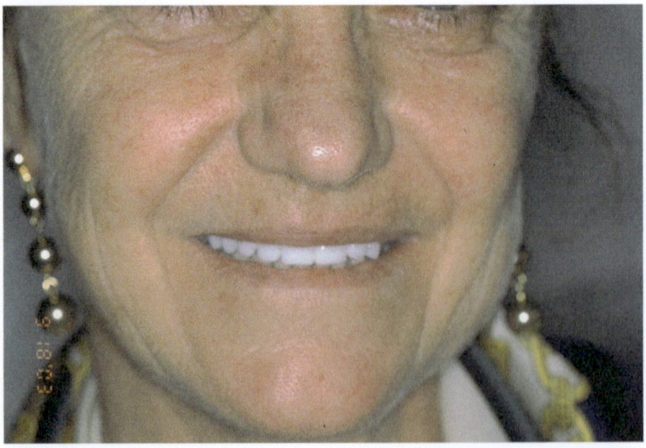

Fig. 12.31 Immediate, screw-secured fixed, highly rigid bridge in place 48 h post-op. Cosmetic result at 1 year post-op (same patient as Fig. 12.21)

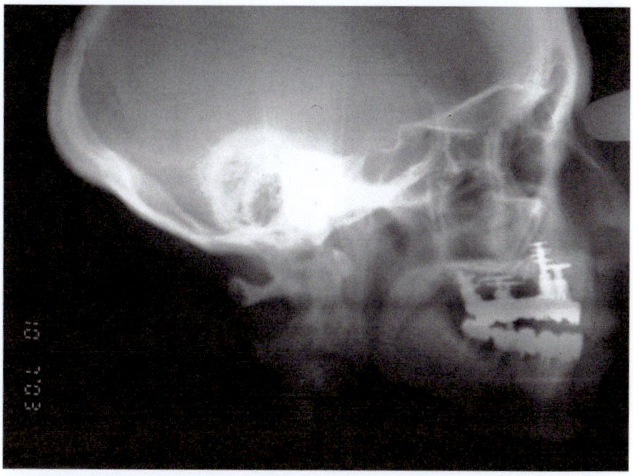

Fig. 12.32 Sagittal view after 8 years showing the basal implants that were installed in the tubero-pterygoid and zygomatic sectors and the premaxilla (same patient as Fig. 12.21)

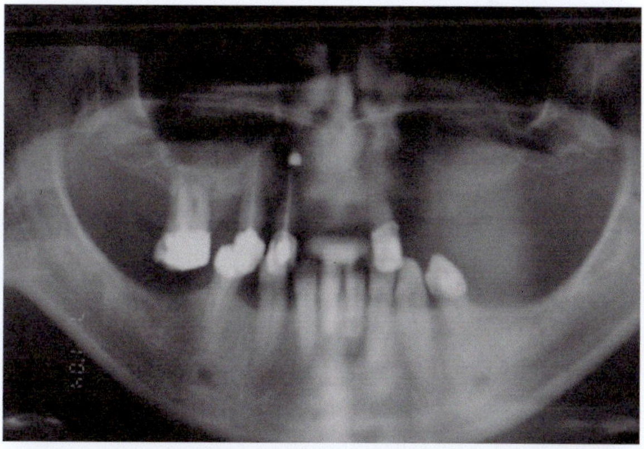

Fig. 12.33 42-year-old patient with aggressive periodontal disease

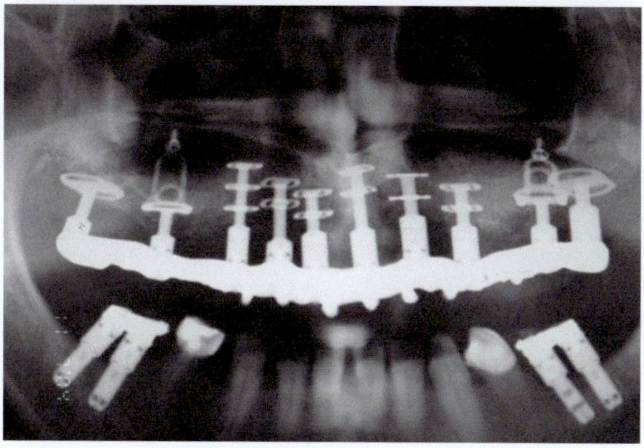

Fig. 12.34 Panoramic view at 9 years: 10 basal Diskimplants® were installed in the maxilla and 4 root-form implants in the posterior mandible (Victory, France) (same patient as Fig. 12.33)

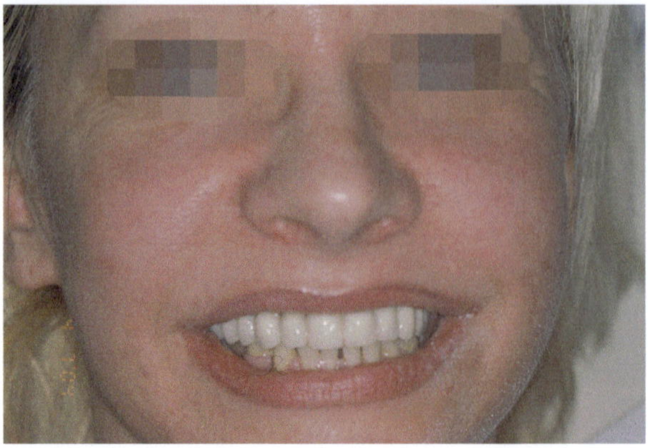

Fig. 12.35 Cosmetic aspect of the rehabilitation (same patient as Fig. 12.33)

A number of guidelines should be followed when implants are planned for totally edentulous atrophic jaws:

- Use manual osseotensors to prepare the recipient bone bed before basal implant placement in the maxilla. This improves the quality of D3 or D4 bone, thereby optimizing initial stability compatible with immediate placement of a fixed, screw-secured-to-implant prosthesis.
- Augment the implant/cortical bone surface contact area by increasing the number of implants, or use multidisk or monodisk implants or plate-form Diskimplants® with a wide base diameter.
- Take advantage of the major cortical skeletal pillars (i.e., canine pillars, zygoma) and tubero-pterygoid sector for solid implant anchorage.
- Administer preoperative Botox® to reduce postoperative stress in patients with strong, hyperactive muscles.
- Guarantee a strong, rigid inter-implant and cross-arch connection with a CrCo screw-secured-to-implant frame acting as an external orthopedic fixator. A transitional transpalatal bar must be added when necessary.
- Reduce masticatory stress by using acrylic teeth.
- Use reduced occlusal surfaces and lingualized occlusion.
- Instruct the patient to eat soft meals for 45 days. A transitional prosthesis should be used for 1 year or more before fabricating the final restoration. This immediately loaded transitional prosthesis can also be kept as the final fixed denture after any necessary corrections have been made.

The Premaxilla and Dental Implants

The alveolar ridge flares outward in the anterior region. Less bone flanks the teeth labially/buccally than palatally, and the root of the incisor is covered by only a very thin plate of bone. Natural buccal alveolar bone fenestration on natural teeth is common in the anterior area. This precludes extensive use of so-called "easy" immediate implantation protocols following tooth extraction. The integrity of the palatal aspect and the buccal bone plate must be examined carefully before implant installation.

The maxillary ridge tends to resorb inwardly and obliquely off the horizontal plane faster than the crest height decreases. The palatal aspect of the residual ridge, usually less adversely affected than the labial/buccal aspect, is thus higher. These resorption patterns are responsible for the knife-edge anatomy common in the edentulous anterior maxilla.

Misconception of the true profile of the hard tissues has had serious implications in implantology. For example, numerous attempts have been made to design an implant shaped like the root of a tooth. Such designs are of limited application because the bone narrows more rapidly than it loses height. The incisive canal must also be taken into account because soft tissue invagination into an implant site can interfere with osseointegration.

Double Diskimplants® present a suitable design for installation in knife-ridge premaxillae when the crest is less than 3 mm in thickness. Otherwise, narrow Fratex® root-form implants can be placed, drilling from the palatal aspect. For flat anterior areas with less than 5 mm of available bone height, a monodisk Diskimplant® is more appropriate.

Some individuals have only a very thin plate of bone separating the crest and the nasal floor. CT scan or cone-beam CT studies can facilitate selection of the most appropriate implant design and dimensions. The premaxilla provides adequate bone of good quality for implant placement. Bone grafts of intraoral origin (mental buccal plate or retromolar mandibular buccal plate) are sometimes required for proper installation of screw-type implants. Bone from the maxillary tuberosity is unsuitable for grafting purposes since it is usually of poor quality. Furthermore, harvesting bone from the tuberosity can compromise ulterior adaptation of a conventional denture should implant failure occur. Following bone grafting, a waiting period of 3 to 9 months is necessary before root-form implants can be inserted. The total waiting period is thus almost 1 year, even with a successful bone graft.

Single, double or plate-form Diskimplants® are an attractive alternative to grafts. They represent a safe and reproducible method for immediate functional loading in patients with a totally edentulous maxilla.

Nasal Cavity

The maxillary and palatine bones separate the oral cavity from the nasal cavity. The anterior, and major, portion of the nasal floor is formed by the palatine process of the hemi-maxillae; the posterior portion is formed by the horizontal process of the palatine bones. The nasal floor is smooth and concave, with that process toward the midline rising to join the process of its bilaterally paired opposite. This prominence serves as a base for the cartilaginous septum that divides the air passage into two fossae. The most anterior part of the prominence, the anterior spine, forms the cleft of the piriform aperture, seen as an upside-down, roughly heart-shaped outline on radiographs. The incisive canal is located posterior to the nasal spine, close to the septum. Within the body of each hemi-maxilla, the canal runs anteriorly and toward the midline until the two canals typically join into a common opening, the incisive fossa.

The relationships between the nasal cavity and the oral cavity interest the surgeon primarily in terms of the amount of bone separating the anterior portion of the cavity from the residual dental crest in the incisor region. In some individuals, the crest of the alveolar ridge is separated from the nasal cavity by only a thin plate of bone. In others, considerable bone exists between the two structures, in which case more support remains for the lip; such generous bone of good density is suitable for a root-form implant. The labial bone below the nose, which extends bilaterally into the canine pillar area, is usually quite dense. In this area, single, double, or triple Diskimplants® can always find sufficient initial cortical support. Should the base of a Diskimplant® protrude on the buccal or palatal aspect, it can serve as a graft holder for autogenous bone chips collected in the vicinity or biomaterial such as hydroxy-apatite (HA) and tricalcium phosphate (TCP) or resorbable membranes such as PRF.

The soft tissues of the nasal cavity (the nasal membrane) are thicker and more richly supplied with blood vessels, nerves, and glands than those of the paranasal sinuses. The vestibule lying in front of the inferior meatus is lined with a continuation of the skin, stratified squamous epithelium, guarded by hairs and lubricated by sebaceous and sweat glands. As the soft tissues pass into the atrium, or beginning of the nose, they become firmly attached to the bone. Perforation of the bone at this point thus nearly always results in perforation of the soft tissues. This can be prevented by intraoral elevation of the nasal floor membrane during implant installation. Bone pushers, bone spreaders, and bone splitting instruments can be used in this area to increase bone volume. However, special training is required for proper manipulation of these manual instruments to avoid fracturing the vestibular bone plate.

Canine Pillars and Plate-Form Diskimplants®

The cuspid is well supported because the strong column of bone in which it is located helps divert occlusal forces upward, away from the dental arch. The labial plate of the cuspid is thicker than that of its mandibular counterpart. The cuspid also flares outward less than the maxillary incisors, and this is an additional security against dislodgement. The cuspid area is anatomically ideal for implant installation in the maxilla, even though mechanical stress and material fatigue must be expected with time. The canine plays a major role during mastication. In some circumstances, part of a canine root may protrude into the sinus area. When bone thickness is at least 3 mm and 12 mm in height, a microthreaded narrow diameter Fratex® root-form implant is advisable. If the alveolar ridge is too thin (less than 3 mm), a double or plate-form Diskimplant® can provide reliable intra- and supra-bony support without the need for a prior bone-grafting procedure.

In most cases of total and partial edentulism, regardless of how the arch appears at visual examination or upon palpation, CT and clinical studies have demonstrated that maxillary bone is initially lost principally from the labial/buccal aspect. The width of the ridge is maintained by the thickening of the submucosal tissues. The patterns of ridge resorption vary considerably. A high, knife-edge ridge precludes the use of root-form implants and requires installation of double Diskimplants®. In contrast, a flat bone plate is more appropriately handled by a plate-form Diskimplant. A compact bone height of 1–2 mm is sufficient to obtain reliable bony anchorage since the base of Diskimplants® is only 0.5 mm thick. Pre-implant bone grafting is not required in such cases.

Maxillary Sinus Region and Zygomatic Basal Implants

Each hemi-maxilla contains a pneumatic sinus that communicates with the nasal cavity and the other paranasal sinuses (frontal, ethmoid, sphenoid). The paired, bilateral paranasal sinuses are rarely symmetrical. The largest of the paranasal sinuses, the maxillary sinus, measures about 34 mm posteriorly, 33 mm supero-inferiorly, and 23 mm laterally and has an average fluid capacity of 15 ml. The maxillary sinus is pyramidal in shape. The base of the pyramid forms the lower wall of the nasal septum; its apex is directed toward the zygomatic arch. One wall of the pyramid faces superiorly, toward the orbital cavity; one faces posteriorly, toward the infratemporal fossa; one faces anteriorly, toward the face; and the last faces inferiorly, toward the dental arch and palate. The walls curve to accommodate other cranial structures and slope to join one another.

The upper molar area is reportedly the most difficult sector to manage with dental implants. Mechanical problems such as implant fracture, microfracture of the peri-implant bone, and subsequent implant loss after 5 years of function are most likely to occur in this region. A failure rate of 44% has been reported in type IV bone in premolar and molar sites equipped with root-form implants of different lengths. In order to avoid such mechanical problems, Diskimplants® or a plate-form Diskimplant® anchored in the dense zygomatic bone are recommended.

Zygomatic root-form implants are a reliable option only if the recipient bone site is at least 6 mm wide and 6 mm high. The maxillary bone crest must also provide 6 mm of good quality bone for crestal anchorage of a zygomatic implant.

Tubero-Pterygoid Site for Microthreaded Pterygoid Implants (Figs. 12.36, 12.37, 12.38, 12.39, 12.40, 12.41, 12.42, 12.43, and 12.44)

Use of manual bone matrix osseotensors 45 days prior to implant surgery is mandatory in order to improve bone quality in this strategic area. When planning implant treatment for the fully edentulous maxilla, the tubero-pterygoid areas should be equipped first. If major difficulties are encountered, it is easy to postpone the implant surgery, suture, put the full denture back in place, and wait 2 months without ruining the future implant site.

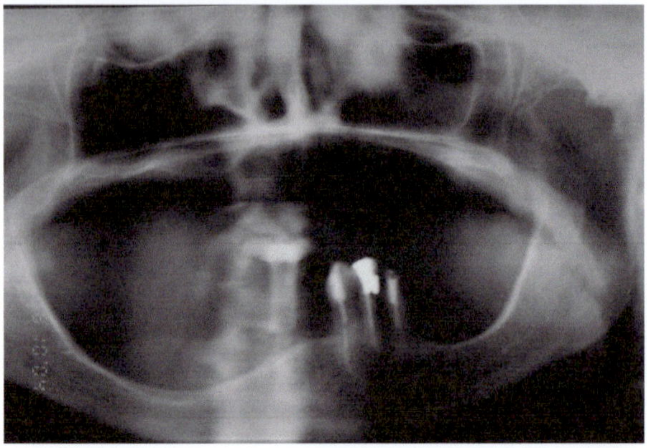

Fig. 12.36 Panoramic view of an extremely resorbed maxilla (patient aged 77 years)

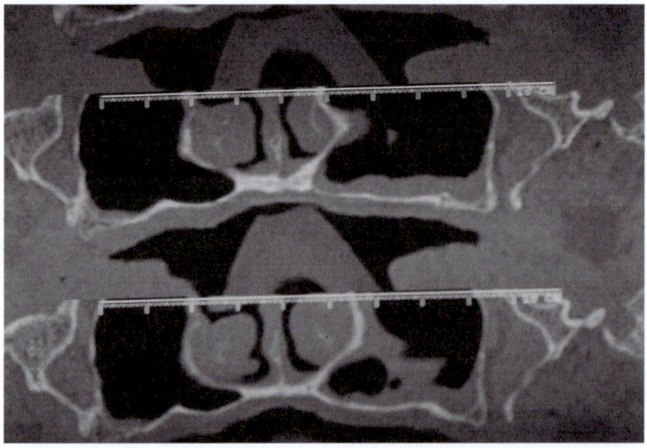

Fig. 12.37 Very little bone was left, even in the premaxilla (eggshell-thin upper jaw). Two sessions of bone matrix osseotensors (Victor, France) were performed 45 and 90 days before surgery to improve the bone quality, augment the blood supply, and promote formation of a callus

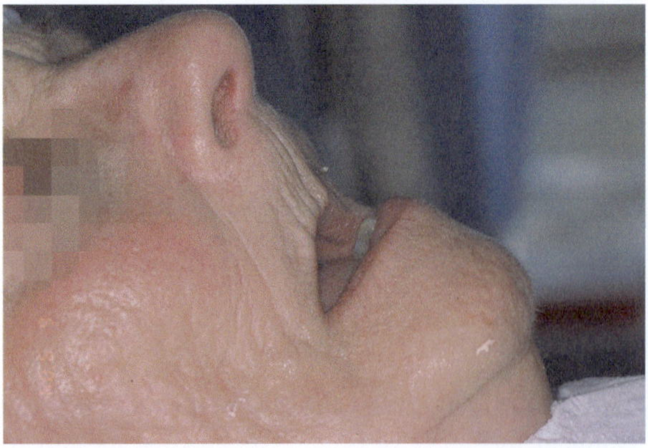

Fig. 12.38 Extraoral aspect ("bird face")

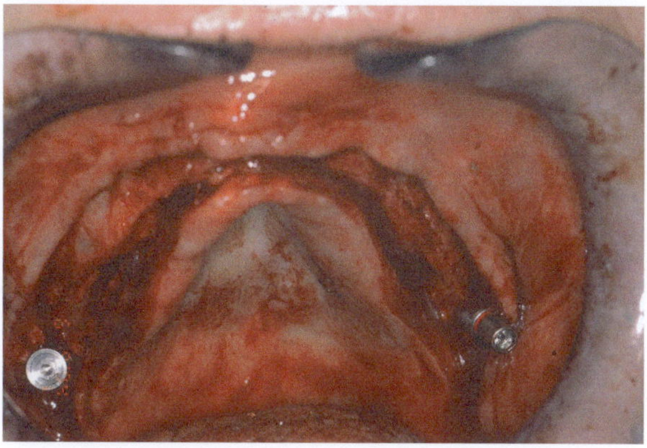

Fig. 12.39 Pterygoid implants in the upper left and upper right maxilla

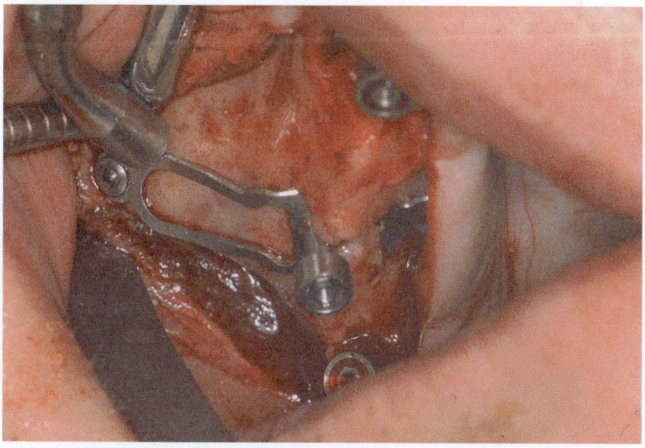

Fig. 12.40 Zygomatic plate-form Diskimplant in place

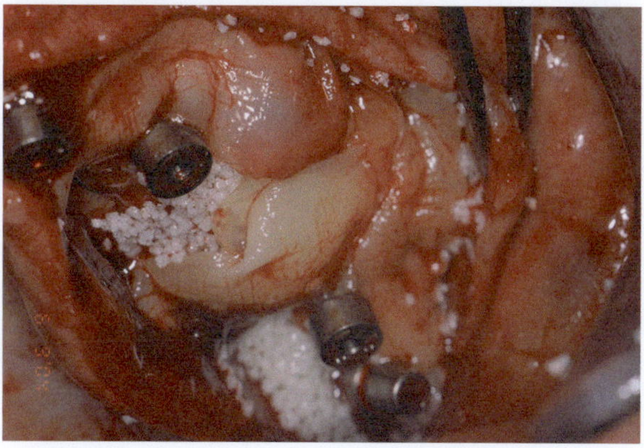

Fig. 12.41 All protruding implant parts are covered with bone substitute material and PRF membranes

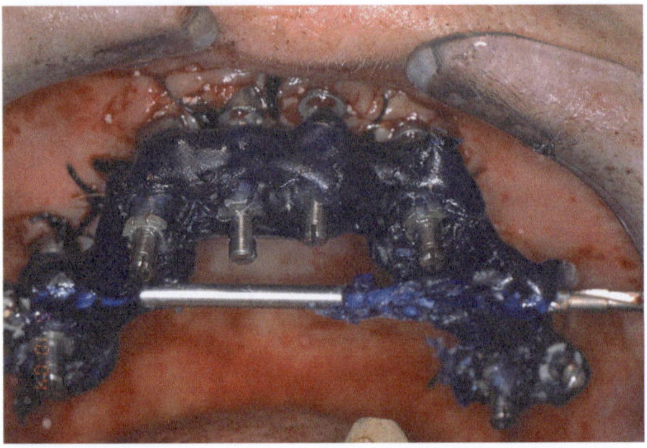

Fig. 12.42 Impression copings screwed onto the implants and held together with resin for an immediate post-op impression

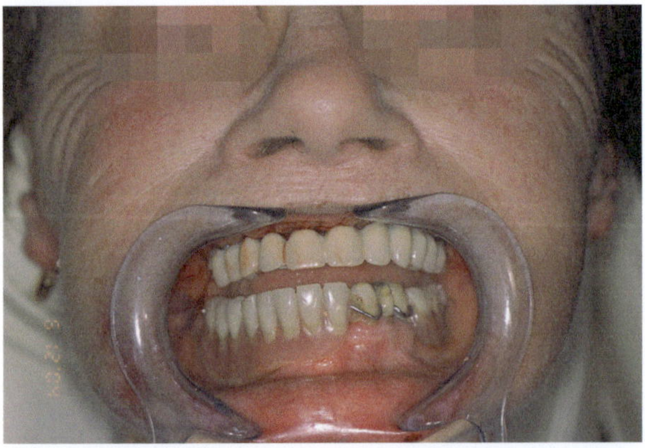

Fig. 12.43 Immediate, screw-secured titanium/Cr-Co bridge with resin teeth (48-hour post-op)

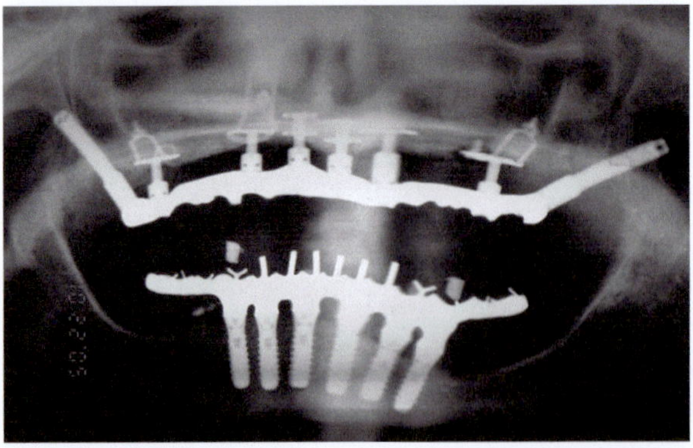

Fig. 12.44 Panoramic view 15-year post-op

The tuberosity joins the pterygoid process of the sphenoid bone. This tubero-pterygoid area usually retains its distinct shape and depth even after extensive alveolar ridge resorption because the pterygoid process is formed by dense, compact bone. Posteriorly, the tuberosity is frequently covered by a layer of compact bone and thus can bear weight. If a microthreaded pterygoid root-form implant or a Diskimplant® can be extended through that portion of the crest below and distal to the sinus wall, it can be anchored in solid bone.

The distinct morphology and dense, pterygoid compact bone structure of the tubero-pterygoid region allow solid anchorage of microthreaded root-form implants (length 20 or 23 mm) or a Diskimplant®. The most apical portion of these tubero-pterygoid implants is anchored in the pterygoid process that forms the posterior wall of the cleft. This area provides the only possible posterior maxillary cortical bone support in a maxilla with a severely ballooned sinus that has invaginated the crest anteriorly and the maxillary tuberosity posteriorly. A pterygoid implant is first gently installed through the pterygoid process, extending forward on the dense palatal aspect of the alveolar crest, and through that part of the tuberosity enclosing cancellous bone, distal to the sinus. If a pterygoid implant cannot be safely installed, a monodisk Diskimplant® (base diameter 9 mm) can be inserted palatally backward, in the thin alveolar crest under the sinus floor, and be connected to anterior implants. This multiunit assembly of interconnected dental implants will bear the prosthesis, so that excessive force is not applied directly to any part of the fragile ridge under the sinus floor. Wide plate-form Diskimplants® (33 or 43 mm in length) are another option. Following elevation of the sinus wall, the Diskimplant® is impacted laterally from the buccal aspect of the tubero-pterygoid area until it reaches the vertical sinus nasal wall (perpendicular plate of the palatine bone). This provides a wide, solid distal support in dense bone for a fixed, implant-supported restoration. This is a reliable alternative for patients who refuse a bone graft and for salvage of failing intrasinusal grafts.

Although very resistant, the pterygoid process can be fractured by application of excessive force with a manual bone spreader for alveolar crest expansion or during dental implant impaction or forceful insertion of a wide, conventional screw-type implant. Microthreaded, self-tapping pterygoid root-form implants are ideal in this region since their design eliminates the risk of bone cracks during implant installation. Implants with larger threads and/or an aggressive, self-tapping apex may be used in selected cases where the pterygoid process is thick and very solid. When conditions dictate the use of single or multidisk Diskimplants®, the base of the disk must be gently impacted laterally into the bone site with a manual seating instrument. Accurate placement of a tubero-pterygoid implant requires exposure of the site. The full-thickness flap incision for exposure of the pterygoid bone should be confined to the crest of the ridge or made 1 mm palatally. A correctly executed incision should parallel the course of the major palatine artery, well away from it. Vestibular angulated transverse releasing incisions are recommended distal to the pathway of the tuberosity vessels. A slight palatal transverse release incision can be made distal to the palatal foramen.

The crestal soft tissue incision should never come near the greater and lesser palatine foramina or their emerging vessels. The greater foramen is located on the hard palate and must remain medial to any crestal incision made for the installation of a root-form implant in the pterygoid region. In soft bone, the use of a manual bone condenser (2 mm diameter) is recommended until a denser area is reached.

The operator should then switch to a specially designed stepped pilot drill mounted on a low-speed handpiece (800 rpm). Use of this drill permits penetration through the cortical plate without cracking or separation of the pterygoid bone from the tuberosity. The osteotomy can then be pursued manually with a 2-mm bone condenser, after which a self-tapping microthreaded tubero-pterygoid Fractal® implant can be gently inserted with using a very-low-speed handpiece. A pterygoid root-form Fractal® implant can also be gently press-fit or tapped into the bone site.

If the major palatine artery is touched just slightly during manual bone site preparation (but not during an incision for flap elevation), placement of the implant body will stop the hemorrhage, and the flap can be sutured safely.

Emergency Procedures

Should the major palatine artery be accidentally severed, local pressure should be applied quickly in the region of the last molar, where the vessel emerges through the greater palatine foramen. Clamping and ligation should follow immediately. If the palatal artery retracts into the bony channel, the hemorrhage must be stopped by filling the bony foramen with resorbable bone wax (Ethicon®). The flap must then be closed and sutured tightly. The patient's former denture is immediately reinserted and maintained in occlusion for 20 minutes. The patient is advised to keep the denture in place for 24 hours, stay on a liquid diet, and then return for a checkup the next day. This is why the two pterygoid implants must be installed first in extremely atrophic maxillae: should a problem occur, it is easy to close the flap and return the patient to an easily retrievable full denture. After flapless verification of bone density with a manual osseotensor 60 days later, the other scheduled implants can be placed in denser bone.

12.2 Basal Implant Therapy for the Completely Edentulous Atrophic Mandible

The use of osseointegrated screw-type dental implants in the completely edentulous mandible is the most documented type of long-term osseointegrated implant therapy. Placement of four or five screw-type implants between the mental foramina using a two-stage method is a reliable and safe means to provide patients with a fixed, implant-supported prosthesis. Nobel Biocare later on introduced the "Brånemark Novum®" concept for rehabilitation of the edentulous mandible with just three wide screws (5 mm diameter, 12 mm long) placed in the anterior mandible to sustain a fixed, screw-retained, immediately loaded prosthesis with 15 mm cantilevers on each side. Thereafter, Paolo Malo developed the "all on four" concept with two distally tilted root-form implants. By reducing the cantilever, these procedures may give predictable results in small, moderately resorbed mandibles in selected clinical situations. However, they are difficult to apply for patients with a strong bite and large mandibles who require reliable molar support to avoid implant loss and mechanical problems due to overload and cantilever with time. Many patients also complain of loss of second molars and may develop TMJ disorders.

In totally edentulous patients, absence of the mandibular second molar has a negative effect on the removable full upper denture. The upper denture must be stabilized by means of molar occlusion, and exclusive anterior and/or reduced mastication should be avoided. Otherwise, the remaining bony structure of the premaxilla may resorb, and the upper denture will have to be constantly relined or remade. Highly atrophic mandibles cannot be handled safely at long term with just three or four screws and a fixed full denture.

Work in applied prosthodontics has clearly demonstrated the mechanical problems encountered with cantilevers over time [1]. In order to avoid fracture of components, fracture of the jaw, and/or loss of osseointegration, distal anchorage in the molar area with wide diameter Diskimplants® (9 mm or 9 × 11 mm) placed in dense bone with a pyramidal bone crest profile is recommended. Only 2–3 mm of bone depth is required for such wide Diskimplant® bases. In more highly resorbed, completely flat bone areas, plate-form Diskimplants® (33 × 9 mm, 43 × 9 mm or 43 × 7 mm models) secured with orthopedic screws and covered with bone substitute material and PRF are recommended. Narrow Fratex® root-form implants can be used providing there are at least 3 mm of crestal bone width buccolingually.

High Knife Ridges (Figs. 12.45, 12.46, 12.47, 12.48, 12.49, 12.50, 12.51, and 12.52)

Double Diskimplants® are particularly adapted for use in completely edentulous high and very thin mandibles and maxillae. A series of several basal implants of this type can be installed and immediately loaded without a cantilever.

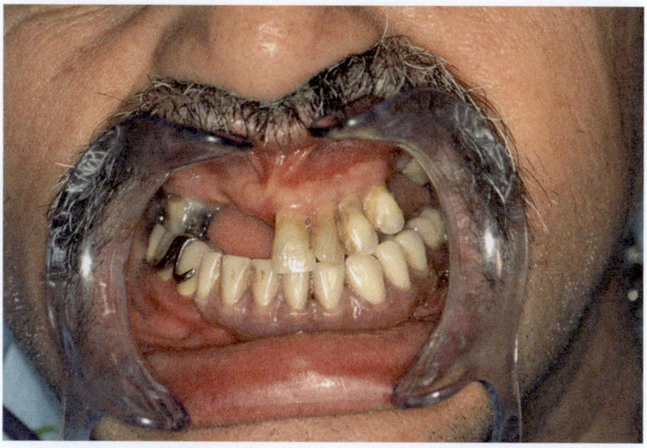

Fig. 12.45 Pre-op extraoral view (1997)

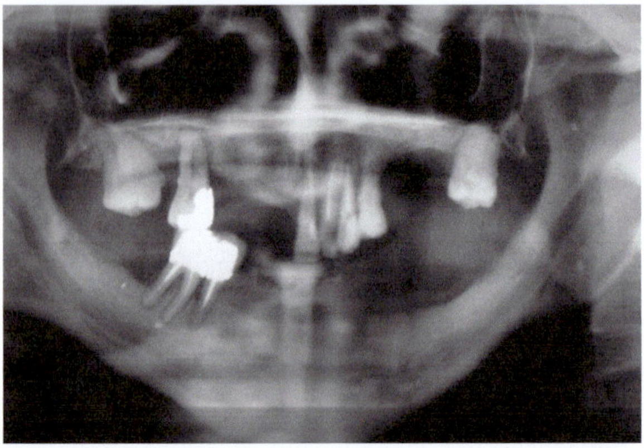

Fig. 12.46 Pre-op panoramic view (same patient as Fig. 12.45)

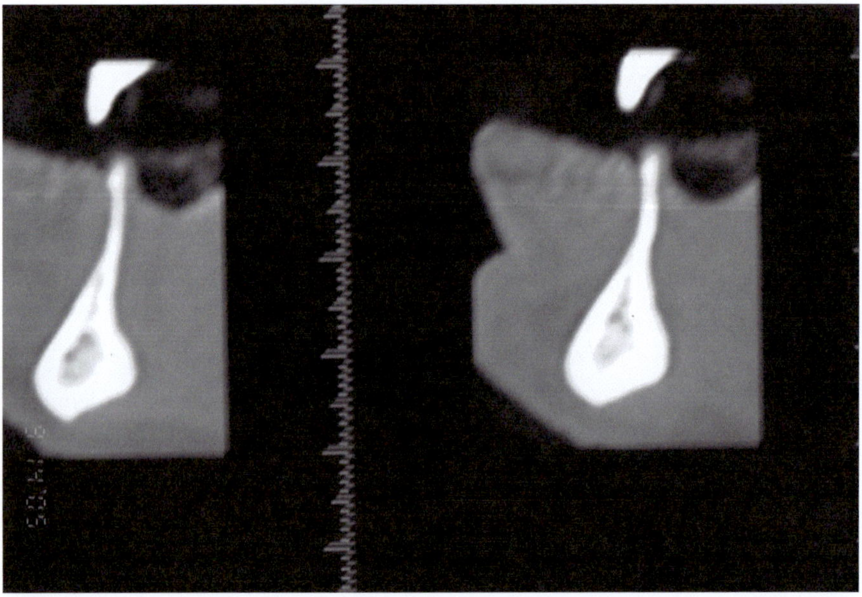

Fig. 12.47 Pre-op CT scan of a high knife ridge (thickness ≤ 2 mm)

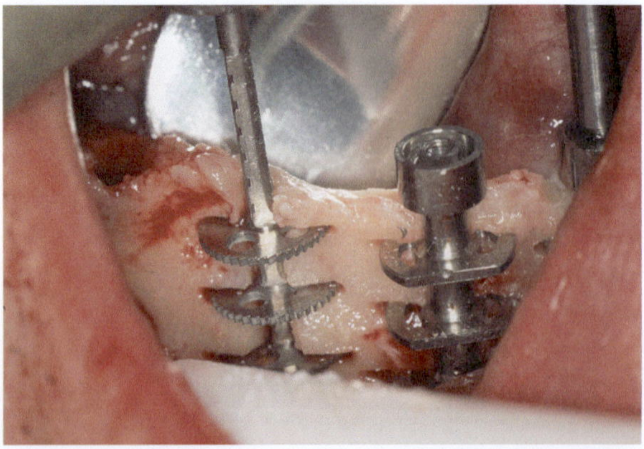

Fig. 12.48 Lateral osteotomy with titanium cutters. The horizontal basal disk can pass from the buccal to the lingual plate (the lingual flap must be protected by a flap holder). The vertical shaft of the cutter should never pass completely through to the other side. Just a small notch is made to maintain the integrity of the lingual bony wall

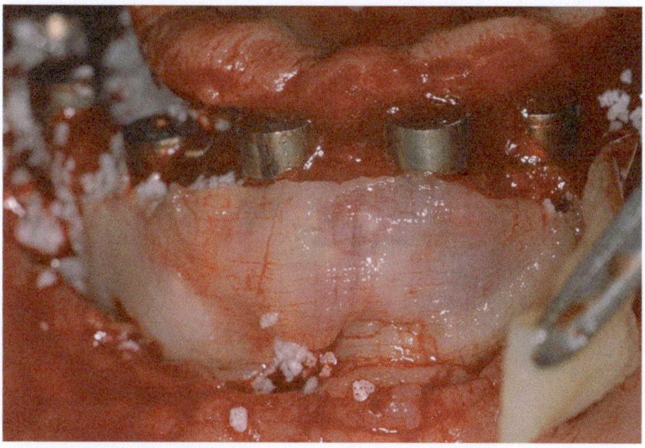

Fig. 12.49 The protruding portion of the disk creates a "tent" with the flap that serves as scaffolding for bone substitute material and PRF

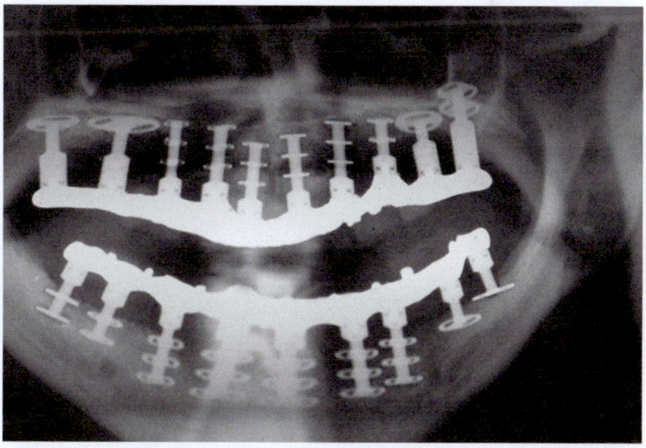

Fig. 12.50 Panoramic view in 2017 after 20 years of service (immediate loading protocol)

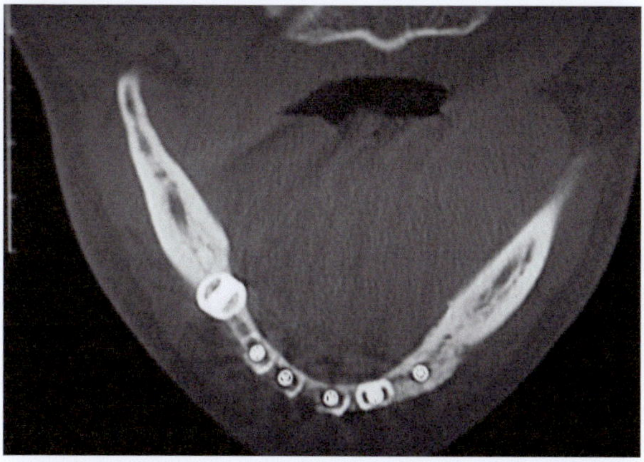

Fig. 12.51 CT scan: occlusal view

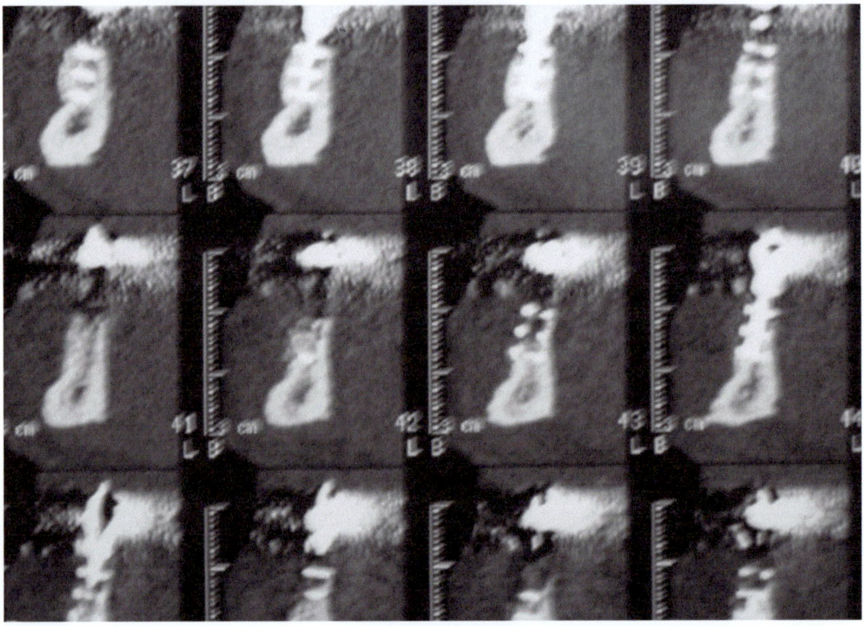

Fig. 12.52 CT scan after 20 years showing the integration of basal Diskimplants® in an extremely high knife bone crest (see Fig. 12.47)

Initial Stabilization of Mandibular Implants

The accurate initial anatomical fit of the Diskimplant® in the receptor site is necessary to avoid fibrosis. The basal plate of the Diskimplant® should always extend from the buccal cortical plate to the lingual plate. Since the atrophic mandible can be highly flexible, especially in the area of the second premolar, primary implant stabilization in dense living cortical bone is essential. This is one reason why the use of Diskimplants® of appropriate diameter is recommended in high knife ridges or when the height of good quality, clinically useful bone is under 8 mm.

Several measures can be used to prevent early basal implant failure in fully edentulous mandibles:

- Place implants in dense buccolingual cortical bone in areas of minimal flexion and torsion, i.e., between the foramina and in the molar areas; avoid the second premolar region in highly atrophic flat mandibles.
- Use an immediate functional loading technique rather than delayed loading. This requires the limitation of implant micromovements during the healing process (less than 100 μm of bone-implant relative motion), otherwise fibrous tissue can develop instead of bone. Adding mini orthopedic fixation screws in order to lock the Diskimplant® base may help to ensure absolute primary stabilization. Installation of a rigid fixed, screw-secured prosthesis 48 hours after surgery immobilizes the endosseous dental implants during function and thus permits subsequent osseointegration. The patient is required to eat a soft diet for the first 45 days after surgery.

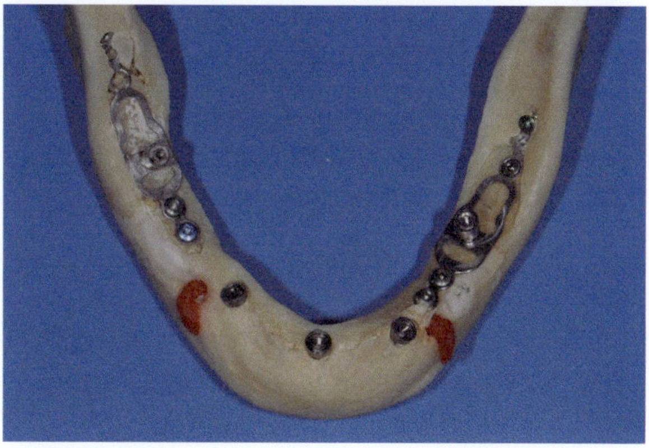

Fig. 12.53 Dry mandible showing the future treatment plan

Pencil Mandible (Fig. 12.53)

In the totally edentulous atrophic flat mandible, installation of dental implants should be avoided in the zone of maximum flexion, i.e., the second premolar area close to the mandibular foramen. Microthreaded root-form implants and Diskimplants® must be distributed in the two areas where flexion and torsion are minimum: the mental area between the foramina and between the molar and the retromolar regions when an immediate loading protocol is used. Wide-diameter (43 × 9 mm) plate-form Diskimplants® are recommended in these areas of dense bone (type I or II) provided the ridge is flat and wide. Double Diskimplants® are reserved for high knife ridges while single-disk implants are used when the ridge is wide and round.

Management of Areas of Dense Bone in the Extremely Atrophic Mandible

Implant placement in dense bone is challenging, especially in pencil mandibles, because of the poor intrabony blood supply that manifests as the absence of bleeding during osteotomy. If an implant is installed despite insufficient blood supply, it may be expelled early on, several days to several weeks after placement.

When planning a root-form implant in the mental sector in combination with basal implants installed in the posterior mandible, the quality of the recipient bed for the root-forms can be improved by the use of a rotary osseotensor. This is the only indication for rotary osseotensors in conjunction with basal implants in the mandible. A single rotary osseotensor impact at each scheduled root-form implant site 1 week before surgery suffices to "soften" hard D1 bone into active D2 bone as the result of the catabolic response initiated by bony penetration of the instrument.

For the mandible, use of a manual osseotensor in basal implantology is limited to tunneling the periosteum 1 week before placement of a Diskimplant® or a plate-form Diskimplant® in the posterior sector in order to promote stem cell activation and improve local blood supply and callus formation at the osteotomy site. For the upper jaw, manual osseotensors are reserved for intrabony penetration of D4 or D3 sites when basal implants or root-form implants are planned.

12.3 Extreme Clinical Situations

Ectodermal Dysplasia (Figs. 12.54, 12.55, 12.56, 12.57, 12.58, 12.59, and 12.60)

This patient was followed up by the family dentist starting at the age of 6 years. In 2003, at the age of 22, basal implants were installed under general anesthesia at the Medical School in Nice, France. The anatomic conditions were so difficult that no root-form implants could be safely installed. The patient received his fixed prosthesis 78 hours post-op. In October 2017, a follow-up examination revealed the absence of any bone loss around the basal implants after 14 years of service.

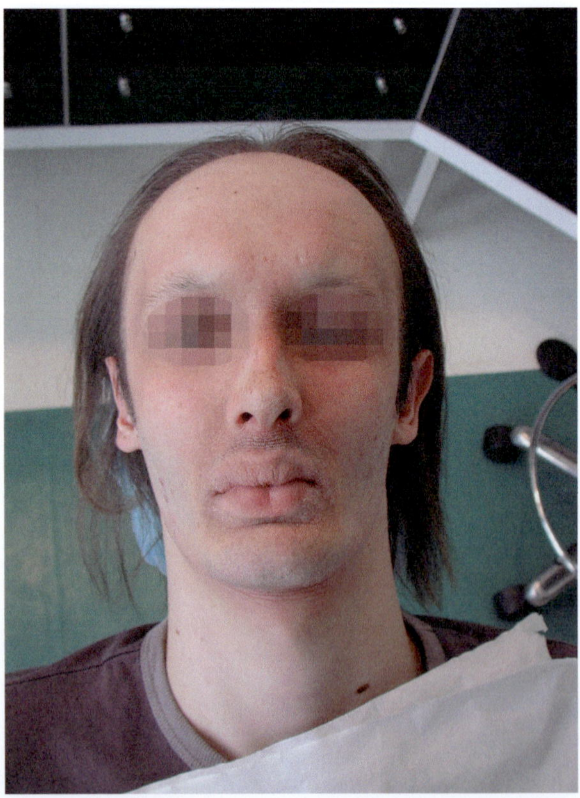

Fig. 12.54 Ectodermal dysplasia: patient aged 22 years (2003)

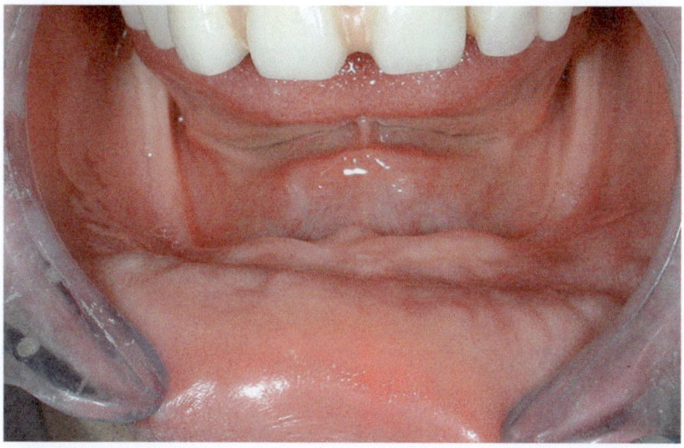

Fig. 12.55 The patient had worn two removable dentures since the age of 7; the appliances were constantly remade as his jaws grew

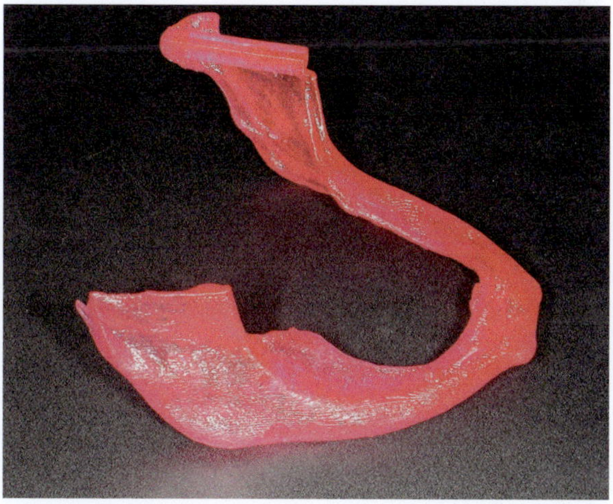

Fig. 12.56 Stereolithographic model of the toothless mandible (ectodermal dysplasia)

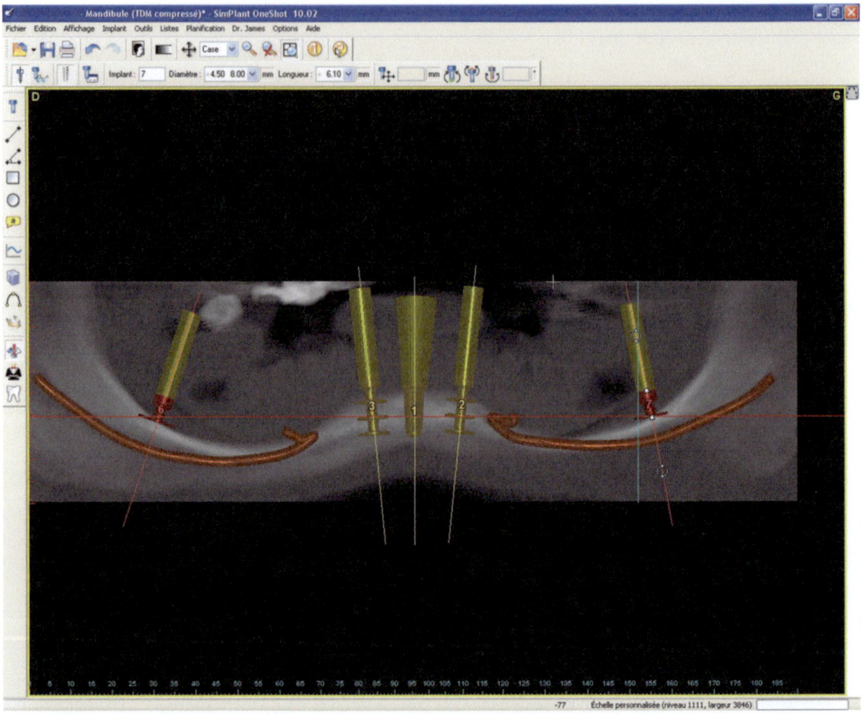

Fig. 12.57 Simulation of the future implant sites using the basal implant library

Fig. 12.58 Intraoral view of the screw-secured, fixed lower prosthesis (same patient as Fig. 12.54)

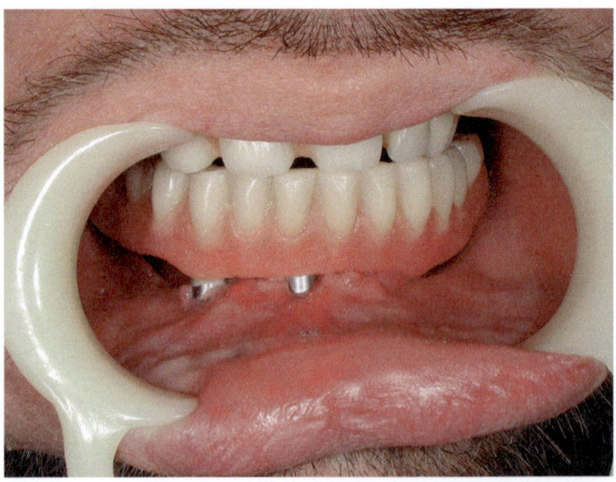

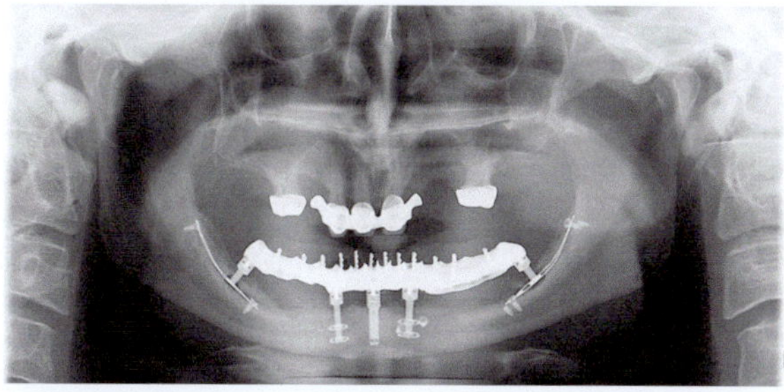

Fig. 12.59 Flat posterior mandible suitable for plate-form Diskimplants®: panoramic view after 14 years of service (same patient as Fig. 12.54)

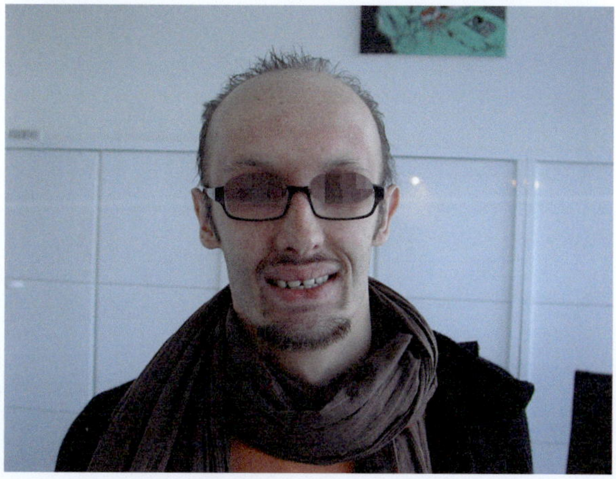

Fig. 12.60 Cosmetic aspect after 14 years (2017); patient aged 36 years (same patient as Fig. 12.54)

Neurofibromatosis ("Elephant Man Disease") (Figs. 12.61, 12.62, 12.63, 12.64, 12.65, 12.66, 12.67, 12.68, and 12.69)

Jean-Marie Donsimoni

Bone Disorders

- Gonial angle 180°; no tuberosity; the upper molars are anchored directly in the orbital floor.
- Forty-four teeth present on the arch or impacted.
- Terebrant infiltrations of the neurofibromatosis lesions in the bone, which meant there was hardly any remaining bone after excision.

Soft tissue disorders : End-stage periodontal disease with extremely voluminous and very hemorrhagic neurofibromatosis lesions. Following excision, edema was so severe that intubation had to be maintained during the 8 days of healing. Surgery was performed under general anesthesia when this male patient was 27 years of age.

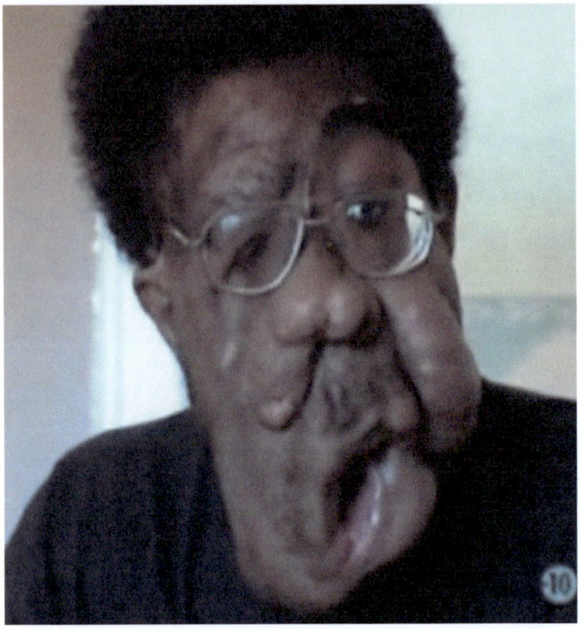

Fig. 12.61 Initial preoperative status of a 27-year-old patient with "elephant man disease" (courtesy Dr. J-M Donsimoni)

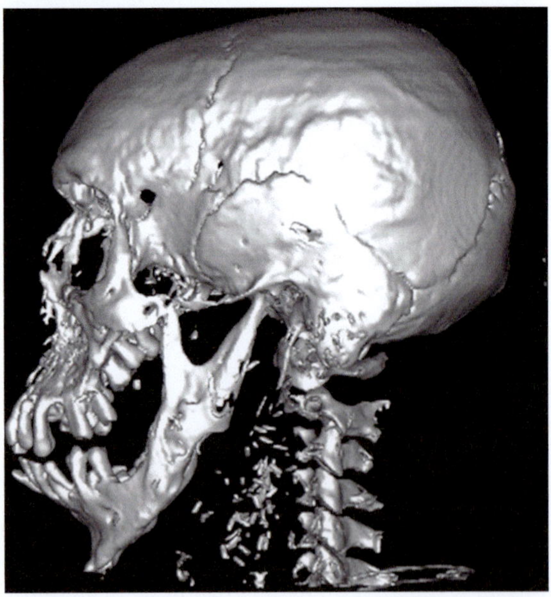

Fig. 12.62 Pre-op 3D reconstruction (lateral view) (same patient as Fig. 12.61)

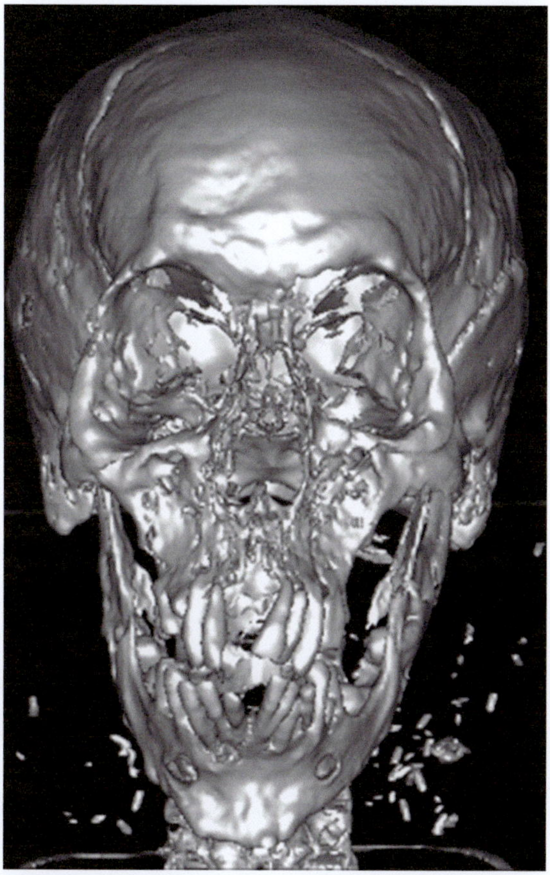

Fig. 12.63 Pre-op 3D reconstruction: front view

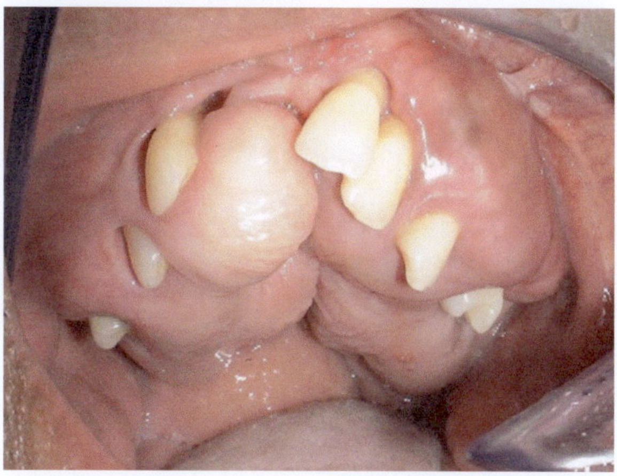

Fig. 12.64 Pre-op intraoral view (maxilla) (same patient as Fig. 12.61)

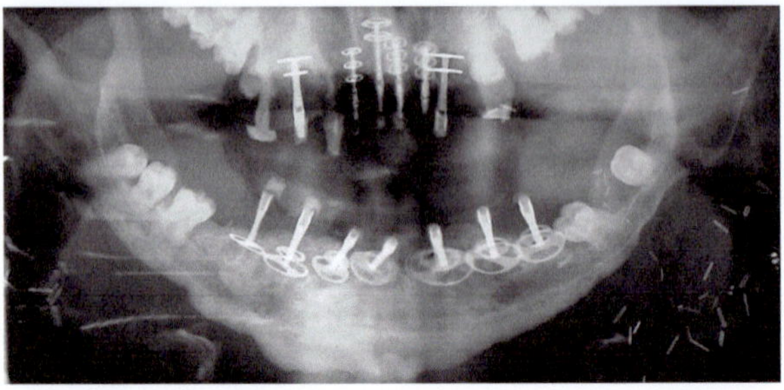

Fig. 12.65 Initial panoramic view after basal implant installation

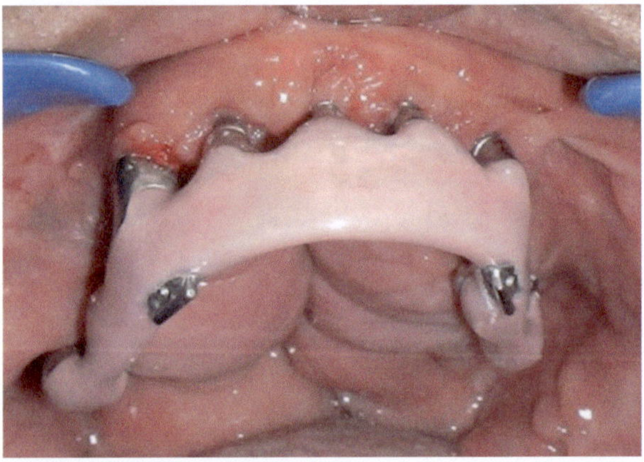

Fig. 12.66 Intraoral view of the screw-secured, ceramic-to-metal bar (maxilla)

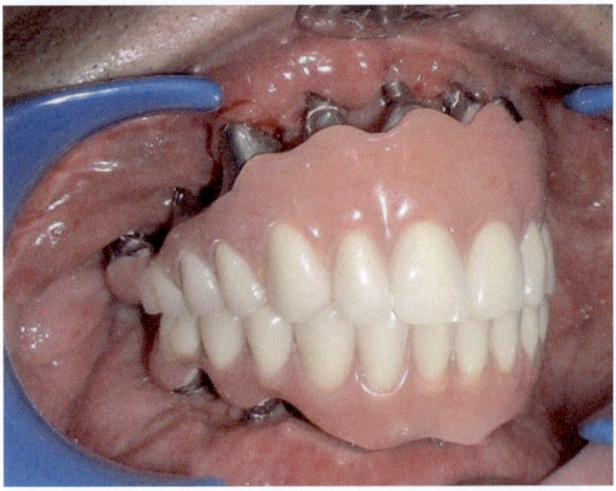

Fig. 12.67 Panoramic view of the upper and lower bridges in place after 14 years of service

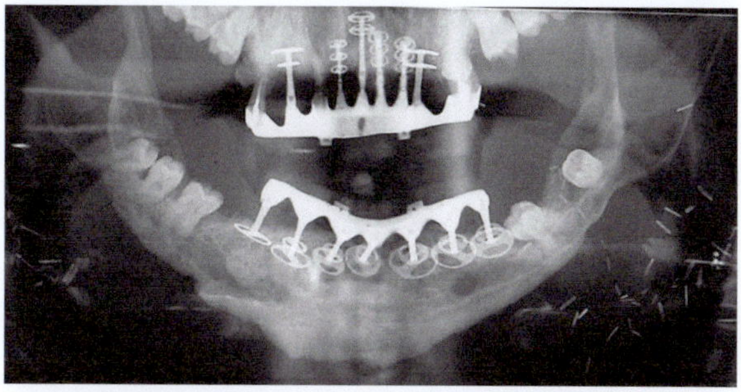

Fig. 12.68 Intraoral view of the final upper and lower prostheses

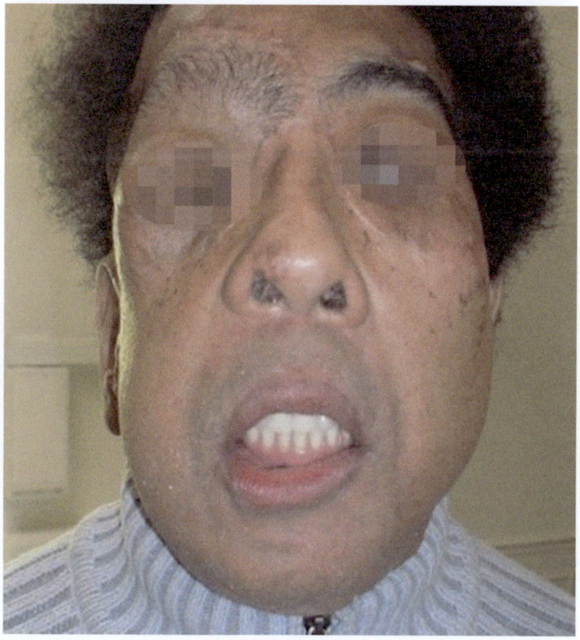

Fig. 12.69 Cosmetic outcome in 2017

After Surgery

To avoid glare on future CT studies, the implants and the prosthetic frameworks were fabricated of pink ceramic on titanium (hence nonmagnetic); the prostheses were fabricated of resin cemented to the frameworks but were retrievable. The small diameter shafts of the Diskimplants® used make them less susceptible to infectious infiltrations. The very wide and high embrasures compensate for the difficulties encountered to reach up this high with a toothbrush (very high vertical dimension); these embrasures also limit the risks of infection. Recurrence of the neurofibromatosis lesions is unlikely in light of the patient's age.

Long-Term Follow-Up (2007–2017)

After nearly 10 years, there have been no complications despite the difficulties for oral hygiene and especially despite the immunosuppressive treatments that can render even the slightest infection critical in only a few days.

12.4 Clinical Evaluation of Immediately Loaded, Screw-Secured Fixed Rehabilitations in Extremely Atrophic Jaws (Figs. 12.70, 12.71, 12.72, 12.73, 12.74, 12.75, 12.76, 12.77, and 12.78)

A series of patients with extremely resorbed, fully edentulous upper and/or lower jaws were rehabilitated with immediately loaded, screw-retained fixed prostheses from February 2000 to November 2017 (Tables 12.1 and 12.2). The age of these 416 patients (female 286, male 130) ranged from 42 to 86 years (mean 64 years). In all, 3428 implants were installed, including Diskimplants® (D), plate-form Diskimplants®

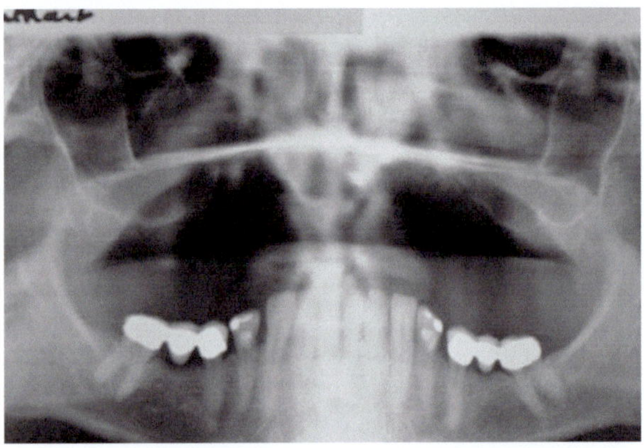

Fig. 12.70 Pre-op panoramic view showing the extremely resorbed maxilla of a patient who had worn a full upper denture since the age of 22

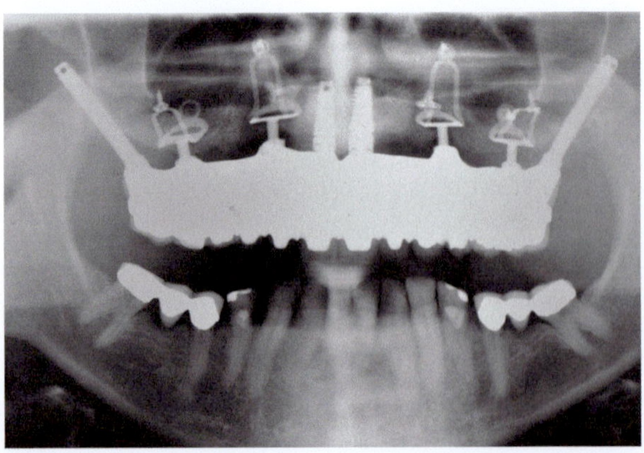

Fig. 12.71 Panoramic view of the final screw-secured ceramic-fused-to-metal prosthesis in 2017 (14 year post-op) (same patient as Fig. 12.70)

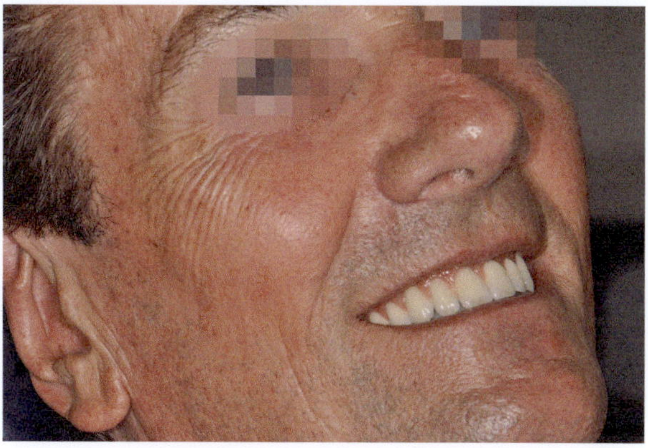

Fig. 12.72 Final cosmetic outcome (same patient as Fig. 12.70)

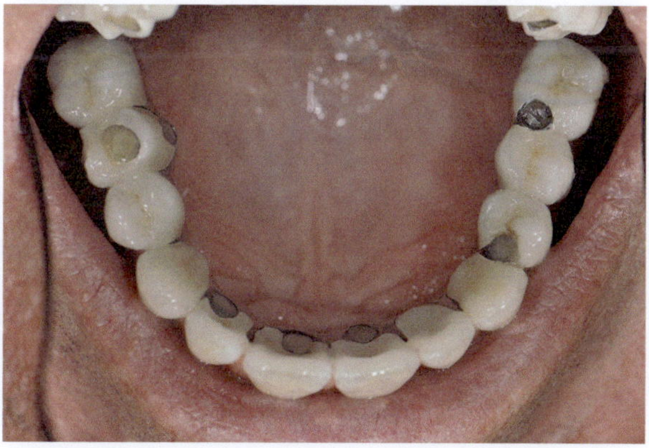

Fig. 12.73 Occlusal view of the rehabilitation (same patient as Fig. 12.70)

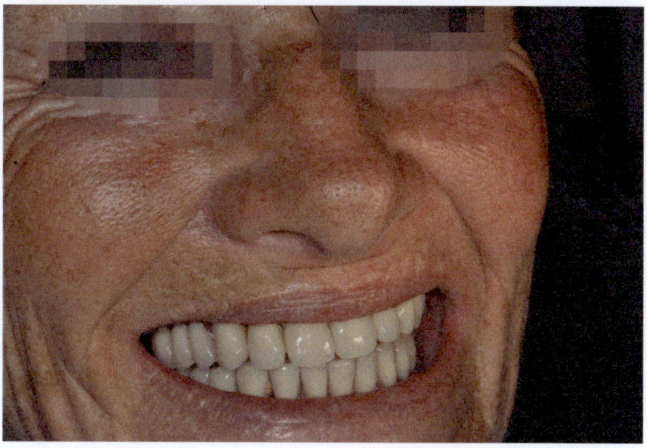

Fig. 12.74 Final cosmetic aspect of a patient with an extremely resorbed maxilla, 6 months post-op

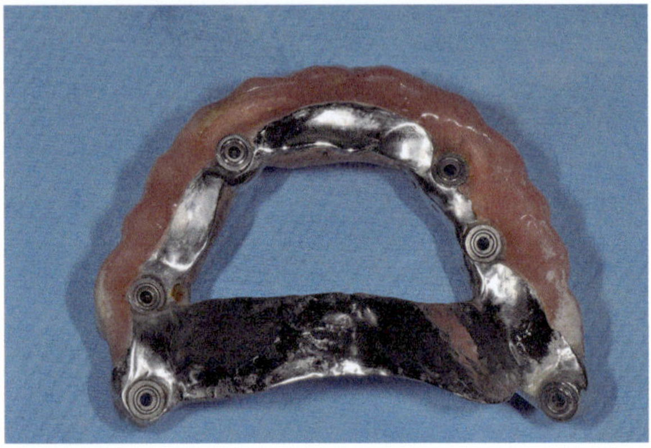

Fig. 12.75 A wide transitional transpalatal bar was made to ensure cross-arch stability for this patient who had lost all of his root-form implants 3 years earlier (same patient as Fig. 12.74)

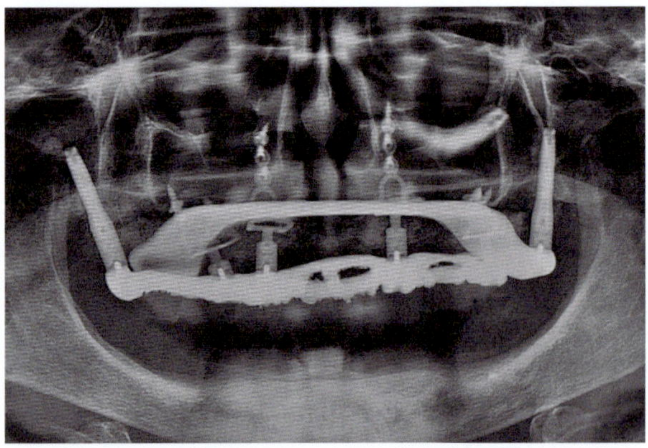

Fig. 12.76 Panoramic view 2 years post-op with the transpalatal bar in place

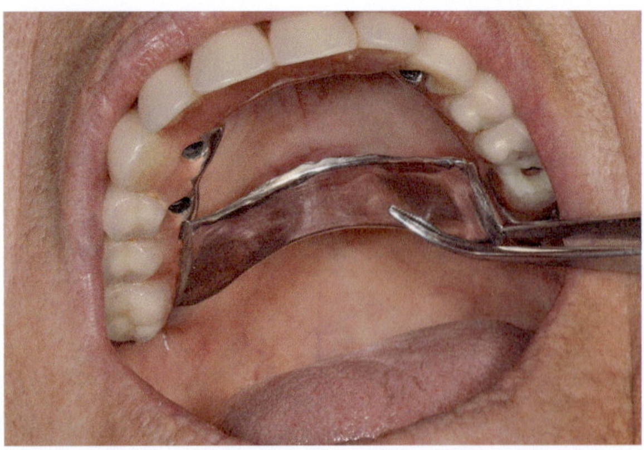

Fig. 12.77 Intraoral view showing removal of the transpalatal bar after 2 years of service

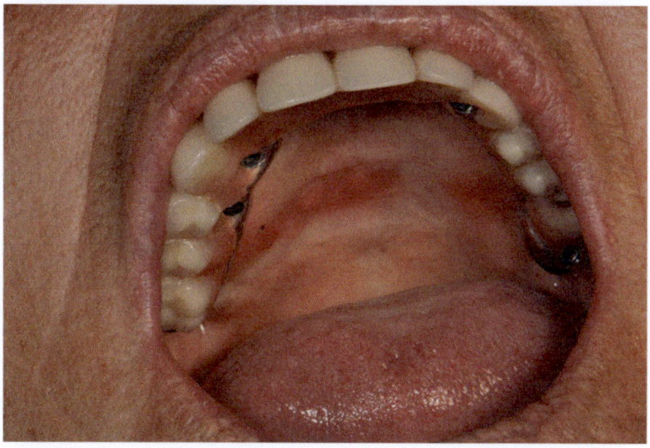

Fig. 12.78 Resin teeth on machined titanium cylinders bonded to the Co-Cr metal frame; this ensures a precise fit of the prosthesis screw-secured on the implants

Table 12.1 Long-term survey of 416 patients with extremely resorbed atrophic jaws managed with basal implants alone or in combination with root-form implants from 2000 to 2017

	Total number of patients (2000–2017) 9 months–18 years Severely atrophic jaws	Total implants placed between Feb 2000 and Oct 2016 (check-up July 2017)—100% immediate, screw-secured-to-implant functional loading procedure	Number of Diskimplants® placed (single, double, triple disk)	Number of plate-form Diskimplants® placed	Number of root-form implants placed R: regular NR: narrow root-form PtR: pterygoid root-form		
	416	3 428	D	Pf D	R	NR	PtR
Female	Maxilla: 159	Maxilla: 1432	Maxilla: 346	Maxilla: 493	213	78	**302**
Age 42–86 years (mean 64)	Mandible: 127	Mandible: 875	Mandible: 101	Mandible: 283	428	63	Max only
Total	**286 patients**	**2307 implants**	**447 Diskimplants®**	**776 Pf D**	**641**	**141**	
Male	Maxilla: 82	Maxilla 697	Maxilla: 106	Maxilla: 252	149	28	**152**
Age 44–82 years (mean 63)	Mandible: 48	Mandible 424	Mandible: 62	Mandible: 94	246	22	Max only
Total	**130 patients**	**1121 implants**	**168 Diskimplants®**	**346 Pf D**	**30**	**50**	
Number of implants lost[a] (2000–2017)	Females	12	2	2	2	3	3
	Males	9	2	1	2	2	2
	Total	21	4	3	4	5	5
		Diskimplants® + root-forms	Diskimplants®		Root-forms		

[a]80% of patients were lost to follow-up over time; see Table 12.2

Table 12.2 Patients lost to follow-up from 2000 to 2017

	Feb 2000	2001	2002	2003	2004	2005	2006	2007	2008	2009	2010	2011	2012	2013	2014	2015	2016	2017
Number of patients/year	20	23	21	24	25	23	23	24	23	24	25	26	27	27	25	29	27	18
Cumulative number of patients operated during the 17 years	20	43	64	88	113	136	159	183	206	230	255	281	308	335	360	389	**416**	July 2017: verification of all patients implanted >9 months earlier (patients operated up until October 2016)
Cumulative number of patients checked annually	20	35	39	45	49	50	53	57	59	63	67	71	75	76	78	80	82	
Cumulative percentage of patients checked annually	100%	81%	61%	51%	43%	37%	33%	31%	28%	27%	26%	25%	24%	22%	21%	20.5%	20%	Nearly 80% of the patients had been lost to follow-up after 17 years
Patients lost to follow-up over time	0	19%	39%	49%	57%	63%	67%	69%	72%	73%	74%	75%	76%	78%	79%	79.5%	80%	

(PfD), Fractal® implants (regular root-form R or pterygoid root-form PtR), and Fratex® implants (narrow root-form, NR). Follow-up varied from 9 months to 17 years.

None of the patients could be managed directly with only root-form implants (not even short, narrow and/or narrow platform blade implants). Anatomic conditions were not favorable for root-form zygomatic implants.

Bone Grafting

Bone grafting and/or sinus lift procedures were not performed for a variety of reasons:

- The patient refused a bone graft and/or sinus lift.
- A graft had already been attempted but failed.
- Extensive bone grafting before implant placement was medically contraindicated in light of the patient's general health status.
- Free bone grafting of the atrophic jaws was not advisable due to the poor quality and quantity of the recipient bone.

Treatment Procedure

Following pre-surgery osteogenic activation, all patients were fully equipped with Diskimplants® (including plate-form Diskimplants®), associated or not with root-form implants. Bone activation was achieved by applying a bone matrix osseotensor to the intended recipient site 2 weeks (mandible, type I bone) to 45–60 days (maxilla, type IV bone) prior to implant placement.

The number of implants installed depended on the anatomic conditions. Treatment for the maxilla consisted in 6 to 12 implants, while mandibles were equipped with 5–9 implants. The immediate functional loading protocol involved placement of a prosthesis screw-secured directly to the implants (with or without transgingival abutments) 48 hours post-op. This transitional prosthesis used titanium bonding cylinders glued into a CrCo framework and commercial composite resin teeth (Premium® by Kulzer/Phonares® by Ivoclar).

Patient Follow-up: Initial verification was performed 48 hours post-op, 1 week post-op, and 45 days post-op.

Six months post-op, the screw-secured prosthesis was retrieved, and all implants were checked individually (panograph, periapical x-rays, cone-beam CT). Thereafter, a checkup was scheduled annually (the screw-secured prosthesis was retrieved only if necessary).

Maintenance instructions consisted in mouthwashes with salt water or bicarbonate, application of Dakin Cooper solution to the gingiva with a cotton swab for the first 45 days, and careful brushing with a soft toothbrush (100 μm). Use of a Waterpik® appliance was permitted after 4 weeks.

12.5 Results

After 1 year, either the transitional prosthesis was conserved (with or without any necessary occlusal adjustments) or a new, definitive prosthesis was fabricated of full zirconia (Zirkonzahn). All but one of the patients declared high or very high satisfaction with the outcome. The exception was a bipolar psychiatric patient with body dysmorphic disorder (BDD) who had not been detected initially and who eventually returned to a full denture. She continuously added acrylic resin to the buccal aspect of the full denture because she felt it improved her esthetic appearance.

Conflict of interest statement Gérard M. Scortecci is the inventor of the Diskimplant and holder of several associated patents that are exploited by the Victory company. He is an unpaid consultant to this firm and a minority shareholder in the company. No money was received from any of the companies mentioned in the book or from any of the companies whose products are mentioned.

Recommended Reading

1. Resnik RR, Misch CE. Avoiding complications in oral implantology. Amsterdam: Elsevier; 2017. p. 90–6.
2. Brown DW. Complete edentulism prior to the age of 65 years is associated with all-cause mortality. J Public Health Dent. 2009;69(4):260–6.
3. Cunha-Cruz J, Hujoel PP, Nadanovsky P. Secular trends in socio-economic disparities in edentulism: USA, 1972-2001. J Dent Res. 2007;86(2):131–6.
4. de Marchi RJ, Hugo FN, Padilha DM, et al. Edentulism, use of dentures and consumption of fruit and vegetables in south Brazilian community-dwelling elderly. J Oral Rehabil. 2011;38(7):533–40.
5. Divaris K, Ntounis A, Marinis A, Polyzois G, Polychronopoulou A. Loss of natural dentition: multi-level effects among a geriatric population. Gerodontology. 2012;29(2):192–9.
6. Dogan BG, Gokalp S. Tooth loss and edentulism in the Turkish elderly. Arch Gerontol Geriatr. 2012;54(2):162–6.
7. Douglass CW, Shih A, Ostry L. Will there be a need for complete dentures in the United States in 2020? J Prosthet Dent. 2002;87(1):5–8.
8. Dye BA, Li X, Thorton-Evans G. Oral health disparities as determined by selected healthy people. 2020 oral health objectives for the United States, 2009–2010. NCHS Data Brief. 2012.
9. Emami E, Freitas de Souza R, Kabawat M, Feine JS. The impact of edentulism on oral and general health. Int J Dent. 2013; 2013:498305,1–7.
10. Eustaquio-Raga MV, Montiel-Company JM, Almerich-Silla JM. Factors associated with edentulousness in an elderly population in Valencia (Spain). Gac Sanit. 2012;27(2):123–7.
11. Felton D, Cooper L, Duqum I, et al. Evidence-based guidelines for the care and maintenance of complete dentures: a publication of the American College of Prosthodontists. JAMA. 2011;142(suppl 1):1S–20S.
12. Fontijn-Tekamp FA, Slagter AP, van der Bilt A, et al. Biting and chewing in overdentures, full dentures, and natural dentition. J Dent Res. 2000;79(7):1519–24.
13. Gotfredsen K, Walls AW. What dentition assures oral function? Clin Oral Implants Res. 2007;18(suppl 3):34–45.
14. Hashimoto M, Yamanaka K, Shimosato T, et al. Oral condition and health status of elderly 8020 achievers in Aichi prefecture. Bull Tokyo Dent Coll. 2006;47(2):37–43.
15. Hatch JP, Shinkai RSA, Sakai S, Rugh JD, Paunovich ED. Determinants of masticatory performance in dentate adults. Arch Oral Biol. 2001;46(7):641–8.
16. Canada H. Report on the findings of the oral health component of the Canadian health measures survey 2007–2009. Ottawa, ON: Ministry of Health; 2010.

17. Kanno T, Carlsson GE. A review of the shortened dental arch concept focusing on the work by the Käyser/Nijmegen group. J Oral Rehabil. 2006;33:850–62.
18. Medina-Solis CE, Perez-Nunez R, Maupomé G, et al. National survey on edentulism and its geographic distribution among Mexicans 18 years of age and older (with emphasis in WHO age groups). J Oral Rehabil. 2008;35(4):237–44.
19. Meningaud JP, Donsimoni JM. Facial allografts and oral rehabilitation. Rev Stomatol Chir Maxillofac. 2012;113(4):350–2.
20. Meningaud JP, Donsimoni JM, Lantieri L. Facial allograft transplantation and basal implantology (cortically-anchored disk-design implants). Rev Stomatol Chir Maxillofac. 2009;110(6):353–8.
21. Millar WJ, Locker D. Edentulism and denture use. Health Rep. 2005;17(1):55–8.
22. Misch CE. Contemporary implant dentistry. Saint Louis: Mosby; 2008. p. 1029–30.
23. Misch CE. Dental implant prosthetics. 2nd ed. Saint Louis: Mosby; 2015. p. 537–43.
24. Mojon P. The world without teeth: demographic trends. In: Feine JS, Carlsson GE, editors. Implant overdentures. The standard of care for edentulous patients. Chicago: Quintessence; 2003. p. 3–14.
25. Mojon P, Thomason JM, Walls AWG. The impact of falling rates of edentulism. Int J Prosthodont. 2004;17:434–40.
26. Muller F, Naharro M, Carlsson GE. What are the prevalence and incidence of tooth loss in the adult and elderly population in Europe? Clin Oral Implants Res. 2007;18(3):2–14.
27. Naik AV, Pai RC. Study of emotional effects of tooth loss in an aging north Indian community. ISRN Dent. 2011;2011:4 (ID 395498).
28. Nieuwenhuizen WF, Weenen H, Rigby P, Hetherington MM. Older adults and patients in need of nutritional support: review of current treatment options and factors influencing nutritional intake. Clin Nutr. 2010;29(2):160–9.
29. Nitschke I, Müller F. The impact of oral health on the quality of life in the elderly. Oral Health Prev Dent. 2004;2(suppl 1):271–5.
30. Odin G, Petitbois R, Cotten P, Philip P. Distraction osteogenesis using bone matrix osteotensors in ectodermal dysplasia: a case report. Implant Dent. 2015;24(5):612–9.
31. Osterberg T, Carlsson GE. Dental state, prosthodontic treatment and chewing ability-a study of five cohorts of 70-year-old subjects. J Oral Rehabil. 2007;34(8):553–9.
32. Osterberg T, Carlsson GE, Sundh V. Trends and prognoses of dental status in the Swedish population: analysis based on interviews in 1975 to 1997 by Statistics Sweden. Acta Odontol Scand. 2000;58:177–82.
33. Osterberg T, Carlsson GE, Sundh V, Mellström D. Number of teeth—a predictor of mortality in 70-year-old subjects. Community Dent Oral Epidemiol. 2007;36(3):258–68.
34. Osterberg T, Dey DK, Sundh V, Carlsson GE, Jansson JO, Mellström D. Edentulism associated with obesity: a study of four national surveys of 16 416 Swedes aged 55-84 years. Acta Odontol Scand. 2010;68(6):360–7.
35. Pelzer K, Hewlett S, Yawson AE, et al. Prevalence of loss of all teeth (edentulism) and associated factors in older adults in China, Ghana, India, Mexico, Russia and South Africa. Int J Environ Res Public Health. 2014;11:11308–24.
36. Prakash N, Kalavathy N, Sridevi J, Premnath K. Nutritional status assessment in complete denture wearers. Gerodontology. 2012;29:224–30.
37. Rich B, Goldstein GR. New paradigms in prosthodontic treatment planning: a literature review. J Prosthet Dent. 2002;88:208–14.
38. Richards W, Ameen J, Coll AM, Higgs G. Reasons for tooth extraction in four general dental practices in South Wales. Br Dent J. 2005;198:275–8.
39. Rodrigues SM, Oliveira AC, Vargas AMD, Moreira AN, Ferreira E. Implications of edentulism on quality of life among elderly. Int J Environ Res Public Health. 2012;9(1):100–9.
40. Saman DM, Lemieux A, Arevalo O, Lutfiyya MN. A population-based study of edentulism in the US. BMC Public Health. 2014;14:65.
41. Scortecci G, Misch CE, Benner KU. Implants and restorative dentistry. London: Martin Dunitz; 2001. p. 241–311.
42. Simunkovic SK, Boras VV, Panduric J, Zilic IA. Oral health among institutionalized elderly in Zagreb, Croatia. Gerodontology. 2005;22:238–41.

43. Srinivasan M, Meyer S, Mombelli A, Müller F. Dental implants in the elderly population: a systematic review and meta-analysis. Clin Oral Implants Res. 2016;28(8):920–30. https://doi.org/10.1111/clr.12898.
44. Sumi Y, Miura H, Michiwaki Y, Nagaosa S, Nagaya M. Colonization of dental plaque by respiratory pathogens in dependent elderly. Arch Gerontol Geriatr. 2007;44(2):119–24.
45. Taji T, Yoshida M, Hiasa K, Abe Y, Tsuga K, Akagawa Y. Influence of mental status on removable prosthesis compliance in institutionalized elderly persons. Int J Prosthodont. 2005;18:146–9.
46. Tallgren A. The continuing reduction of the residual alveolar ridges in complete denture wearers; a mixed-longitudinal study covering 25 years. J Prosthet Dent. 1972;27(2):120–32.
47. Tramini P, Montal S, Valcarel J. Tooth loss and associated factors in long-term institutionalized elderly patients. Gerodontology. 2007;24(4):196–203.
48. Tsakos G, Herrick K, Sheiham A, Watt RG. Edentulism and fruit and vegetable intake in low-income adults. J Dent Res. 2010;89(5):462–7.

Multicenter Clinical Applications 13

Gérard M. Scortecci

13.1 Multicenter Application of Basal Implants

The following case studies illustrate the excellent results achieved by implant specialists and general practitioners trained in basal implant dentistry. These private practitioners or full-time hospital or university staff generally carried out all stages of the therapeutic plan (treatment planning, basal implant surgery, and prosthodontics). All had received specific training in the use of Diskimplants®, the majority at the University of Nice-Sophia Antipolis postgraduate program in basal implantology or in practical courses organized by the Implantoral Club International (ICI) since 1984 (Table 13.1).

A comprehensive medical and dental history was obtained from each implant candidate, followed by clinical examination and 3D imaging studies. Written informed consent was obtained in all cases after the patient had been thoroughly informed of the nature of basal implant therapy and other treatment options (conventional prosthetic approach, bone grafting, etc.). Approximately 90% of the patients underwent flapless treatment with a bone matrix osseotensor to improve the recipient bone bed 10–45 days before implant installation.

Delayed loading or immediate functional loading protocols were executed according to the inclusion/exclusion criteria described elsewhere in this book:

- All basal plate-form Diskimplants® were completely covered by bone substitute material and PRF membranes.

G. M. Scortecci (✉)
University of Nice-Sophia Antipolis Medical School, Nice, France

New York University, New York, NY, USA

University of Southern California, Los Angeles, CA, USA

Private Practice, Nice, France
e-mail: scortecci@wanadoo.fr

© Springer Nature Switzerland AG 2019

G. M. Scortecci (ed.), *Basal Implantology*, https://doi.org/10.1007/978-3-319-44873-2_13

- When the submerged technique was used, the implant sites were allowed to heal 6 to 8 months, depending on bone quality and the individual appointment schedule.
- When an immediate functional loading protocol was used, the highly rigid fixed, implant-supported screw-secured titanium/CrCo/resin prosthesis was installed 48–72 hours after implant placement.

All prostheses were fabricated by commercial dental laboratories familiar with the use of basal implant components. The final prosthetic options included:

1. Continued use of the transitional titanium/CrCo denture with resin teeth
2. Ceramic-fused-to-metal with machined titanium copings bonded to the frame
3. 3D machined titanium frame (resin or ceramic teeth)
4. 3D machined CrCo framework (resin or ceramic teeth)
5. Full zirconia technology (e.g., Zirkonzahn, Prettau)

Table 13.1 European versus US tooth positions

Maxilla	**Upper right**								**Upper left**							
USA	1	2	3	4	5	6	7	8	9	10	11	12	13	14	15	16
Europe	18	17	16	15	14	13	12	11	21	22	23	24	25	26	27	28
Mandible	**Lower right**								**Lower left**							
USA	32	31	30	29	28	27	26	25	24	23	22	21	20	19	18	17
Europe	48	47	46	45	44	43	42	41	31	32	33	34	35	36	37	38

Case Study 1: Edentulous Resorbed Mandible

Dr. Alain Ansel, Thionville, France (Surgery and Prosthodontics)
Follow-Up: 2015–2017

Female, 71 years old at implant placement

Non-smoker, good general health

Atrophic posterior mandible, knife ridge anterior mandible, loss of teeth in the incisor-canine sectors

Oral mucosa: Healthy

Oral hygiene: Good, check-up every 6 months, no problems noted at last visit

Preop management:

- Osseotensor treatment of the mandible
- Relief of the lower denture

Surgical and prosthetic procedures: Local anesthesia, immediate functional loading 96 hours post-op of five Diskimplants® (two plate-form Diskimplants® covered by bone substitute material and PRF membranes, three double Diskimplants®) and two Fractal® root-form implants with a fixed, screw-secured highly rigid prosthesis

X-rays/imaging: Panoramic radiographs, CT scan (Figs. 13.1 and 13.2)

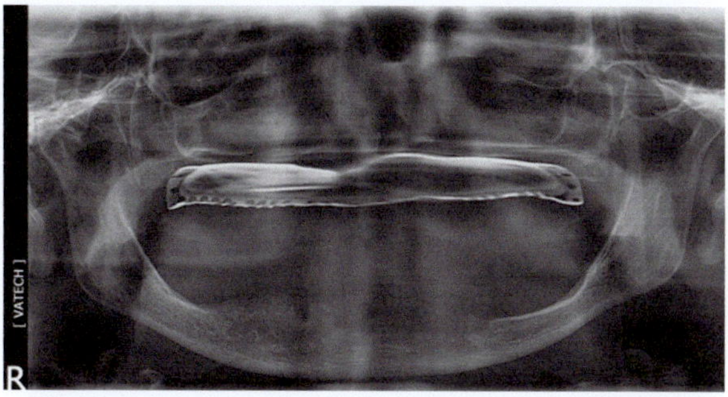

Fig. 13.1 Initial panoramic radiograph. April 30, 2015

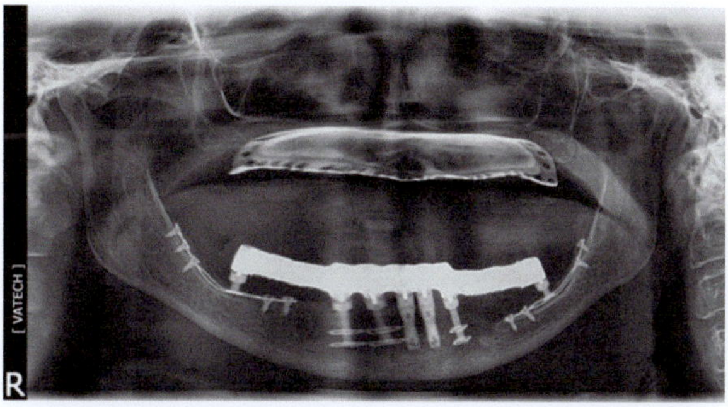

Fig. 13.2 Bridge installed. Oct. 16, 2015

Case Study 2: Complete Maxillo-mandibular Implant Rehabilitation

Dr. Philippe Cotten, Barcelona, Spain (Surgery and Prosthodontics)

Follow-Up: 2011–2018

Female, 46 years old at implant placement

Atrophic posterior mandible on both sides

Mandibular nerves exposed

Correspondents in Bogota, Colombia: Dr. Carolina Castiblanco, Dr. William Romero

Oral hygiene	Dental visits	Days lost from work
Satisfactory	17	15 days

Occlusion: Stable group function

Surgical and prosthetic procedures (3):

Maxilla (2 surgeries):

Sept. 9, 2011: Local anesthesia, oral sedation

Implants placed in positions 18 and 28 (2 pterygoid Fractal® root-form implants, dia. 3.3 mm, length 16 mm)

Sept. 12, 2011: General anesthesia

Placement of four Fractal® root-form implants (dia. 3.75 mm, length 11 mm) in the premaxilla and two zygomatic plate-form Diskimplants® (43 × 9/9G2-DP), immediate loading protocol

Mandible: Aug. 28, 2012, local anesthesia and oral sedation

Extraction-implantation, immediate loading protocol.

Four Monobloc root-form implants (dia. 3.75 mm, length 11 mm) and two ramus plate-form Diskimplants® (43 × 9/9G2-DP).

All plate-form Diskimplants® were completely covered by BSM and PRF.

Progress:

Maxilla: Transitional bridge with a metal framework; the final zirconia bridge was placed 4 years later (April 19, 2016).

Mandible: Transitional bridge with a metal framework and resin teeth placed 3 days after surgery; the final zirconia bridge was placed 3 years later (April 19, 2016).

Subsequent treatment: Annual check-ups in Mexico

X-rays/imaging: Panoramic (10), full-mouth CT scan (1), stereolithographic model (maxilla and mandible)

Follow-up as of February 2018: The patient was satisfied and had no complaints (Fig. 13.3).

In 2006, a LeFort procedure with osteosynthesis plates was completed by an iliac bone graft and installation of six cylindrical root-form implants in the maxilla. The bridge was placed 9 months later.

In 2010, the patient began to notice that the bridge was mobile; she lost her anterior implants and returned to a removable maxillary denture.

She first presented at our consultation in June 2011 (Figs. 13.4, 13.5 and 13.6).

On Sept. 9, 2011, a first surgery was performed under local anesthesia. Two pterygoid Fractal® root-form implants (ref. 3.3 h16-MF4) were placed in the pterygoid processes (positions 28 and 18) under radiologic guidance.

The other maxillary implants were installed on Sept. 12, 2011, under general anesthesia:

- Two zygomatic plate-form Diskimplants® (ref. 43 × 9/9G2-DP) in the right and left infra-sinus regions
- Four root-form implants (ref. 3.75 h11) in the anterior maxilla

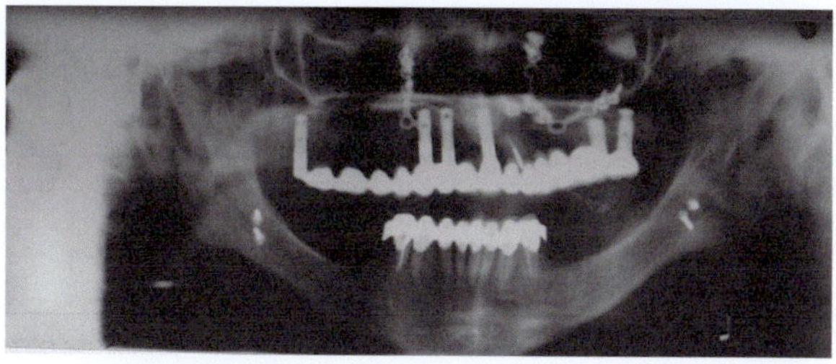

Fig. 13.3 May 18, 2006

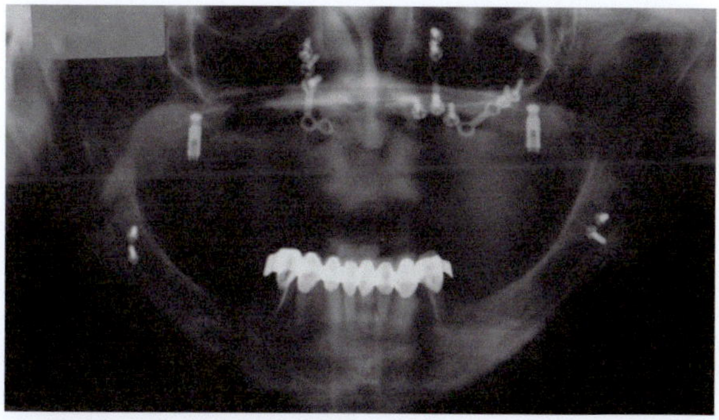

Fig. 13.4 June 17, 2011

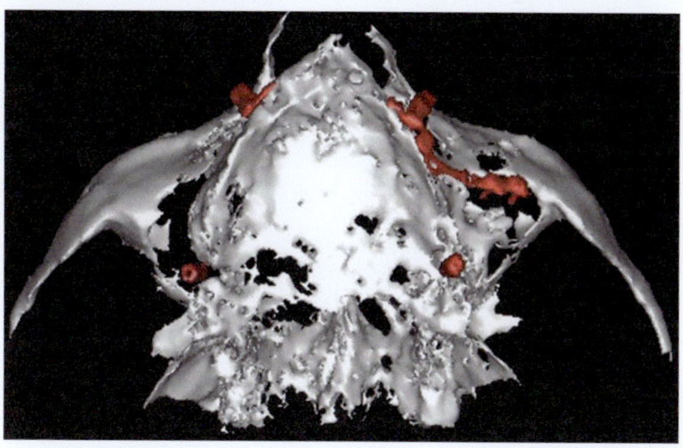

Fig. 13.5 CT scans revealed the locations of the osteosynthesis plates and the amount of residual bone following loss of the implants. Occlusal view

– Sept. 14, 2011: Immediate loading with a highly rigid transitional titanium/chromium-cobalt/resin bridge and a cross-palate bar

Aug. 28, 2012: Complete implantation of the mandible after removal of the anterior bridge and the residual roots

– Installation of four Monobloc root-form implants (ref. 3.75 h11)
– Two ramus plate-form Diskimplants® (ref. 43 × 9/9G2-DP).

Aug. 30, 2012: Immediate loading of the highly rigid, transitional titanium/chromium-cobalt/resin bridge.

The transitional bridges were left in function for 4 years before fabrication of full-arch maxillary and mandibular prostheses (Prettau zirconia technique) (Figs. 13.7, 13.8 and 13.9).

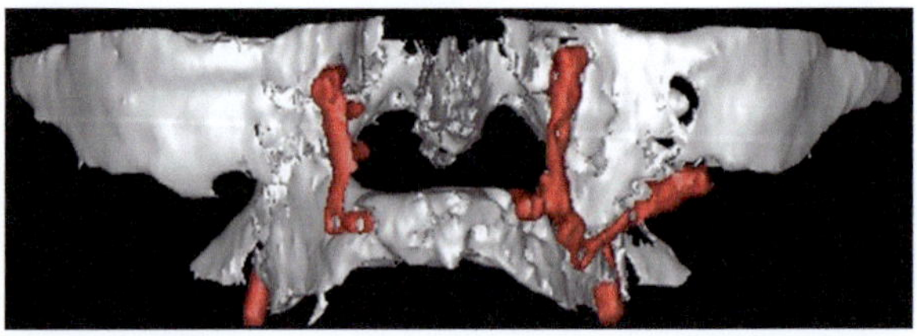

Fig. 13.6 CT scans revealed the locations of the osteosynthesis plates and the amount of residual bone following loss of the implants. Front view

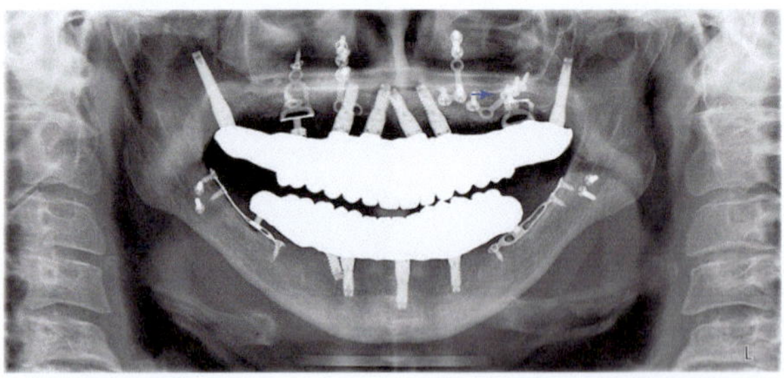

Fig. 13.7 April 19, 2017

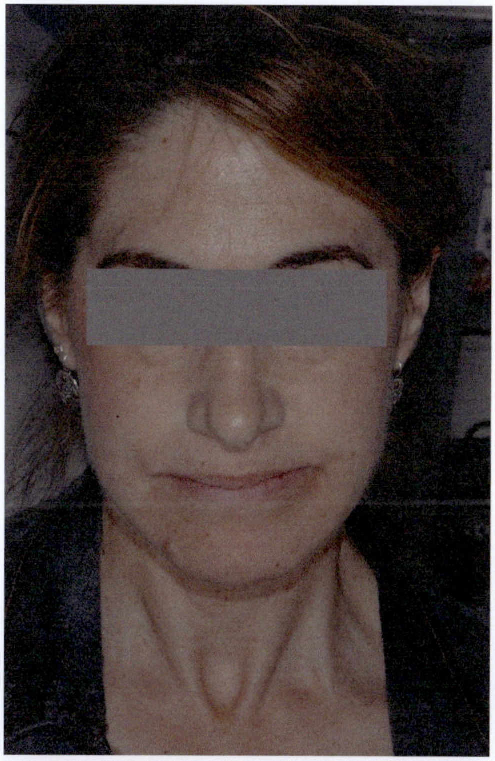

Fig. 13.8 June 17, 2011

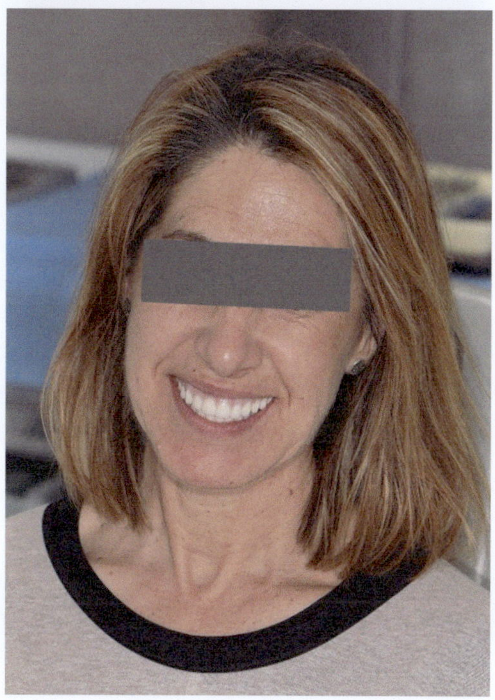

Fig. 13.9 June 20, 2017

Case Study 3

Dr. Louis Dagnelie, La Hulpe, Belgium (Surgery and Prosthodontics)
Follow-Up: 2008–2017.

Male, 66 years old at implant placement

Advanced periodontal disease

Oral hygiene: Fair

Preop management:

- Extraction of upper teeth (periodontal disease)
- Full upper denture worn for 3 months

Surgical and prosthetic procedures: Local anesthesia

Five double Diskimplants®, two triple Diskimplants®, and one single-disk Diskimplant® placed and loaded immediately with a fixed, screw-secured CrCo-resin bridge

X-rays/imaging: Panoramic, CT scan (Figs. 13.10 and 13.11)

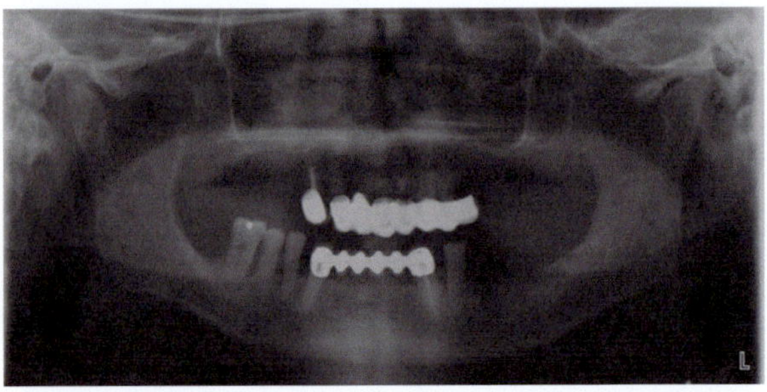

Fig. 13.10 2008

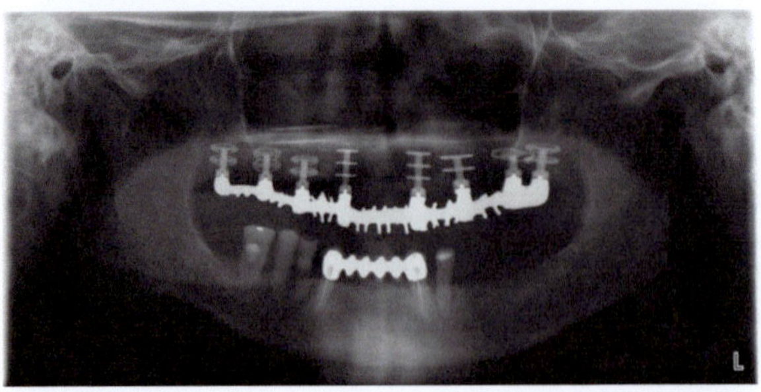

Fig. 13.11 2017

Case Study 4: Maxillary Implant Treatment

Dr. Hassan Idrissi Ouedghiri, Casablanca, Morocco (Surgery and Prosthodontics)

Follow-Up: 2014–2017

Male, 43 years old at implant placement

Atrophic maxilla

Oral mucosa: Healthy

Oral hygiene: Fair

Preop management:

- Sinus lift and bone graft substitute, extraction of lower right molar

Surgical and prosthetic procedures: Local anesthesia and oral sedation; immediate loading protocol; fixed bridge screw-secured to two zygomatic plate-form Diskimplants®, two pterygoid Fractal® implants, and six root-form implants in the premaxilla

Progress: Final ceramic-baked-to-metal fixed bridge

X-rays/imaging: **Panoramic, CT scan** (Figs. 13.12, 13.13 and 13.14)

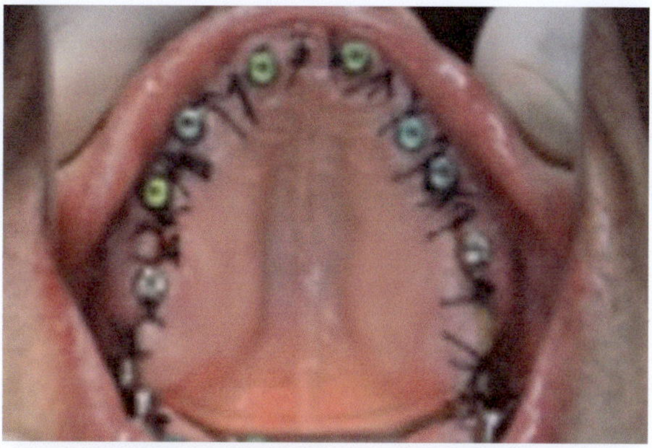

Fig. 13.12 Post-op occlusal view

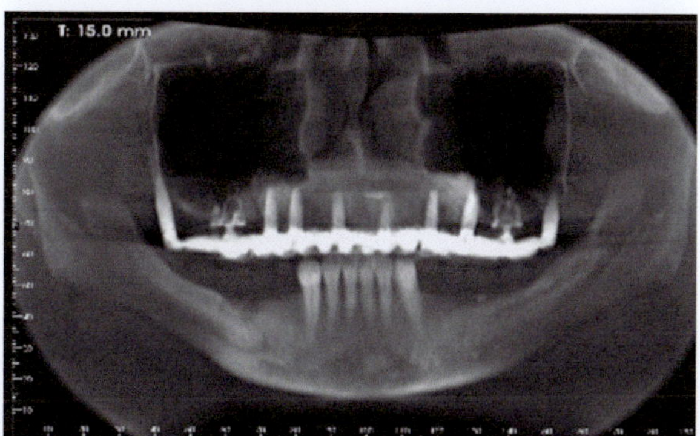

Fig. 13.13 Immediate functional loading of the fixed screw-secured bridge (same patient as Fig. 13.12)

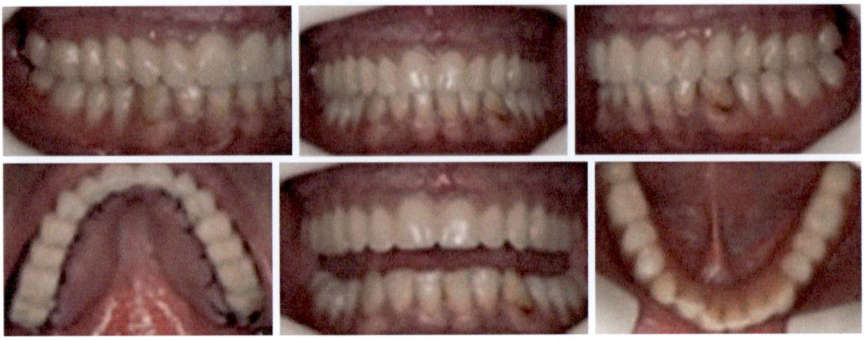

Fig. 13.14 2017

Case Study 5

Dr. Charles Minoyan, Chojnice, Poland (Surgery and Prosthodontics) Follow-Up: 2014–2017

Female, 54 years old at implant placement

No health problems

Bridge 34–38 mobile, roots of 38 carious

Oral hygiene: Satisfactory

Preop management: 38 removed; for financial reasons, the bridge was sectioned to conserve 34, which was only slightly mobile.

Surgical and prosthetic procedures:

Two monodisk Diskimplants® and one double Diskimplant® were installed; bridge fabricated from a block of PMMA.

X-rays/imaging: Panoramic radiograph (Figs. 13.15 and 13.16)

Fig. 13.15 2014

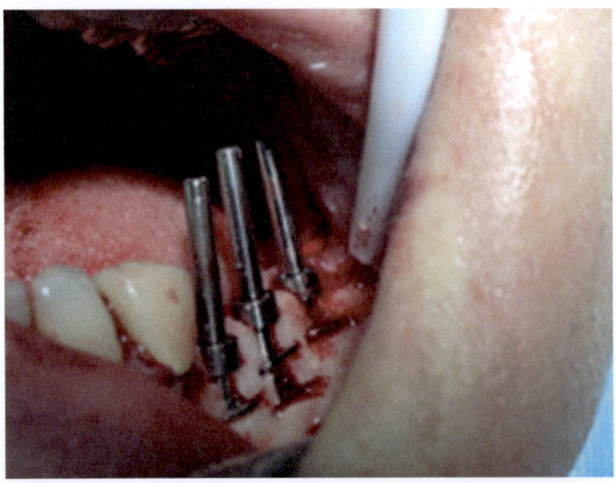

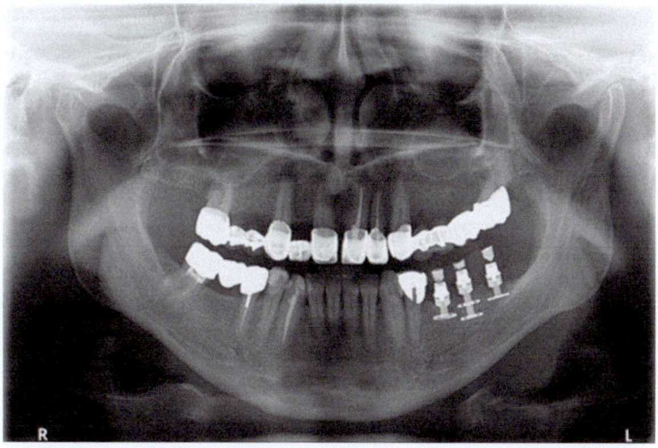

Fig. 13.16 2016

Case Study 6: Maxillo-mandibular Implant Treatment

Dr. Pierre Monsarrat, Albi, France (Surgery and Prosthodontics)
Follow-Up: 2010–2017

Female, 56 years old at implant placement

No longer wanted to wear the full denture she had had for 20 years but waited 18 months before deciding to proceed with implant placement.

Non-smoker

Oral mucosa: Healthy, no inflammation

Oral hygiene: Fair.

Surgical and prosthetic procedures: General anesthesia; immediate loading protocol

Maxilla: One Fractal® implant 3.75 h8-MF1

Two zygomatic plate-form Diskimplants® (33 mm)

Two canine pillar plate-form Diskimplants® (43 mm)

Two pterygoid Fractal® implants (3.3 h16-MF4)

Mandible: Six Fractal® implants dia. 3.75 mm (8 mm and 11 mm)

Transitional prostheses replaced 8 months later with the final prostheses:

Maxilla: Ceramic to metal with titanium bonding cylinders

Mandible: Zirconia prosthesis

X-rays/imaging: Panoramic, CT scan (Figs. 13.17, 13.18 and 13.19)

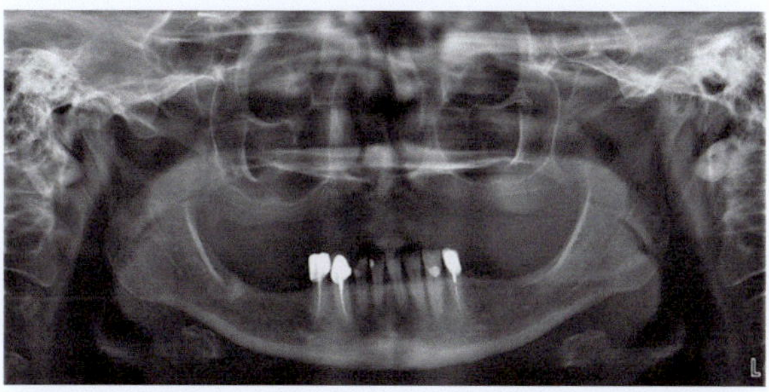

Fig. 13.17 Oct. 19, 2010: Preop panoramic radiograph

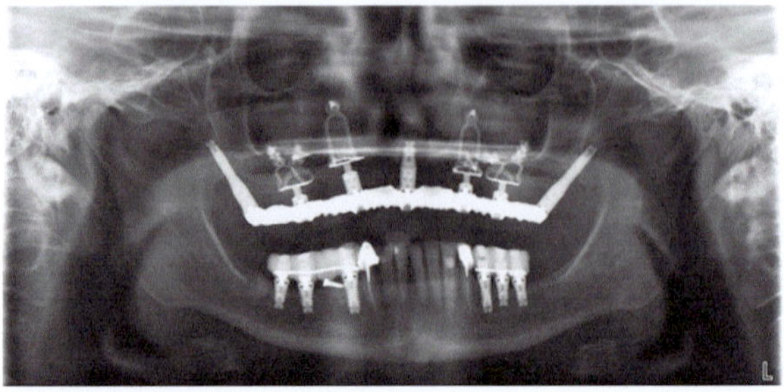

Fig. 13.18 May 31, 2017

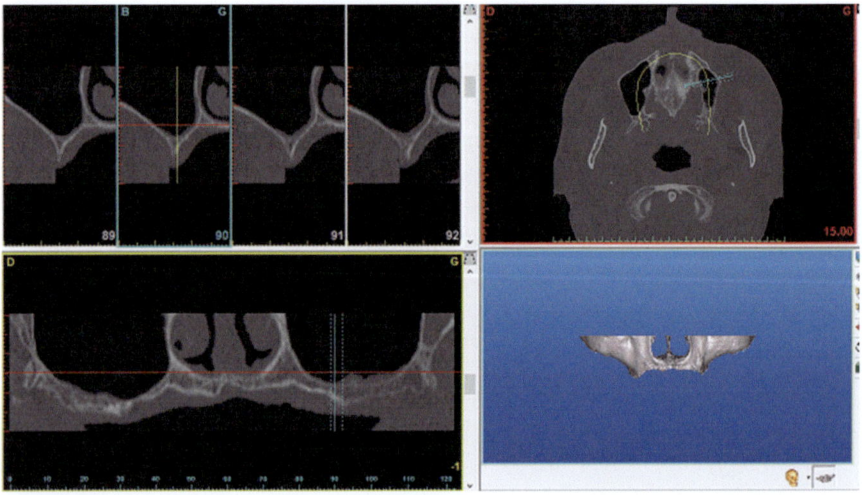

Fig. 13.19 Pre-op study

Case Study 7: Maxillo-mandibular Implant Treatment

Dr. Renaud Petitbois, Antibes, France (Surgery and Prosthodontics)

Follow-Up: 2002–2017

Male, 45 years old at implant placement

Maxillary knife ridge

Oral mucosa: Advanced periodontal disease

Oral hygiene: Average

Preop management: Extraction of periodontally affected teeth

Surgical and prosthetic procedures:

Maxilla: Immediate loading of eight root-form implants, two double Diskimplants®, two single-disk Diskimplants®, four triple Diskimplants®, and one pterygoid Fractal® implant

Mandible: Delayed loading protocol (3 months) for the five root-form implants

X-rays/imaging: Panoramic, CT scan (Figs. 13.20 and 13.21)

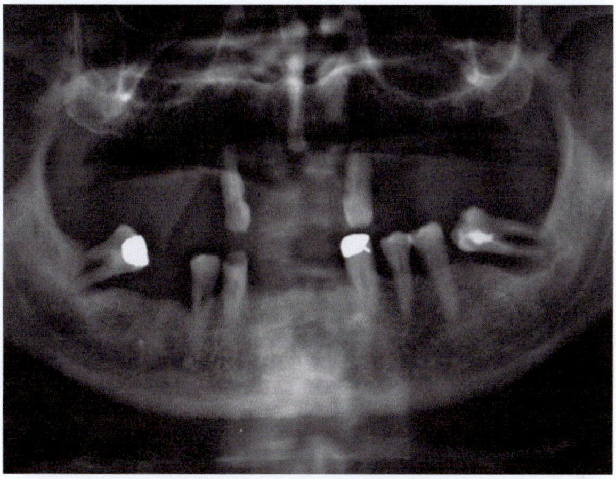

Fig. 13.20 2002: Initial panoramic radiograph

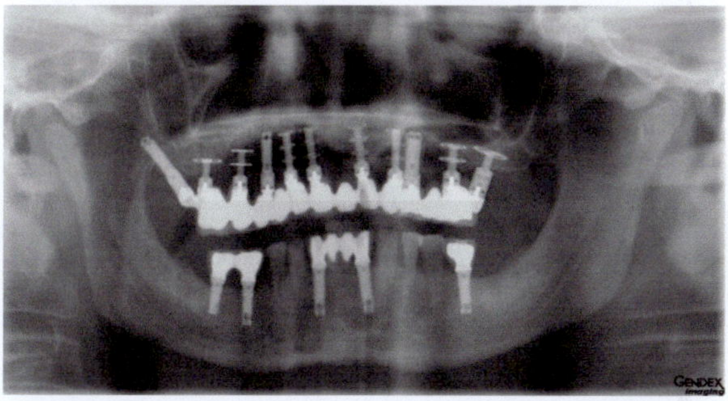

Fig. 13.21 2017

Case Study 8: Maxillary Implant Treatment

Dr. Lari Sapoznikov, Basal Implant Center, Tel Aviv, Israel (Surgery and Prosthodontics) Follow-Up: 2011–2017

Female, 60 years old at implant placement

Extremely atrophic maxilla

Full upper and lower dentures

Heavy smoker, quit 1 month before implant surgery

Oral mucosa: Healthy

Oral hygiene: Good

Preop management: Osseotensor 45 days before basal implant placement

Surgical and prosthetic procedures: Local anesthesia and IV sedation; immediate fixed acrylic prosthesis screw-secured to two zygomatic plate-form Diskimplants®, two canine pillar plate-form Diskimplants®, and three root-form implants 24 hours post-op; ceramic/composite-fused-to-metal bridge placed 10 days later. She remained with her full lower denture.

X-rays/imaging: **Panoramic, CT scan** (Figs. 13.22 and 13.23)

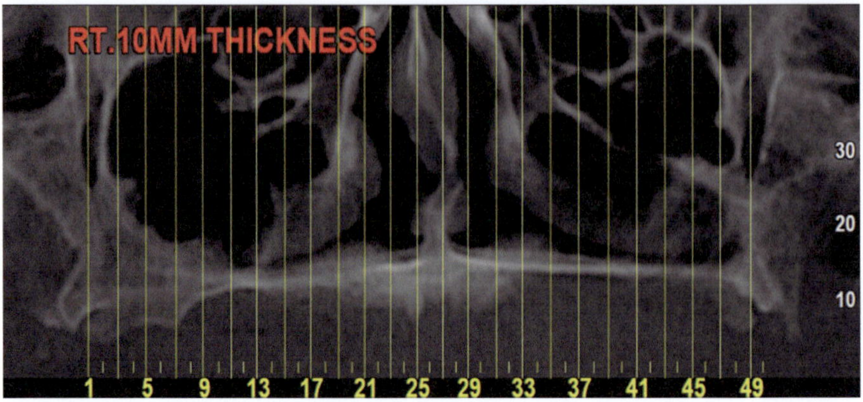

Fig. 13.22 2011: Preop CT scan

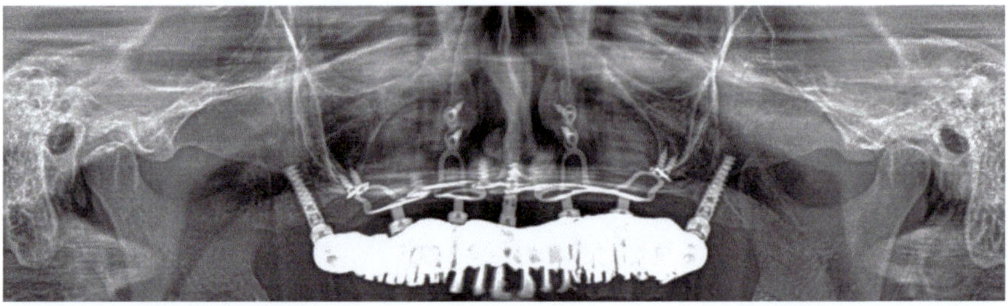

Fig. 13.23 2017: 3 years post-op

Case Study 9: Maxillary Implant Treatment

Dr. Martin Schweppe, Telgte, Germany (Surgery and Prosthodontics)

Follow-Up: 2006–2017

Female, 66 years old at implant placement

Atrophic maxilla

Oral mucosa: Advanced periodontal disease

Oral hygiene: Good

Preop management: First consultation in 2005

Surgical and prosthetic procedures:

Local anesthesia; immediate loading of two pterygoid Fractal® implants, two zygomatic plate-form Diskimplants®, three triple Diskimplants®, two double Diskimplants®, and two single Diskimplants® placed in 2006; full zirconia bridge placed in 2008

X-rays/imaging: Panoramic, CT scan, control panoramic in 2016 (Figs. 13.24, 13.25, 13.26, 13.27, 13.28 and 13.29)

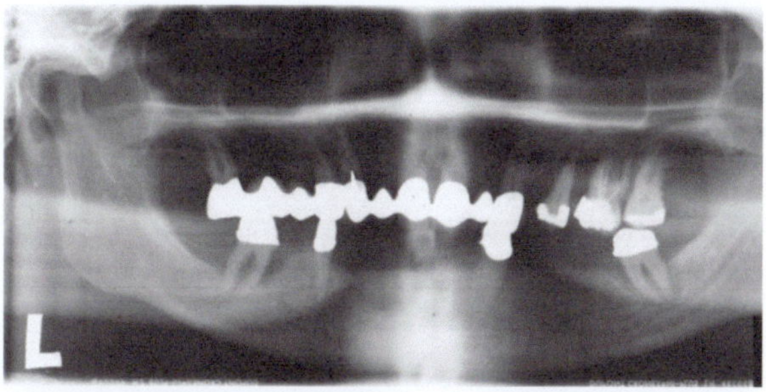

Fig. 13.24 2005: Initial panoramic radiograph before implant placement

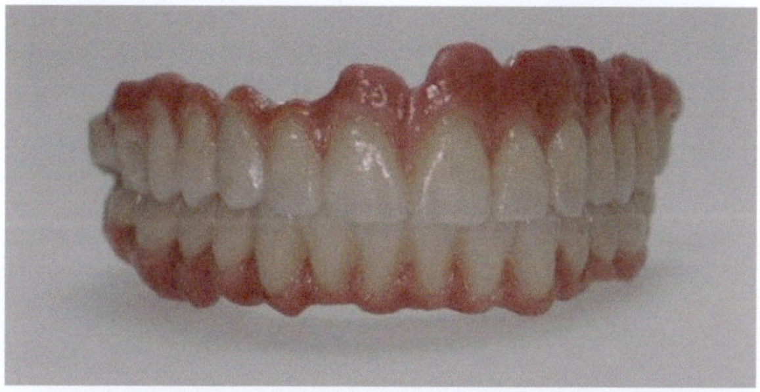

Fig. 13.25 Full implant-supported Zirkonzahn rehabilitation

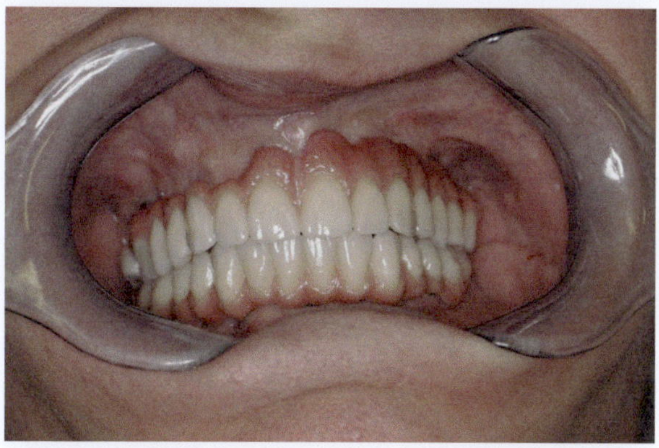

Fig. 13.26 Intraoral situation 2 years post-op. Front view

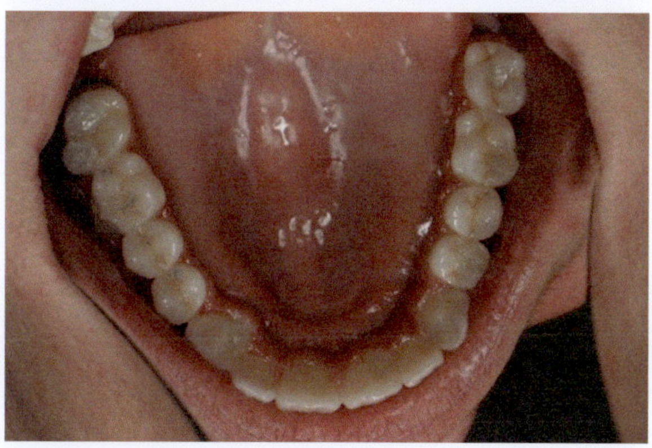

Fig. 13.27 Intraoral situation 2 years post-op. Occlusal view

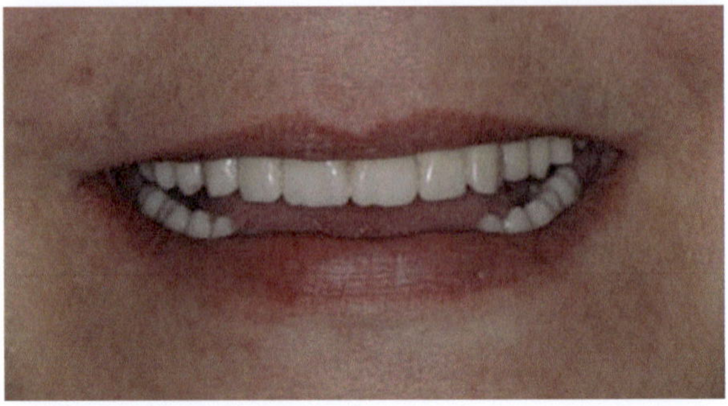

Fig. 13.28 Situation in 2017

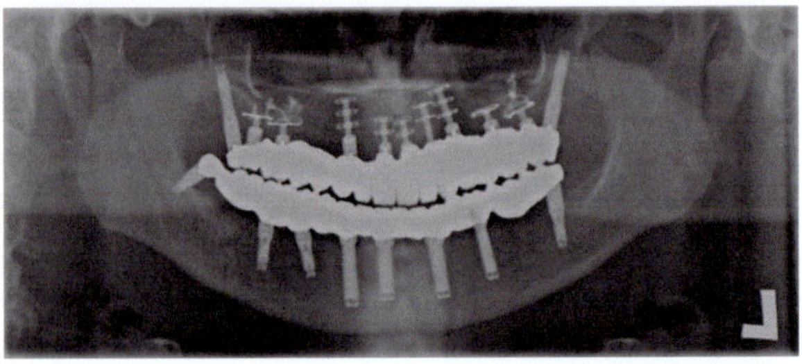

Fig. 13.29 Panoramic view in 2017

Case Study 10: Maxillo-mandibular Implant Treatment

Dr. Jacques Vermeulen, Flumet, France (Surgery and Prosthodontics)

Follow-Up: 2004–2017

Female, 37 years old at implant placement

Oral mucosa: Healthy

Oral hygiene: Good

Preop management:

- New upper and lower full dentures
- 3D Simplant® treatment planning

Surgical and prosthetic procedures: Immediate loading protocol

Maxilla: seven root-form implants (two in the pterygoid processes), one Diskimplant®, one double Diskimplant®

Mandible: two Diskimplants®, two ramus plate-form Diskimplants®, four root-form implants

X-rays/imaging: Panoramic, CT scan

Days lost from work: 1 week (Figs. 13.30, 13.31, 13.32 and 13.33)

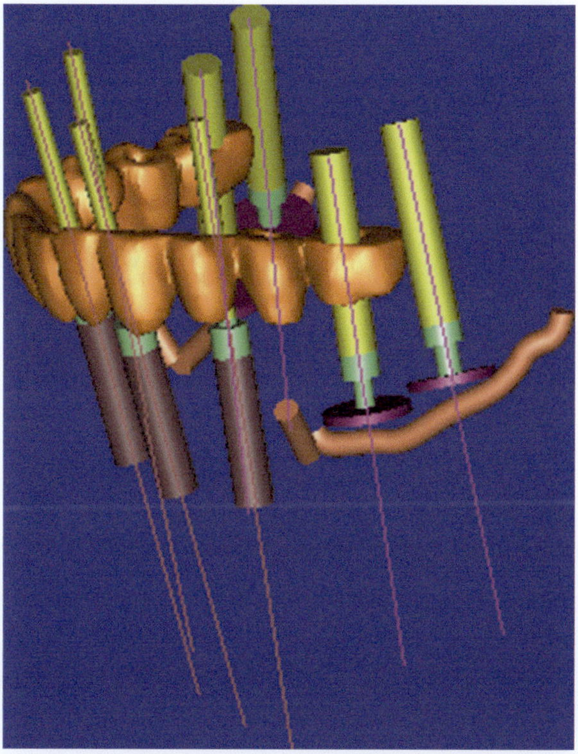

Fig. 13.30 2004: lateral view

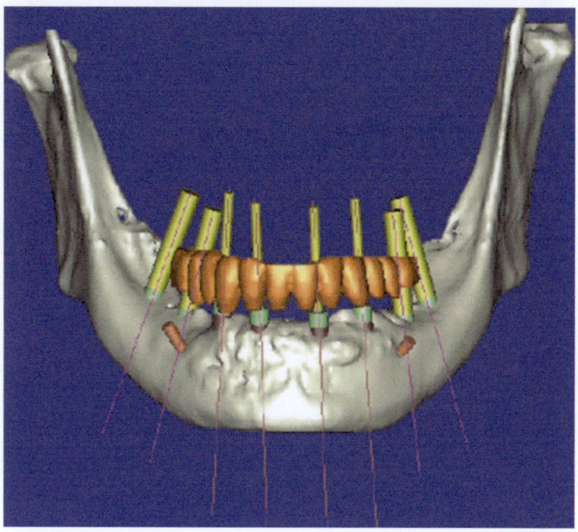

Fig. 13.31 2004: front view

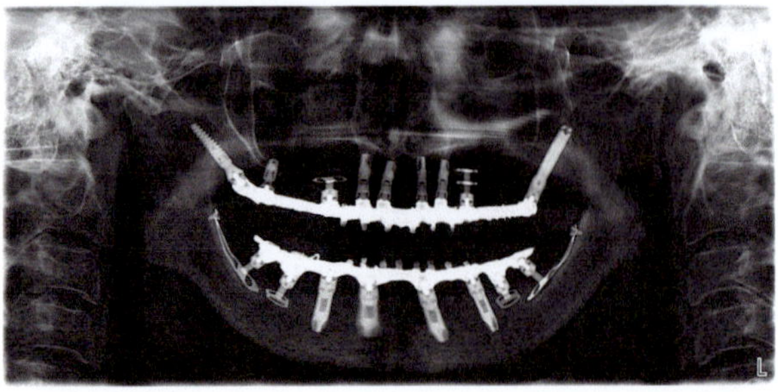

Fig. 13.32 Follow-up radiograph 8 years post-op (2012)

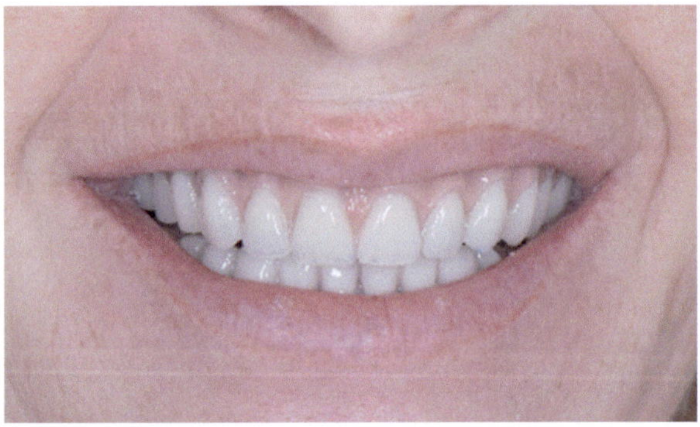

Fig. 13.33 Esthetic outcome 12 years post-op (2016)

Conflict of interest statement Gérard M. Scortecci is the inventor of the Diskimplant and holder of several associated patents that are exploited by the Victory company. He is an unpaid consultant to this firm and a minority shareholder in the company. No money was received from any of the companies mentioned in the book or from any of the companies whose products are mentioned.

Recommended Reading

1. Ihde S. Principles of BOI. Heidelberg: Springer; 2004.
2. Resnik RR, Misch CE. Misch's avoiding complications in oral implantology. Amsterdam: Elsevier; 2017.
3. Scortecci GM, Misch CE, Benner KU. Implants and restorative dentistry. London: Martin Dunitz; 2001.
4. Spiessl B. Internal fixation of the mandible. Heidelberg: Springer; 1989.

Complications: Prevention, Correction, and Maintenance

14

Gérard M. Scortecci and Guillaume Odin

14.1 Prevention

The best treatment of complications is prevention. This can be achieved, to a great extent, by appropriate diagnosis and treatment planning following adequate surgical and prosthetic training, appropriate oral hygiene, daily maintenance, and annual checkups. However, even the most "successful" implant systems and well-trained teams can encounter problems due to medical conditions or accidents. Despite the proven biocompatibility of titanium Diskimplants®, a number of recommendations should be respected:

- Follow training courses on Diskimplant® placement, use of associated prosthetic components, avoidance of pitfalls, and management of potential complications.
- Start with simple cases in non-smokers and psychologically stable patients; extensive reconstructions are difficult even for experienced dentists.
- Carefully review the patient's dental history (tobacco or substance abuse, caries, periodontal disease, oral infections, sinusitis, allergies, bisphosphonates, neuralgia, tooth fractures, bruxism, wear, etc.).
- Check to be sure that occlusal, periodontal, and oral hygiene conditions are favorable.

G. M. Scortecci (✉)
University of Nice-Sophia Antipolis Medical School, Nice, France

New York University, New York, NY, USA

University of Southern California, Los Angeles, CA, USA

Private Practice, Nice, France
e-mail: scortecci@wanadoo.fr

G. Odin
ENT and Maxillo-facial Surgery Department, Institut Universitaire de la Face et du Cou, University of Nice-Sophia Antipolis Medical School, Nice, France
e-mail: odin.g@chu-nice.fr

© Springer Nature Switzerland AG 2019

G. M. Scortecci (ed.), *Basal Implantology*, https://doi.org/10.1007/978-3-319-44873-2_14

- Ensure thorough prosthodontic evaluation using models mounted in occlusion, wax-up, and preparation of a surgical guide prior to implant surgery.
- Carefully determine the available bone volume and quality. Respect the size requirements for the basal implant. Check bone quality during pre-surgery osteogenic activation with bone matrix osseotensors.
- Place the basal implants in a prosthetically useful position with the aid of a simple surgical guide made in the dental lab or with 3D technologies. Respect the concept of absolute primary implant stability in dense living bone.
- For single-tooth replacements with Diskimplants®, immediate loading is to be avoided except in very specific conditions.
- For partial edentulism (including single-tooth replacements), delayed loading with a 6-month waiting period is advisable if the clinical situation cannot guarantee long-lasting absolute primary stability during function. Always verify that the removable denture does not damage the implants during the waiting period.
- For total edentulism, immediate functional loading is the safest approach with basal implants.
- Passive fit, rigidity, and precision of the fixed, basal implant-supported superstructure are mandatory. Ensure primary stability of the bone-anchored basal implants using passive, highly rigid, and strong fixed implant-supported prosthetic superstructures: their elaboration must take into account the principles of occlusion, mechanics, and hygiene maintenance. Numerous failures in implantology result from poorly designed (imprecise, fragile) or defective prostheses, associated or not with malocclusion, overload, and lack of maintenance and/or inadequate oral hygiene [1, 2].
- Should a problem occur (screw or cement loosening, fracture of components or an implant body, etc.), take immediate action to minimize or avoid additional deterioration.
- Following implant placement, patients should be given a document listing all details required for identification of the implant(s) and all prosthetic components used, plus the address of the professional who managed the case.

14.2 Preoperative Precautions

Allergy to Titanium (Figs. 14.1 and 14.2)

Although titanium is generally well accepted in the human body, there have been reports of allergic reactions. A titanium disk placed on the skin by a dermatologist can help to make a preoperative diagnosis when an allergy is suspected.

Anticipation of Mechanical and Biological Problems (Figs. 14.3 and 14.4)

Poor management of temporary prostheses in heavy smokers: in the case illustrated here, all implants were lost.

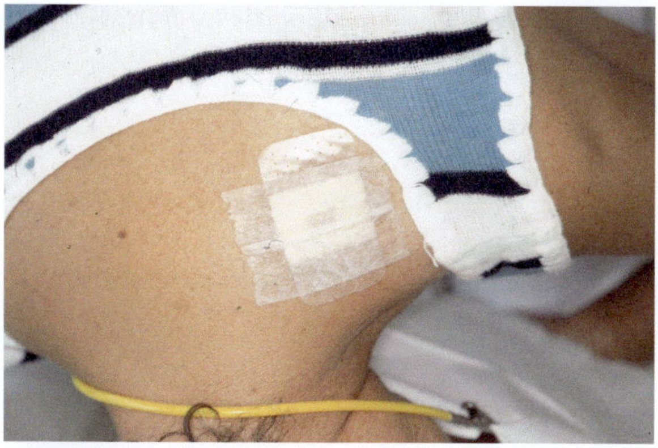

Fig. 14.1 Cutaneous test for titanium allergy: titanium disks placed on the shoulder of a patient who claimed a history of multiple metal allergies

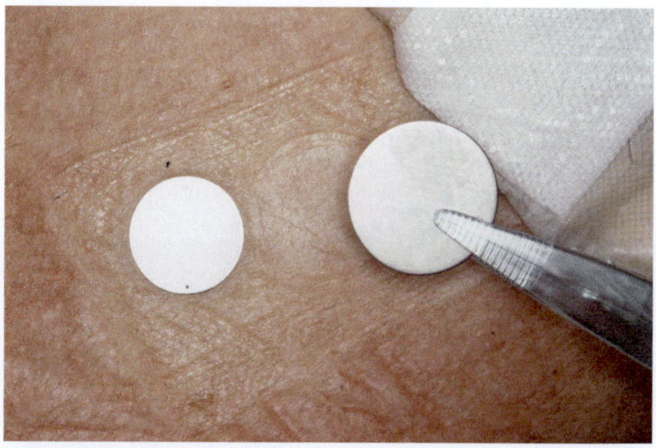

Fig. 14.2 Verification on day 5: the absence of redness or any irritation indicative of an allergy to titanium meant that titanium implants could be safely installed (same patient as Fig. 14.1)

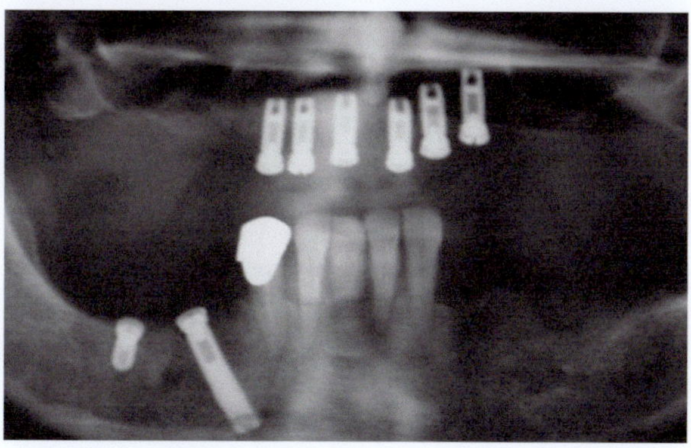

Fig. 14.3 Early loss (after 4 months) of all root-form implants in a 52-year-old woman who was a heavy smoker

Prevention of Peri-implantitis by Avoiding Rough Surfaces (Figs. 14.5, 14.6, 14.7, 14.8 and 14.9)

Non-modified, machined surfaces are preferable because they have the longest history of functional osseointegration in human jaws [3]. While rough surfaces may provide an immediate advantage in terms of primary stability, they are the source of

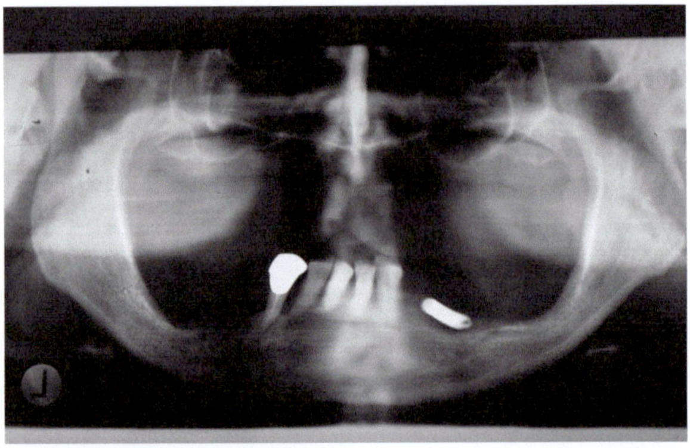

Fig. 14.4 After implant loss, the surgeon attempted to place another implant in the lower left mandible, but it also failed (same patient as Fig. 14.3)

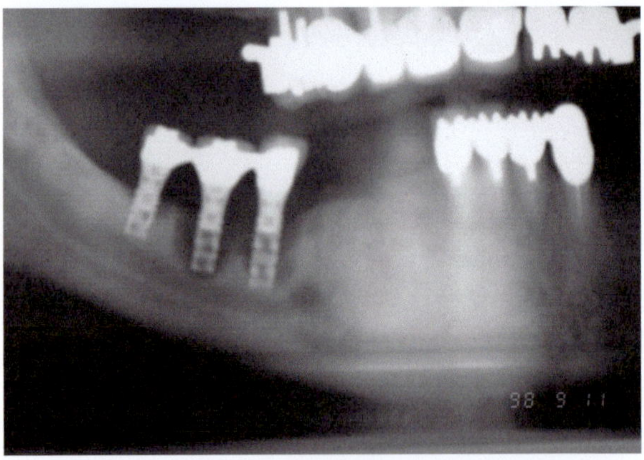

Fig. 14.5 Peri-implantitis around plasma spray-coated root-form implants after 6 years of service

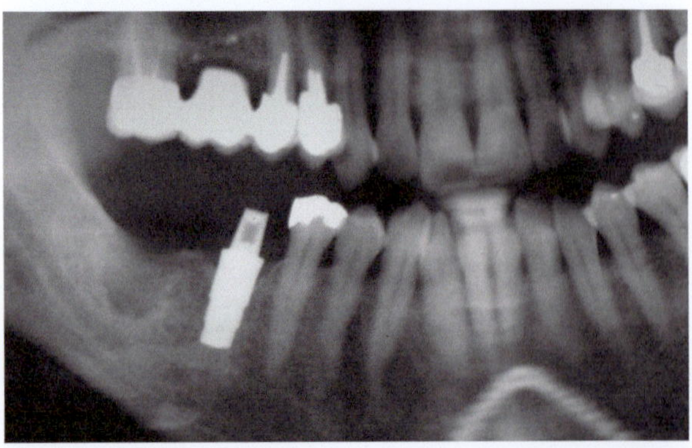

Fig. 14.6 Removal of the cemented bridge and the posterior root-form implant

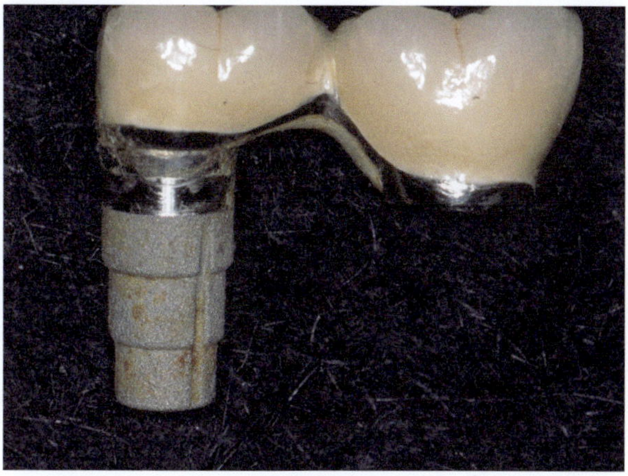

Fig. 14.7 Late loss of an osseointegrated implant with a plasma spray coating after 8 years

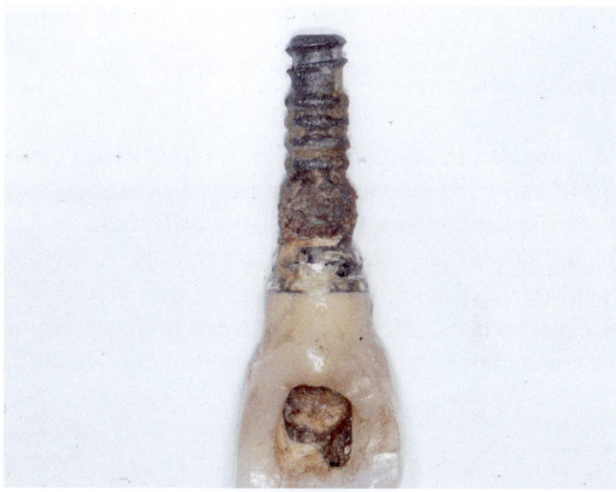

Fig. 14.8 Early loss (after 8 months) of a single-tooth replacement that had been placed in function immediately

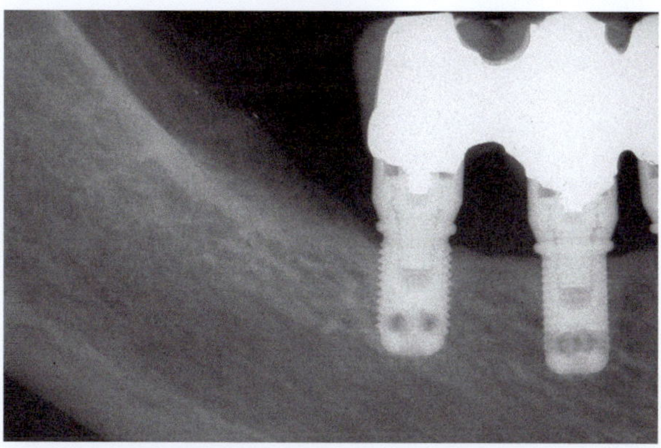

Fig. 14.9 Short (6 mm) root-form implant with a non-modified surface state (Structure® implant, Victory, France) after 21 years of service (patient aged 81 years). No bone loss or peri-implantitis

considerable metal release during function. Furthermore, should bone retraction occur, it is impossible to adequately clean an exposed rough implant surface [4].

Consensus on the Prevention of Bacterial Endocarditis

Surgery and invasive diagnostic procedures always carry a risk of introducing bacteria into the bloodstream. This is usually of little consequence unless the patient has a severe deformity of the endocardial surface. The American Heart Association recommends that patients at risk receive prophylactic antibiotics prior to dental and other surgical procedures.

- Standard regimen: 3 g amoxicillin per os 1 h before surgery
- Patients allergic to penicillin: 600 mg clindamycin per os 1 h before surgery or 500 mg clarithromycin per os 1 h before surgery or 500 mg azithromycin per os 1 h before surgery

Bisphosphonates (Figs. 14.10, 14.11, and 14.12)

As high-dose IV bisphosphonates can rapidly put a patient at risk of osteonecrosis of the jaw, such individuals are not candidates for any type of implant, including basal implants. Some patients have had dental implants for years, however, and require bisphosphonates for cancer therapy. A thorough checkup of oral status is mandatory. All teeth and implants at risk should be removed before starting IV bisphosphonates. Should the bone and implants become exposed, failing implants must be removed with a minimum of trauma.

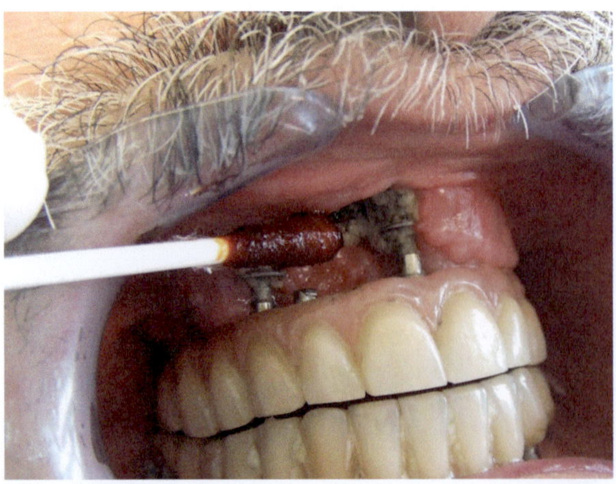

Fig. 14.10 Maxillary bone exposure 3 months after bisphosphonate administration for treatment of bone metastases. Povidone iodine is applied daily to reduce local infection by actinomycetes

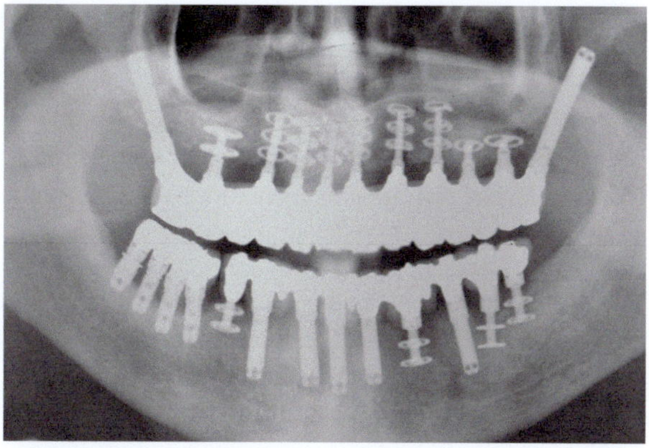

Fig. 14.11 Initial status before bisphosphonates (the implants had been installed 18 years earlier)

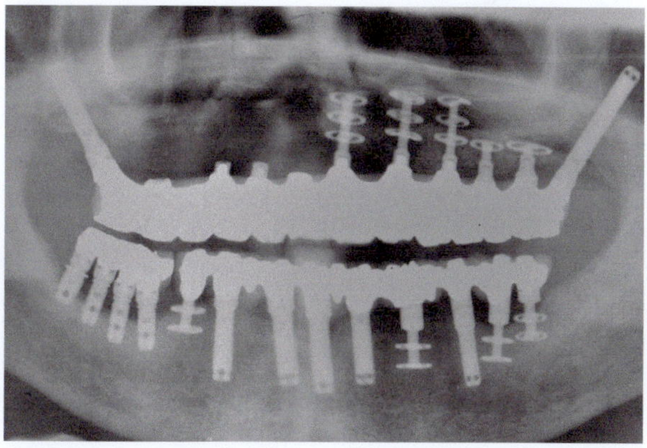

Fig. 14.12 Four Diskimplants® were retrieved in the upper right quadrant. The fixed bridge on basal implants was maintained for 4 years. The patient died at age 86 years old from generalized cancer; the fixed implant-supported bridge was still in service at the time of death

14.3 Anesthesia and Sedation

Anticipation of Pharmacologic Complications and Related Problems

Most basal implant surgery can be performed in a specially organized dental office. The need for general anesthesia in a hospital or clinic is generally reserved for extremely complex cases and phobic patients.

Sedation

When intravenous sedation is used in the dental office, it must be administered by a well-trained professional. A prior consultation with the anesthesiologist is mandatory. Should a problem occur, all necessary equipment must be in good working order and all necessary drugs readily available. Patients should refrain from liquids and solids for

6 h prior to administration of the drugs. When oral sedation is planned, patients should be instructed to eat breakfast or a light lunch in order to avoid the potential risk of hypoglycemia. Oral sedatives should be given in the dental office. It is irresponsible to assume that all patients and all clinical situations can be managed using only oral sedation. If the patient becomes nervous under oral sedation, it is better to stop the procedure, suture, and give another appointment, at which time more sophisticated sedatives or anesthetics can be used. In some cases, general anesthesia is required.

Sedation and acute retrograde amnesia provided by most benzodiazepines (Valium® 20 mg) are beneficial for preoperative use but establish the need for postoperative assistance. This means that patients must be accompanied and have proximal assistance for at least 24 h after surgery. Hydroxyzine (Atarax® 100 mg) given 20 min before surgery is a valuable adjunct. This antihistamine (H1 blocker) exerts a sedative effect by central blockade of the excitation transmitters acetylcholine and histamine. When combined with Valium®, the effects of both drugs are potentiated. Their anticholinergic and antiemetic actions may have both prophylactic and therapeutic uses. Hydrazine is also effective for the prevention of allergic reactions. It is important to emphasize the positive effects of low-dose adrenaline (1:200,000, articaine, Dentsply) in local anesthetics against respiratory depression and anaphylactic shock.

Local-Regional Anesthesia

Many patients can be treated solely with local anesthesia, without sedation. Although the toxicity of local anesthetics has been described in numerous comprehensive reports, life-threatening reactions are virtually inexistent when they are given following recommended dosage guidelines.

In the USA, profound intraoral anesthesia is most commonly induced using a 2% lidocaine 1:100,000 epinephrine formulation characterized by rapid onset (1–3 min) and a duration of 60–90 min (safe maximum number of cartridges, 8–14). In Europe and Canada, articaine (Alphacaine, Dentsply) 4% and 1:200,000 adrenaline (vasoconstrictor) give the same results for longer anesthesia (safe maximum number of cartridges, 8–12). Bupivacaine (Marcaine) 0.5% with epinephrine 1:200,000 provides 6–9 h of long-lasting local anesthesia (safe maximum number of cartridges, 10). Mepivacaine 3% alone, without a vasoconstrictor, is usually not recommended for oral implant surgery because it is safer to have some adrenaline, even a low concentration, in the tissues (safe number of cartridges, 6–9).

14.4 Complications During Surgery

Intraoperative Bleeding (Figs. 14.13, 14.14, and 14.15)

Any intrabony bleeding that occurs after osteotomy can be easily stopped by impacting the Diskimplant®, closing then suturing the flap, and afterwards having the patient bite down for 20 min on an appropriate surgical pack. Bleeding can be prevented by always making a mid-crestal full-flap incision into the attached gingiva.

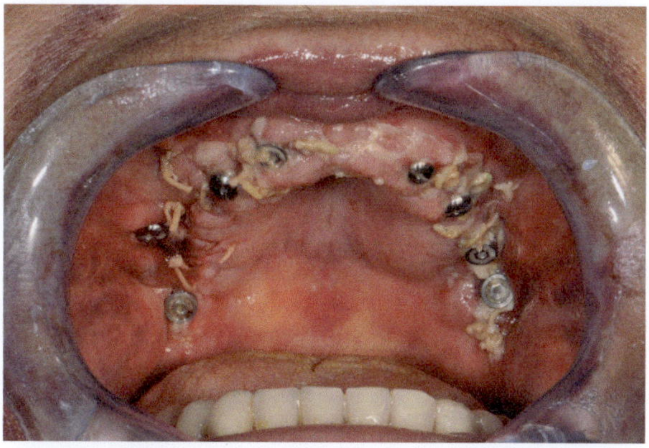

Fig. 14.13 Postsurgical hematoma; intraoral view 48 h post-op

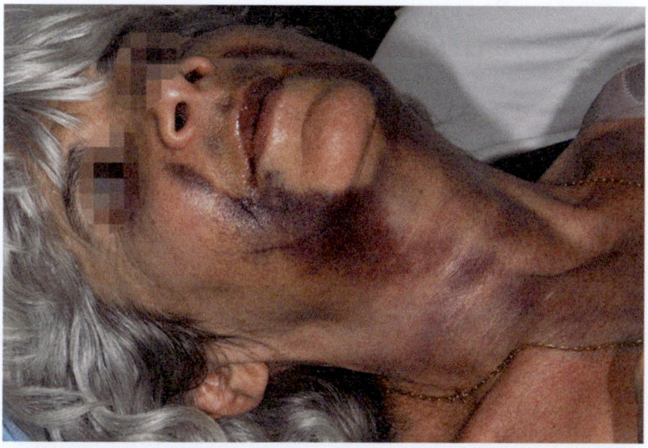

Fig. 14.14 Extraoral view of an extensive hematoma after basal implant surgery. The patient had no pain and was not particularly worried

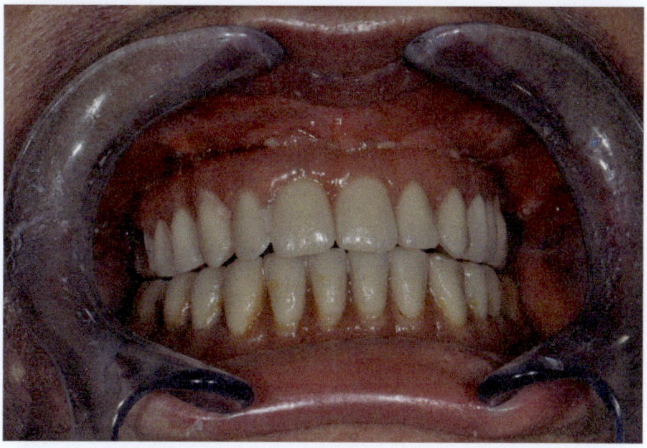

Fig. 14.15 The fixed, screw-secured prosthesis was installed on basal implants 3 days after surgery. Antibiotic therapy was maintained until complete resolution of the hematoma (10 days)

Straight vertical incisions should be avoided in the muscle. A horizontal or angulated posterior or anterior release incision is preferable. Gently elevate a full-thickness flap lingually and buccally, taking care not to damage the periosteum (use of a sterile gauze to "push" the tissues back is recommended).

Mandibular Nerve Injury

The most common neurologic problem is injury of the mandibular nerve. Mechanically related injury can occur as the result of stretching, compression, partial resection, or total transection during flap elevation or drilling procedures. The incision line is of paramount concern. For basal implant installation, crestal incisions must always remain in the middle of the attached gingiva. Alterations in the blood supply owing to local hematoma or thermal injury can also affect the nerve. Should this occur, implant installation should be postponed; a basal implant can be placed after complete resolution of all local signs. If the patient continues to complain of pain and/or anesthesia in the lower lip 2 weeks after uneventful implant installation, remove the implant, and wait for total clinical relief before attempting new implant surgery. Normally, healing occurs within several weeks. Never wait for implant integration if neuralgia persists.

Lingual Nerve Injury

Injury to the lingual nerve is impossible to identify radiologically and may last for years, with only partial and unpredictable recovery. This nerve may be damaged during extraction of mandibular wisdom teeth. Patients commonly report paresthesia and a burning sensation in the lateral part of the tongue. Injury of this type has also been reported in connection with placement of root-form implants in the molar area through the lingual plate. This complication can easily be prevented by avoiding any type of release incision in the lingual direction. Incisions should always be crestal, with vestibular release incisions. Full-thickness flaps on the lingual side must be elevated carefully, in continuous tight contact with the bone. A flap holder should be secured safely against the exposed lingual bone plate during lateral osteotomy because the nerve remains within the full mucosal flap. A partial-thickness flap should never be elevated in this highly critical area.

Injury of the Infraorbital Nerve

Injury to this nerve can cause partial anesthesia or dysesthesia of the upper lip. This complication can be avoided by careful handling of the full-thickness flap using sterile gauze to push back the tissues. During osteotomy, a large, rigid plastic suction tube should be held firmly against the buccal bone plate under the infraorbital nerve foramen.

Treatment of Neuralgia (See Also Sect. 14.10)

Minor nerve damage can heal spontaneously in several days to several months (generally 3 months). The recovery time depends on the extent and type of injury and the blood supply (scar tissues heal slowly). Administration of clonazepam (Rivotril®), carbamazepine (Tegretol®), pregabaline (Lyrica®), or pyridoxine (vitamin B_6) is often recommended for treatment of more severe injuries. Microsurgery with 9/0 or 11/0 sutures performed under a microscope may succeed in repairing a mandibular nerve sectioned during major maxillofacial surgery, but healing is unpredictable. For acute mandibular nerve neuralgia or causalgia, injection of specific drugs around the stellate (cervicothoracic) ganglion in the cervical area may provide relief, but the response to such therapy is also unpredictable. Since neuralgia is so difficult to treat, prevention is essential. In complex situations, the patient should be referred to a specialized pain management facility.

Fracture of the Severely Atrophic Mandible

The mechanical strength of the mandible is reduced, at least temporarily, by multiple implant site preparations. Fracture can occur with bone site preparations or, later on, as a result of late infection and excessive stress during mouth opening (yawning) and/or function. Numerous cases of spontaneous fatigue fracture under full mandibular dentures have also been reported in pencil mandibles, even without implant installation. Extreme caution should thus be exercised when dealing with the thin mandible, which is particularly vulnerable to thermal injury and infection owing to its dense cortical nature and extremely poor intrabony blood supply.

Mandibular fracture may be prevented as follows:

- Bilateral Botox® injection into the temporal and masseter muscles 1 week pre-op.
- Patients should be cautioned to limit stresses to the jaw during the prolonged healing period (soft diet for a minimum of 45–60 days).
- Use of Diskimplants® or microthreaded self-tapping, small diameter root-form implants (Fratex®) that require just a single drill, rather than standard root-form implants requiring a series of drills.

Management of a Mandibular Fracture (Figs. 14.16, 14.17, 14.18, 14.19, 14.20, and 14.21)

Fracture of a severely atrophic edentulous mandible is always a challenge because of the diminished central blood supply, decreased bone vitality, and dependency on the periosteal blood supply. The situation is aggravated when multiple implants are present: little bone is available for customary screw-and-plate repair, and additional periosteal reflection is undesirable. Treatment possibilities include:

- Immediate implant retrieval from the fractured zone followed by immediate placement of plate-form Diskimplants® on both sides, with rigid intraoral connection to osseointegrated implants in the mental area. A screw-retained prosthesis should be used as a rigid external fixator in order to obtain immediate initial stability.

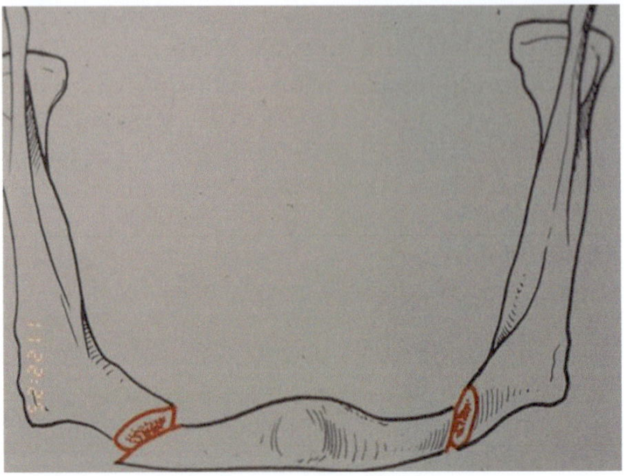

Fig. 14.16 Fractured pencil mandible

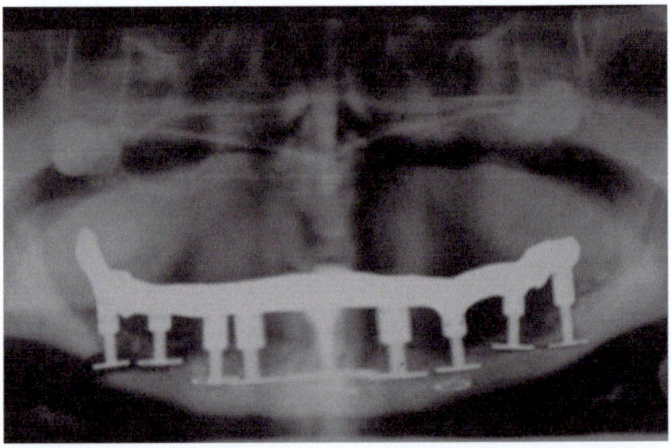

Fig. 14.17 In December 2000, this 64-year-old woman fractured her right posterior mandible 2 years after Diskimplant® installation. Interestingly, she experienced very little pain and just thought that a screw securing her fixed appliance had come loose

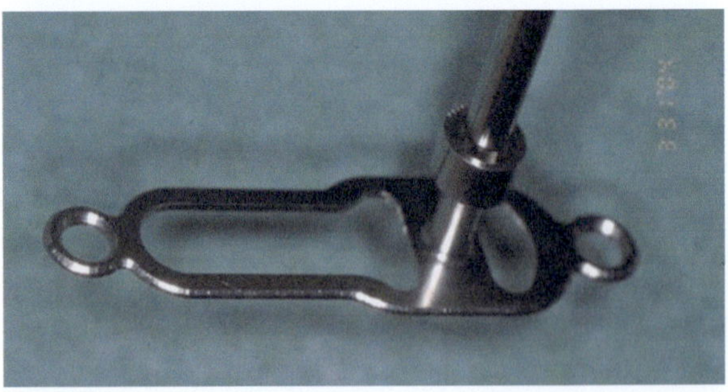

Fig. 14.18 In February 2001, the first plate-form Diskimplant® was developed to provide a rapid solution for this extreme situation, because the patient was at risk of losing her entire horizontal mandibular arch (the left side was also at risk) (same patient as Fig. 14.18)

- Stabilization of the fractured zone with mini plates, in which case the patient must wait several months before receiving a new prosthesis.
- In all cases, the patient should be instructed to stay on a soft diet for 45 days. Critical situations may require maxillo-mandibular immobilization with special intraoral or extraoral appliances.

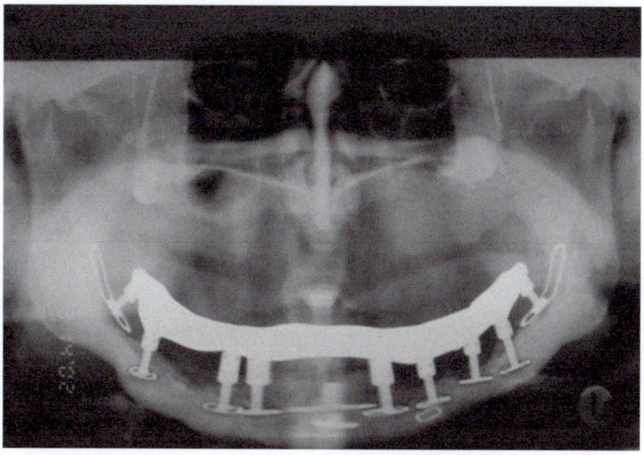

Fig. 14.19 Complete resolution after 6 years thanks to immediate, absolute immobilization of the fractured mandible. A bone gain was obtained on both sides (same patient as Figs. 14.17 and 14.18)

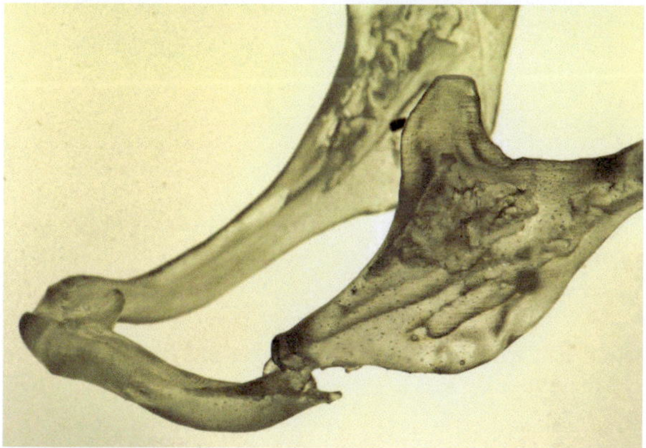

Fig. 14.20 Spontaneous fracture of the mandible under a removable denture

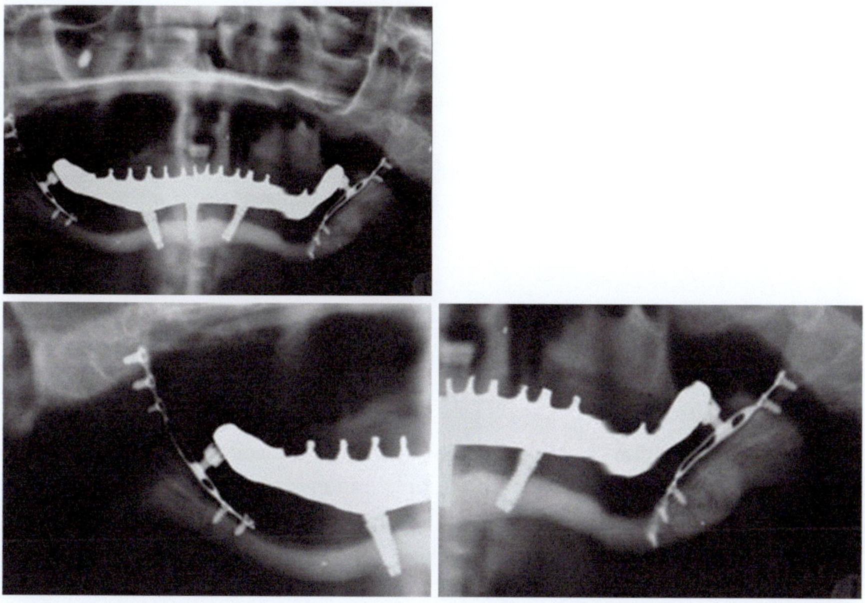

Fig. 14.21 Fixed rehabilitation of the fractured mandible (8 years post-op) (same patient as Fig. 14.20)

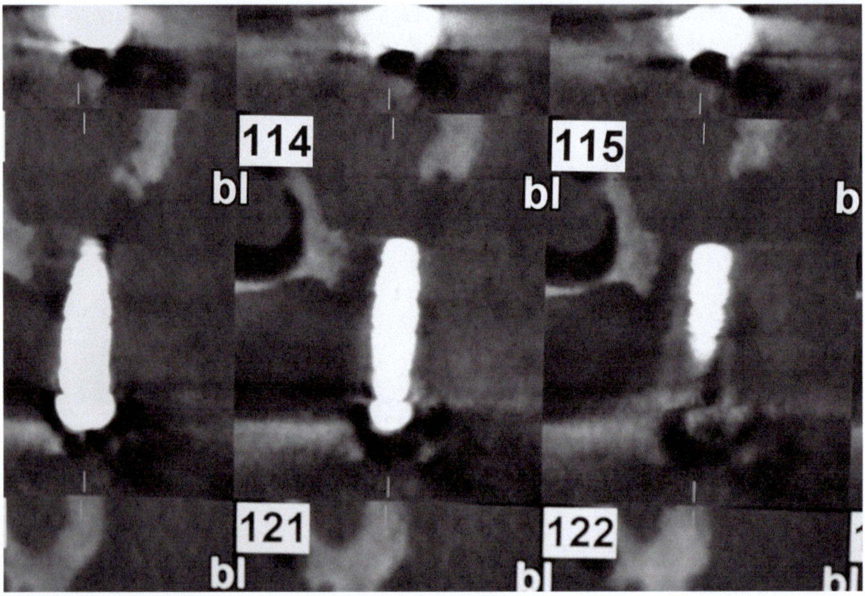

Fig. 14.22 Extensive maxillary bone loss with a large oro-antral communication in a heavy smoker after failure of an all-on-four procedure 9 months post-op

Maxilla: Penetration of the Nasal Floor and/or Sinus Floor (Fig. 14.22)

Thorough preoperative investigations (cone beam CT or a stereolithographic model) should provide the clinician with enough information about the adequacy of bone volume and density under the nasal and sinus floors. When bone height and density are limited, apical anchorage of an implant in the dense bone of the nasal floor or sinus floor cortex is technically acceptable as this provides initial stability without complications. A Diskimplant® can be safely installed to avoid a bone graft when bone height is under 7 mm. A nasal membrane lift and/or a sinus membrane lift can be performed at the time of basal implant installation. Bone substitute materials and PRF must be placed between the membrane and the implant.

Oro-antral Communication (Figs. 14.23, 14.24, 14.25, 14.26, 14.27, 14.28, and 14.29)

Small oro-antral communications can be managed with a palatal pedicle graft. Large communications subsequent to multiple implant removals and/or failure of a sinus lift require referral of the patient to a maxillofacial or ENT Department for surgical treatment and closure with a pedicle fat pad.

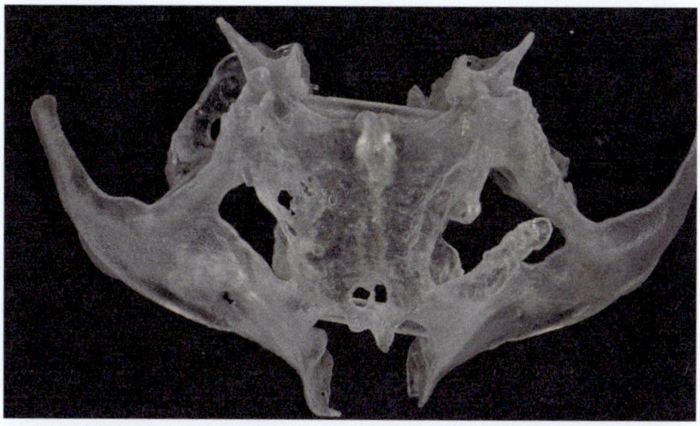

Fig. 14.23 Stereolithographic model showing the large bone defect on both sides

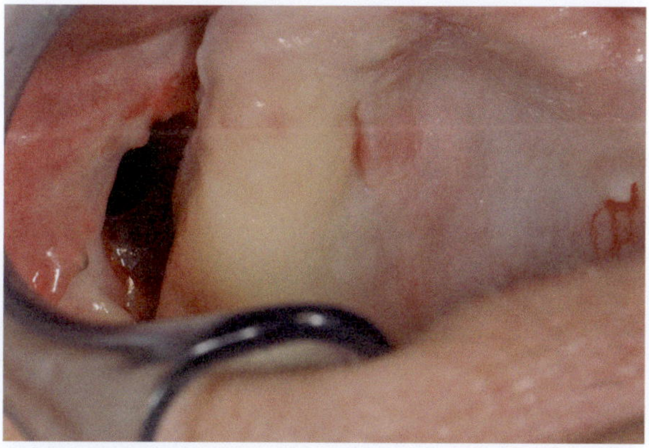

Fig. 14.24 Intraoral view of an oro-antral communication 2 years after implant loss

Improper Basal Implant Placement

Whether the result of inadequate planning, poor judgment, or loss of spatial orientation during surgery, basal implants are sometimes installed in positions or at angulations that are less than ideal for the intended prosthetic purpose. They may be placed too far buccally or labially and impinge on the soft tissues of the lip or cheek. When placed too far lingually in the mandible, implants may irritate the thin, mobile, and vulnerable mucosa of the floor of the mouth and cause problems during speech. This may be the result of bone being locally deficient in volume or unsuitable in density, factors that were perhaps not adequately appreciated preoperatively. When basal implants are too close together, it is difficult to maintain adequate hygiene and the health of the mucosa suffers. One of the most common errors is implant placement too far buccally. This inevitably leads to exposure of part of the basal implant and difficulties in obtaining a satisfactory soft tissue environment and acceptable cosmetic outcome.

Initial cortical support is mandatory for Diskimplants®, especially in low-density bone. If the disk diameter is not wide enough to engage both cortical plates (buccal and lingual or palatal), poor osseo-adaptation and loss of integration under excessive stress must be expected, especially with type IV bone (Misch classification D4).

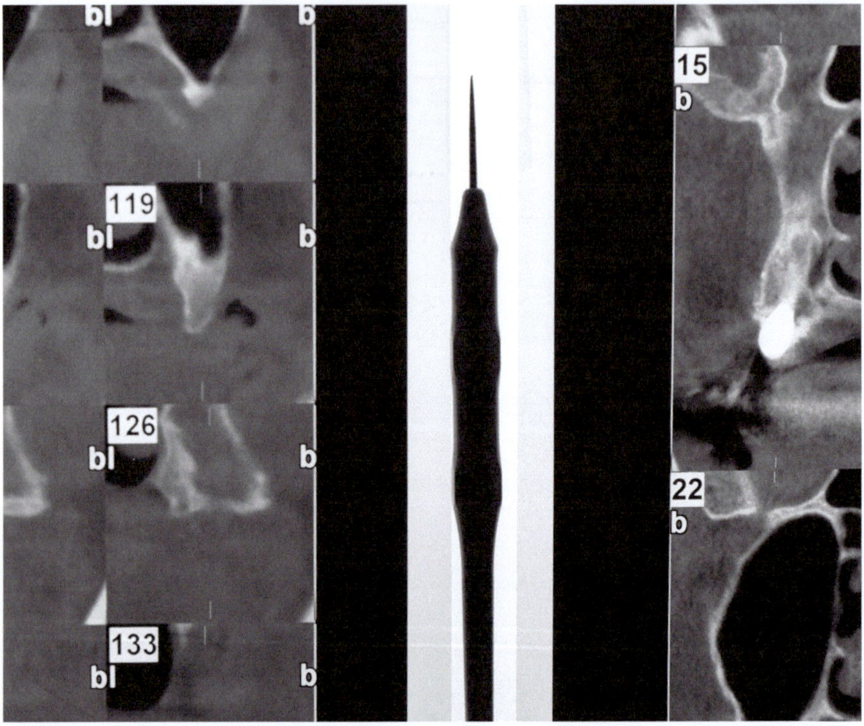

Fig. 14.25 Bone matrix activation with a manual osseotensor in order to stimulate blood supply 90 days before surgical closure of the oro-antral communication

Fig. 14.26 60 days after osseotensor application, the oro-antral communication had already reduced in size (compare to Fig. 14.24)

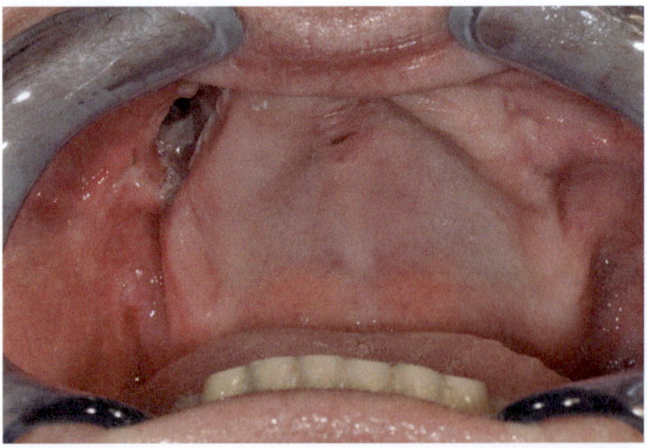

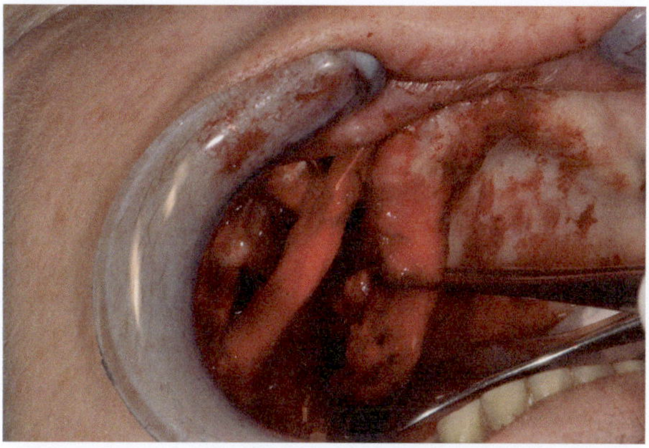

Fig. 14.27 PRF, a bone substitute material (CoreBone®), and collagen membranes were placed using a multilayer approach. A vascularized maxillary fat pad is mandatory in such situations to complete the closure of the defect

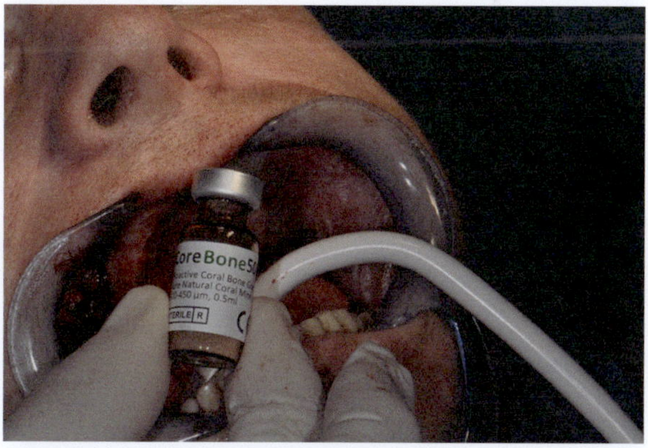

Fig. 14.28 Collagen membranes and CoreBone® were added with PRF

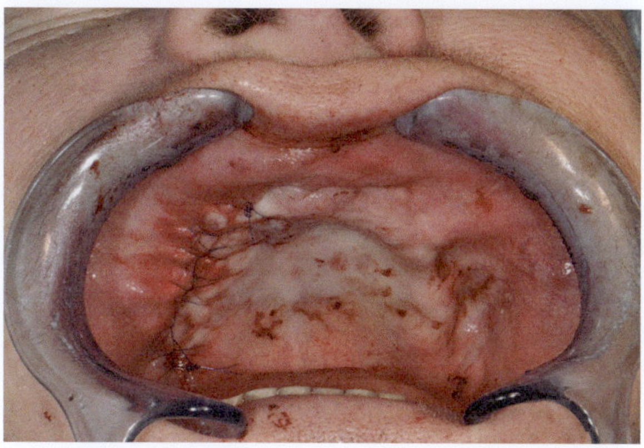

Fig. 14.29 The full-thickness flap was closed without tension

Basal Implant Placement in the Sinus

This problem can be prevented by careful preoperative planning, including 3D cone beam investigation, pre-surgery application of bone matrix osseotensors, wax-up, and joint consultation with the prosthodontist. Care must be taken not to mistake the projection of the hard palate for the floor of the sinus on a panoramic radiograph. Bone measurement with calipers on a stereolithographic model and cone beam 3D simulation allow selection of the optimum base diameter for placement in the densest available bone. In soft bone, the largest diameter possible should be used. If a small opening is observed in the sinus during osteotomy with a cutter, the sinus membrane should be gently elevated by pushing PRF membranes and bone substitute material through the opening into the sinus. A large diameter, monodisk implant can be placed safely, provided that its position between the buccal plate and the palatal plate guarantees multicortical anchorage. For more difficult situations, a plate-form Diskimplant® is mandatory. A non-osseointegrated Diskimplant® in the sinus can easily be removed through a lateral bone window.

Accidental Swallowing or Inhalation of Components and/or Instruments

When coated with saliva, small implant components and the instruments used for their manipulation may escape the clinician's grip and fall into the oropharynx, where reflex swallowing may take the item out of sight almost immediately. The item may be ingested or, even worse, inhaled. This is a particular risk with recumbent patients. Should this occur, immediately turn the patient's head in order to stop the swallowing reflex, then place him or her in a head-down position and attempt to recover the lost component. If this proves impossible, the practitioner should accompany the patient (placed in a head-low position) to the hospital and give all necessary information to the emergency medical team. Endoscopic removal may prove necessary for larger components that are ingested or inhaled. Ingestion of very small components such as screws or veneers is usually less serious and requires only that the patient be placed on a high-fiber diet.

Manual screwdrivers and similar instruments should always be equipped with a safety line of dental floss (minimum length 10 cm). Small components such as transgingival abutments should be handled using purpose-designed titanium drivers.

14.5 Postoperative Complications

Management of Postoperative Swelling, Hematoma, and Pain

The best results are obtained by application of an ice pack immediately after surgery. When necessary, the following corticoid regimen can be administered: 60 mg Solupred® per os post-op *plus* 60 mg per os the day after surgery and *then* 60 mg per os the second day after surgery. For extensive hematomas, antibiotic therapy (amoxicillin 2 g/day) should be maintained until complete resolution is achieved. Painkillers (paracetamol 1000 mg) and anti-inflammatory drugs plus an ice pack are the best means to reduce pain after surgery.

Incision Line Opening

The main cause of this complication is soft tissue suturing with tension at surgery. To prevent the incision line from opening due to the pull of the muscles, an internal release incision should be made in the periosteum with a scalpel or soft brushing; this will ensure passive positioning of the flaps at suturing. This is particularly important when using basal implants together with bone augmentation (GBR). If the design of the removable interim prosthesis is the cause, it must be modified extensively so as not to exert force on the area of basal implant exposure. The patient should not wear the denture for 3 days after suturing and, thereafter, just for cosmetic reasons, and must stay on a soft diet for 45 days.

Attempting to resuture a flap that opens after 3 or more days is both useless and painful. Allow the wound to heal by secondary intention, which takes about 3 weeks. The site must be gently rinsed with physiological saline three times a day.

Subgingival Plaque Associated with Peri-implant Complications

The microbiota associated with successful basal implants and that associated with peri-implant complications are basically similar to those associated with periodontal health and disease, respectively. Bacteria-host interactions suggest that patients with osseointegrated basal implants could benefit from preventive measures. Claims that mechanical debridement every 3 months can maintain peri-implant health for osseointegrated implants are simply not true. Such so-called prevention can actually result in peri-implant mucositis and/or peri-implantitis.

Plastic scalers and rubber cups are generally recommended for professional cleaning of natural teeth but should be avoided with "healthy" and calculus-free dental implants. This cleaning technique may actually increase contamination by opening the hemi-desmosomal biologic seal between the highly polished titanium surface of Diskimplants® and the surrounding soft tissues, with subsequent risk of fistula formation. In the case of transgingival abutment contamination with fistula formation, surgical debridement of infiltrated soft tissues and removal of the existing abutment is recommended, after which a new, sterile transgingival component should be installed.

Patients with recurrent saliva-related calculus buildup may benefit from screw-retained full zirconia prostheses (Figs. 14.30, 14.31, 14.32, 14.33, and 14.34) because calculus does not adhere to highly polished zirconia surfaces.

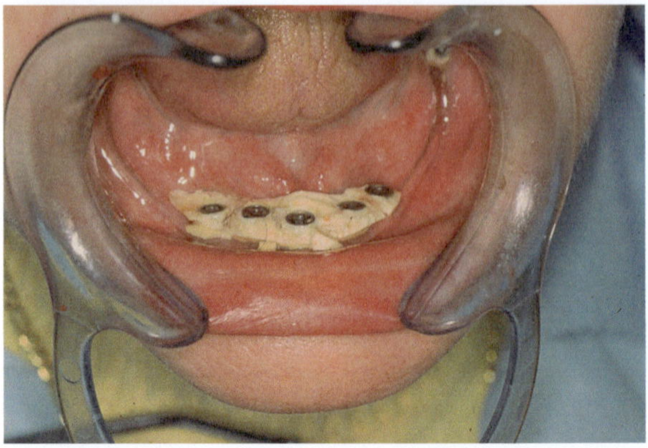

Fig. 14.30 Ultrarapid calculus buildup required bridge retrieval every 3 months

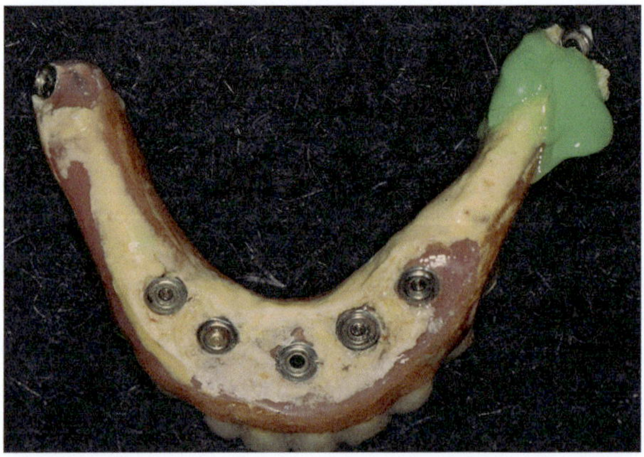

Fig. 14.31 The calculus covered the entire internal surface of the lower screw-secured denture

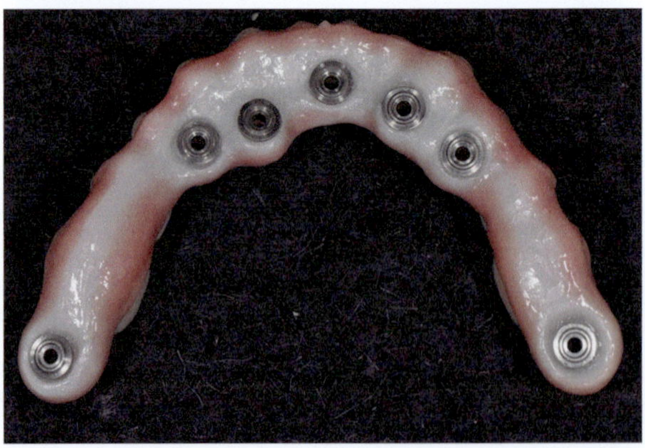

Fig. 14.32 Full zirconia without pink ceramic under the pontic was mandatory to prevent the adhesion of calculus

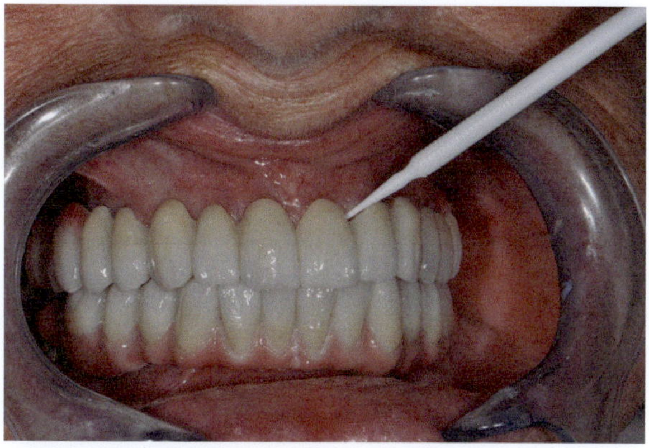

Fig. 14.33 Upper and lower full zirconia prostheses (Zirkonzahn)

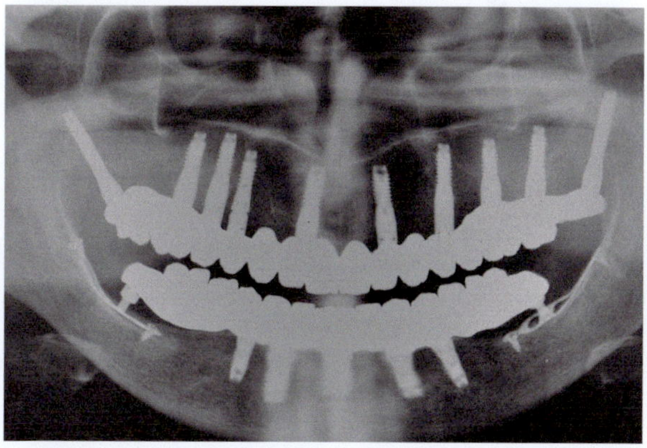

Fig. 14.34 Panoramic radiograph 12 years post-op (same patient as Fig. 14.33)

Protrusion of a Portion of an Osseointegrated Diskimplant®

Occasionally, the base of a Diskimplant® protrudes slightly into the oral cavity through the alveolar mucosa after years of function. Patients generally feel no pain, but the professional detects the protruding titanium disk at annual checkups. This portion of the disk must be eliminated without flap elevation to avoid soft tissue contamination by metal particles.

Following local injection of an anesthetic around the protruding disk, a round diamond bur mounted on a high-speed turbine can be used to remove it under copious irrigation. On rare occasions, the entire disk of a triple or double Diskimplant® lies exposed above the gingival level as the result of bone resorption. The exposed disk can be eliminated by cutting the metal connecting it to the central vertical shaft with a diamond or carbide bur. Preparation of a 2 mm space around the external portion of the disk allows lateral retrieval of the circular base. Use of long shaft, double Diskimplants® (7G5-DDM or 7G5-DDM5) instead of triple disk versions avoids this problem. Should a portion of a mandibular plate-form Diskimplant® protrude lingually, it can be removed but only if the remainder of the implant is osseointegrated. If not, the entire plate-form Diskimplant® must be removed and the defect filled in with bone substitute material and PRF (Figs. 14.35, 14.36, and 14.37).

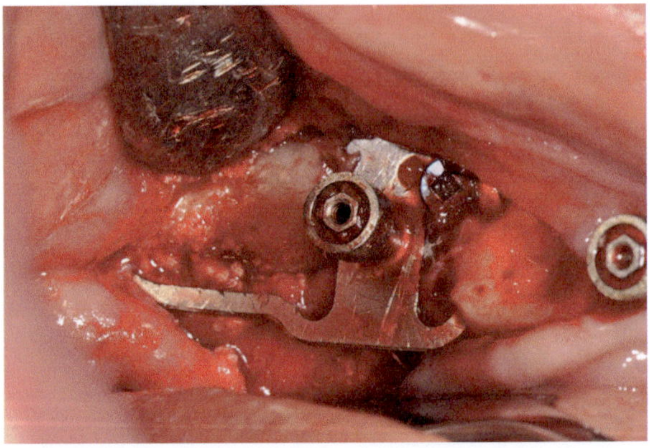

Fig. 14.35 Full-flap exposure of the lingual aspect of a plate-form Diskimplant® in the posterior left mandible. Partial bony coverage of the plate is visible

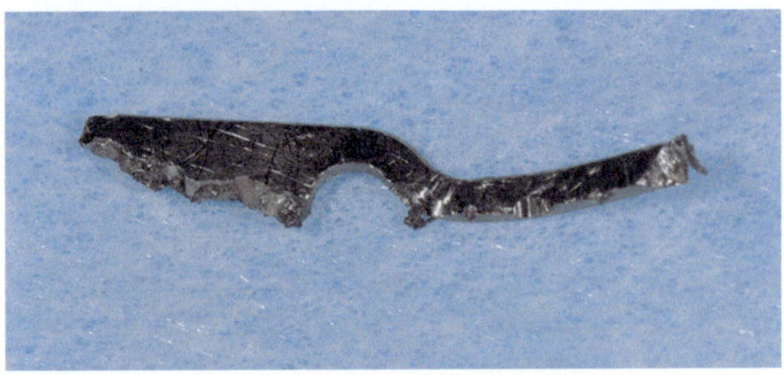

Fig. 14.36 The protruding portion of the plate was cut off with a carbide bur under copious irrigation. The remainder of the plate was completely embedded in the mandibular bone. Aspect of the retrieved titanium lingual bar

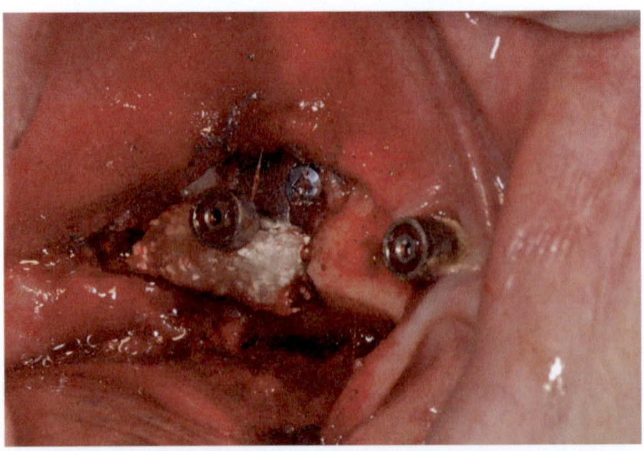

Fig. 14.37 Bone substitute material (CoreBone®) plus PRF were used to cover the defect. The full-thickness flap was then sutured without tension

Peri-implantitis

Peri-implantitis is infrequent (less than 0.1%) with Diskimplants®, even in periodontally compromised patients. The machined, vertical shaft of the Diskimplant® is narrower (approx. 2 mm) than conventional screw-type implants, a feature that minimizes iatrogenic trauma to the alveolar crestal bone. In certain cases, minimally invasive peri-implant surgery, including soft tissue removal and laser treatment, may prove helpful.

Exposure of a Plate-Form Diskimplant®

Should a plate-form basal implant become partially exposed during the healing period, no attempt should be made to cover it by resuturing the flap.

- Exposure of a small portion of a non-painful and nonmobile plate-form Diskimplant® implant at the crestal emergence will slowly heal and be covered by the mucosa in several weeks.
- If a small area of exposure remains on the buccal aspect after 45 days, light anesthesia permits the exposed metal to be impacted using a flapless procedure. The fixed, screw-secured prosthesis must be left in place during impaction. The patient should merely clean the exposed surface with saline solution on a disposable cotton swab. The problem can be corrected later on, after osseointegration.
- If a large portion of a plate-form Diskimplant® becomes exposed through the tissues, the implant should be rapidly removed. To avoid this problem, make sure that the basal implant fits tightly into and/or onto the bony bed (maintained in intimate contact with the recipient bone by preparation of the site with a cutter) and is completely covered by an adequate layer of bone substitute material and PRF.

Strategy When Faced with Apparent Failure of a Diskimplant®

A failing (mobile and/or painful), non-osseointegrated basal implant must be removed as soon as possible. When conditions are favorable, a larger-diameter Diskimplant® can be installed immediately in the existing implant site. However, so long as the prosthetic restoration is stable and the patient is comfortable, without pain or infection, Diskimplants® can often be left in place. This is particularly true in edentulous patients. A Diskimplant® that is slightly mobile (movement less than 0.5 mm) but not painful can be left in place if the implant-supported prosthetic restoration is highly rigid and provides overall stability. Flapless placement of a 5- or 6-mm-long orthopedic fixation screw against the disk under local anesthesia may provide additional stability. This should be done with the screw-secured prosthesis in place. In favorable occlusal conditions, reintegration of Diskimplants® is also possible provided the prosthetic rehabilitation is absolutely stable.

Sometimes, apparent implant failure is actually due to fracture of the prosthetic framework (Figs. 14.38, 14.39, and 14.40). Fabrication of a new, rigid, and much stronger fixed bridge often allows complete healing at the bone/implant interface after 6 months.

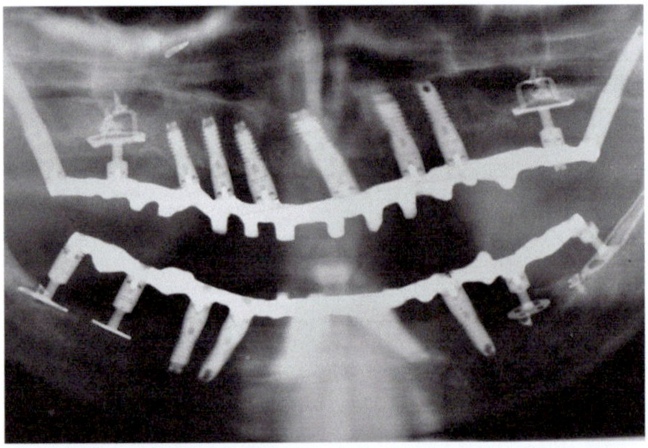

Fig. 14.38 Immediate loading of full upper and lower rehabilitations. Unfortunately, the lower left framework was too thin and fractured after 7 months

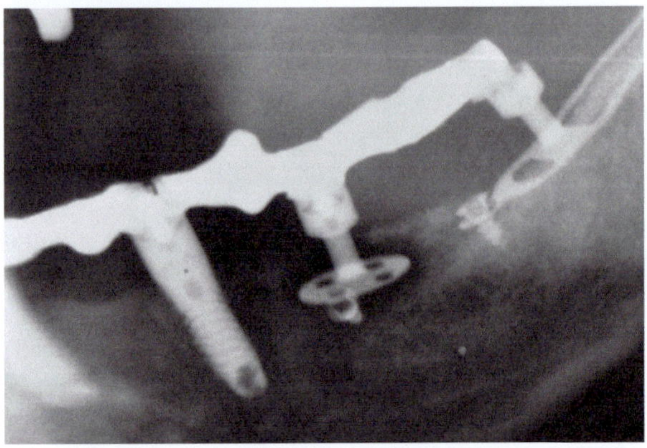

Fig. 14.39 The lower left Diskimplant® started to lose its osseointegration but was not painful and there were no signs of infection, just slight mobility

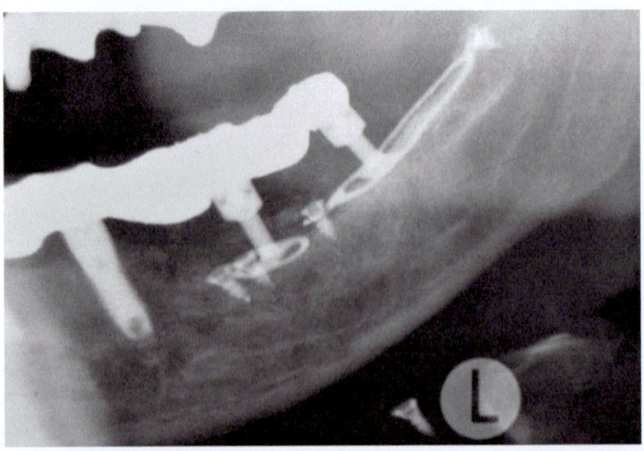

Fig. 14.40 A completely new, stronger, and highly rigid framework was made. Six years post-op, clinical examination and radiological studies demonstrated complete recovery

Retrieval of a Failing Diskimplant®

A Diskimplant® that fails to osseointegrate owing to an error in selection of the base diameter or poor positioning in cancellous bone without initial multicortical support must be removed as soon as possible if painful and highly mobile. Removal of a non-osseointegrated Diskimplant® involves minimal bone loss owing to the small dimensions of the osteotomy. Furthermore, the shallow depth of bone used for anchorage (usually 3–5 mm) favors subsequent healing and repair and reduces the risk of permanent injury. Traumatic block section removal should be avoided.

When necessary, Diskimplants® can be retrieved using the same lateral pathway as for insertion:

- If the initial osteotomy has already been filled in by bone tissue, use the corresponding titanium cutter to reopen the T-shaped site. A carbide bur may be utilized to reduce bone destruction. A sharp bone scissors is used to grasp the base of the Diskimplant®.
- If the initial T-shaped osteotomy has been filled in by fibrous tissue rather than bone, a No. 11 blade and a carbide bur suffice to free the Diskimplant®.
- A piezotome may prove helpful for retrieval of a failing basal implant.

14.6 Management of Mechanical Problems

The mechanical problems encountered with basal implants are similar to those seen with root-form implants and should be taken care of as soon as possible. Recommendations for correction of potential problems are listed below:

- Never let the situation deteriorate. Mobile implant-supported teeth, pain, and infection should always be treated first.
- Prepare a realistic plan to manage the complication (including the possibility of implant removal) after a frank discussion with the patient. If the implant(s) were placed by another practitioner, he or she should be contacted as well. Alternative conventional solutions must also be discussed.
- Correction is not always a straightforward procedure and may involve risky and/or expensive restoration. Inform the patient of all potential problems and costs before any work is performed.
- If unfamiliar with the implant system used, suggest that the patient return to the professional originally in charge of the restoration. If the patient is reluctant to do so, or if this is not feasible, obtain advice from other professionals and/or the implant manufacturer so as not to compromise the patient's initial oral status and entail unnecessary expenses.

Prevention of Mechanical Problems

- Never under-equip a patient with a strong bite or a heavy grinder with a history of dental and prosthetic fractures.
- Avoid a cantilever whenever possible.
- Use a highly rigid, screw-secured titanium framework with a transitional transpalatal bar for patients with extremely atrophic, completely edentulous jaws.
- Stable inter-arch dental relationships are mandatory.
- A night guard can reduce stress in compromised clinical situations.
- Botox® injections may prove useful for heavy grinders.
- Use transitional commercial teeth mounted on a solid metal framework before fabricating a final prosthesis in order to reduce the initial occlusal stress during the first 6 months after functional loading.

Fracture of Cosmetic Components

- Check the occlusion.
- Determine the cause of the fracture.
- A resin fracture can be repaired chairside with acrylic resin and a denture tooth or composite restoration.
- Ceramic fracture: grind the remaining ceramic down to the metal frame, then take an impression of the prepared sector to make an individual telescopic ceramic or full zirconia crown. Make a chairside resin temporary for use during fabrication of the final tooth. An occlusal metal surface may be required for patients with a strong bite with little space. Cement the ceramic crown back on with resin cement; remove all excess with the liquid monomer and a sharp instrument. Check the occlusion.
- A night guard is mandatory for patients who clench or grind; bilateral Botox® is indicated for difficult cases.
- Full zirconia can be a reliable option for heavy grinders who can destroy conventional ceramic-to-metal prostheses (Figs. 14.41, 14.42, 14.43, and 14.44).

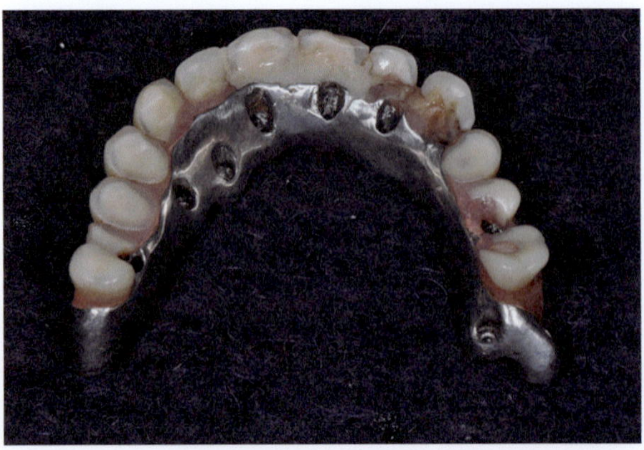

Fig. 14.41 Implant placed in 1991. Severe bruxism and clenching led to multiple fractures of the resin cosmetic elements. Botox®, a night guard, and increase of the vertical dimension reduced ongoing fractures for a limited period

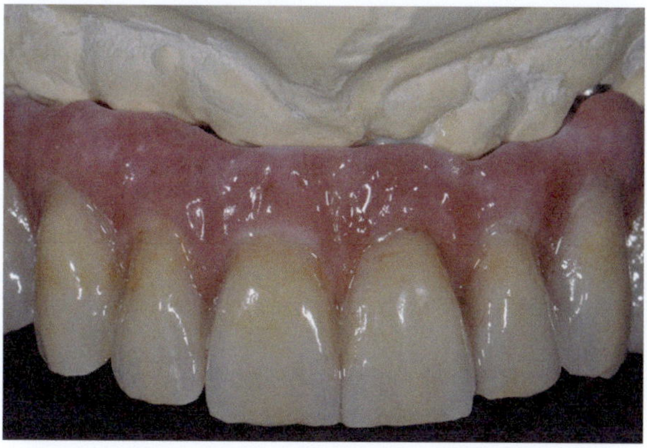

Fig. 14.42 In 2005, it was decided to replace the gold/resin bridge with a full zirconia (Zirkonzahn) rehabilitation screw-secured on basal implants (same patient as Fig. 14.41)

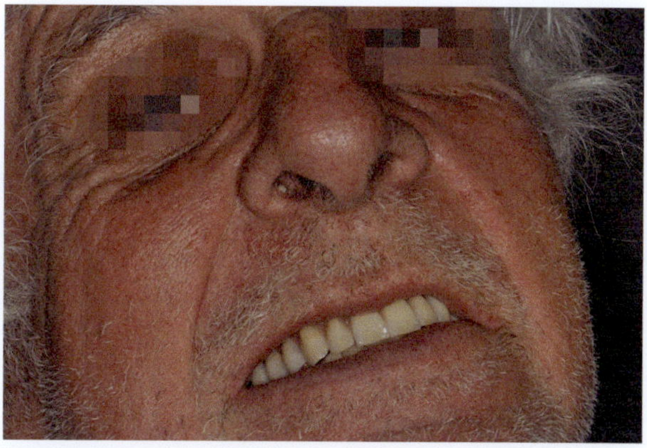

Fig. 14.43 Cosmetic outcome (same patient as Figs. 14.41 and 14.42)

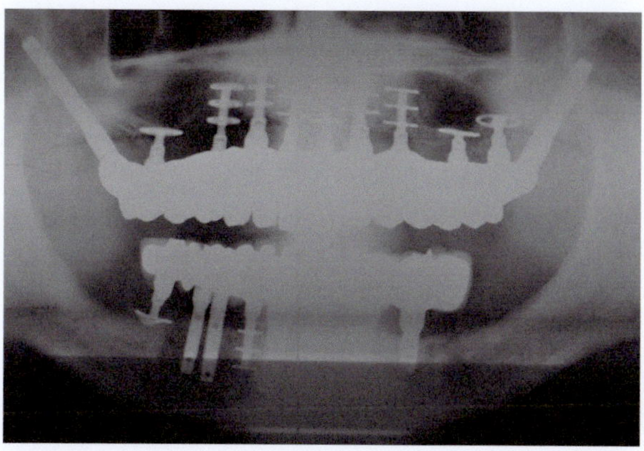

Fig. 14.44 Panoramic radiograph taken in April 2017 (26 years post-op: 1991–2017). No visible fracture of any cosmetic elements (same patient as Figs. 14.41, 14.42, and 14.43)

Loosening of a Prosthetic Retaining Screw

Repeated loosening of a retaining screw is a warning sign of future screw fracture. In most cases, this is caused by poor fit of the prosthesis at the implant/abutment interface that is aggravated by occlusal stress, unilateral mastication, malocclusion, under-equipment necessitating placement of an additional implant, and bruxism. In some cases, the prosthesis must be entirely redone, and/or additional implants must be planned. A night guard is advisable.

Management depends on when loosening occurs:

1. Early screw loosening, less than 6 months after prosthesis installment: gold M1.4 screws can merely be retightened at 10–15 Ncm following verification of the occlusion.
2. Late screw loosening, more than 6 months after placement of the prosthesis: Never try to retighten loose screws in this situation as they may break and become impossible to retrieve. Use of a new screw is recommended. Check the occlusion.
3. Very late screw loosening, many years after prosthesis installment, is more likely related to metal modification with time, elongation, wear, and metal compression. When a prosthetic restoration becomes loose after years of service, all screws should be replaced and retightened after 24 h, and the occlusion must be rechecked.

In all cases, prosthetic retaining screws should be retightened 24 to 48 h after placement (in one day, teeth come into contact 1000 to 1500 times, and even more often in case of bruxism).

Screw Loss

- When possible, check the patient's records to be sure that the proper retaining screw was used.
- Install a new screw. Gold M1.4 screws should be tightened to 10–15 Ncm; larger-diameter M2 screws must be tightened to 20–30 Ncm.
- Have the patient return the next day to retighten the screw and recheck the occlusion.

Fracture of an Abutment Screw or a Prosthetic Retaining Screw (Figs. 14.45 and 14.46)

Fracture of an abutment screw requires replacement of the entire abutment. Check the accuracy of fit at the prosthetic interface with a periapical radiograph, and verify the occlusion before replacing it. If a retaining screw breaks, it must also be replaced. When retrieving the fractured portion of a retaining screw, the primary

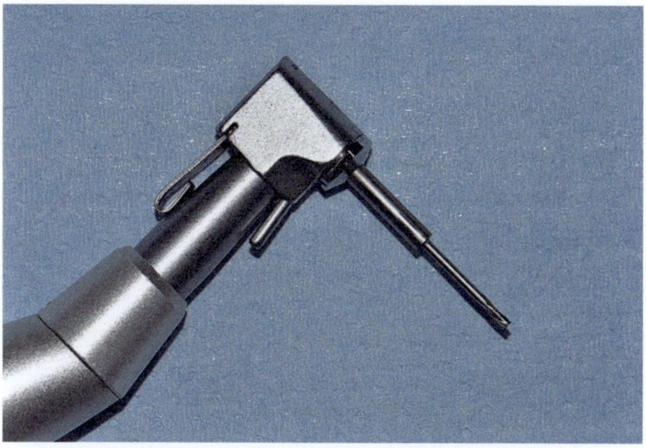

Fig. 14.45 Specially designed instrument operated in reverse with a high-power, slow-speed handpiece (60–80 rpm) for retrieval of fractured screws

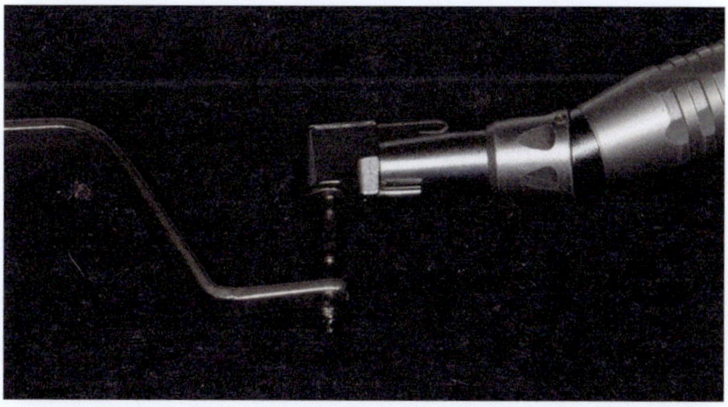

Fig. 14.46 A cylindrical tube is used to help maintain the correct direction

rule is "never aggravate the situation." This means *do not* use ultrasound devices. Proceed as follows:

- Take a periapical radiograph to localize the fractured part.
- Always lubricate the screw access hole before attempting to remove a fractured screw. A drop of eugenol can be used as a lubricant.
- The fractured portion of the screw is usually not flat but somewhat jagged. Using a rigid dental probe, push down against the uneven surface and turn counterclockwise. The broken portion generally unscrews easily. A very thin, brand-new diamond flame bur mounted on a contra-angle disconnected from the unit and activated manually in reverse, as with a probe, may prove helpful. Be careful not to damage the internal threads of the implant. After removal of the fractured piece, verify the implant threads with a manual tap. Take a digital retroalveolar radiograph before activating the tap to ensure that it is correctly positioned in the axis of the implant in order not to damage the threads. A cylindrical pickup type impression coping can be used as a guide when activating the tap.
- If retrieval of a fractured screw proves difficult or impossible with the above approach, use a screw-removal instrument mounted on a low-speed (60–80 rpm), high torque handpiece operated in reverse. Alternately, after lubrication of the

fractured screw, push down on the surface with a cotton swab and turn counter-clockwise; the cotton fibers wrap around the remaining screw threads and may allow removal.

Gold prosthetic retaining screws are generally recommended to avoid creation of a cold solder as can occur with titanium screws. The latter are sometimes impossible to retrieve if they break.

Loosening of a Transgingival Abutment

- Unscrew the abutment retaining screw to retrieve the prosthesis secured to the transgingival abutment.
- Retighten the transgingival abutment after checking to be sure it is not damaged; otherwise use a new abutment.
- Replace the prosthesis and secure it with the appropriate retaining screw.
- Check the occlusion.
- A night guard is recommended.

Loosening of Cement-Retained Prostheses

Should a screw-secured hex abutment post become loose, retrieve the cement-secured bridge by gently pulling on it with a dental crown extractor. If the metal prosthetic components have formed an undetachable cold solder as the result of high masticatory forces, it may be necessary to completely cut and open the restoration at the abutment post site and fabricate a new prosthesis.

14.7 Management of a Fractured Diskimplant® (Figs. 14.47, 14.48, 14.49, 14.50, 14.51, 14.52, 14.53, 14.54, 14.55, 14.56, and 14.57)

An aggressive bone block section to retrieve a fractured Diskimplant® should be avoided because much less invasive solutions exist as a function of the clinical context:

- Non-osseointegrated Diskimplant®: removal can be performed easily along the path of initial insertion using a scalpel and a 700 XXL carbide bur.
- An osseointegrated Diskimplant® can be left in place and:
  (a) A conventional prosthetic appliance can be fabricated if the patient is reluctant to undergo new implant placement.
  (b) A new Diskimplant® can be placed mesially and/or distally.
  (c) Another Diskimplant® can be installed above or below the initial site. Start the lateral osteotomy; when the titanium cutter touches the fractured disk, replace it with a carbide bur in order to pass through the titanium base of the

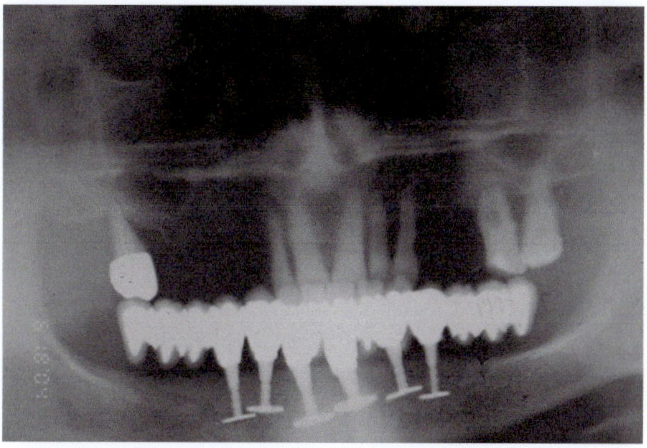

Fig. 14.47 The excessively long cantilevers created mechanical problems

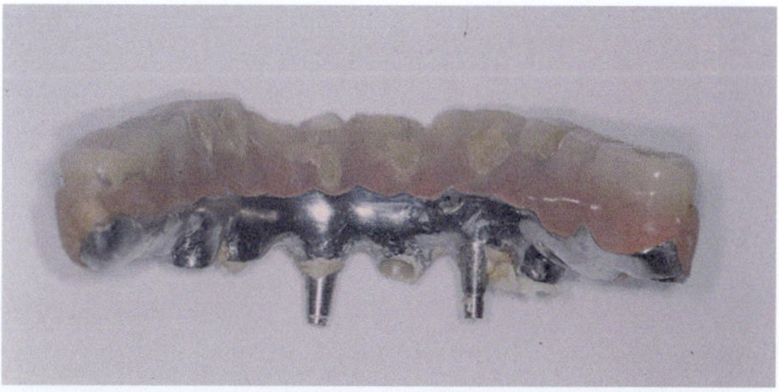

Fig. 14.48 Multiple fatigue fractures of older generation, externally threaded Diskimplants® after 11 years of function

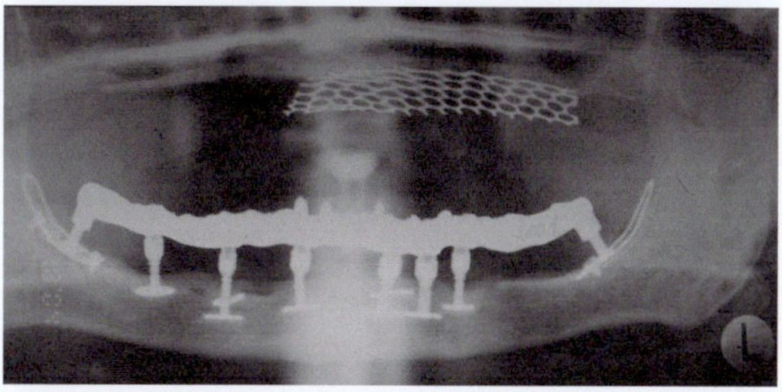

Fig. 14.49 A plate-form Diskimplant® was placed posteriorly on each side, and new Diskimplants® were installed in the mental sector to replace those that had fractured. Panoramic radiograph after 13 years

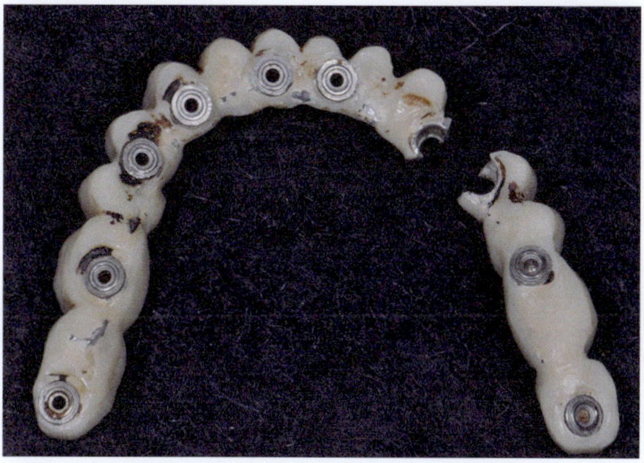

Fig. 14.50 Fractured, screw-secured bridge (fracture occurred at the weakest point of the metal framework)

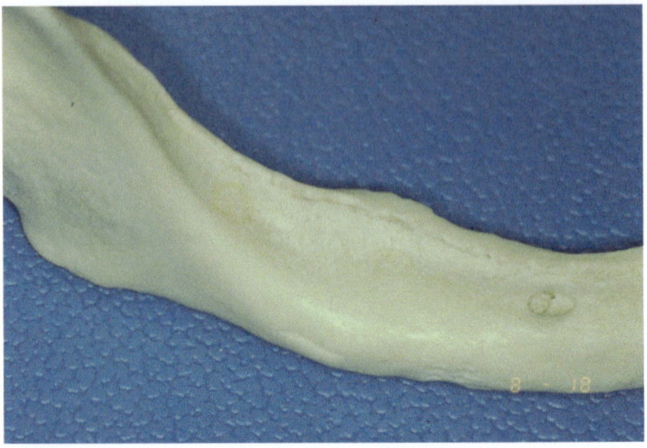

Fig. 14.51 Highly atrophic dry posterior mandible. The mental foramen is located on the crest

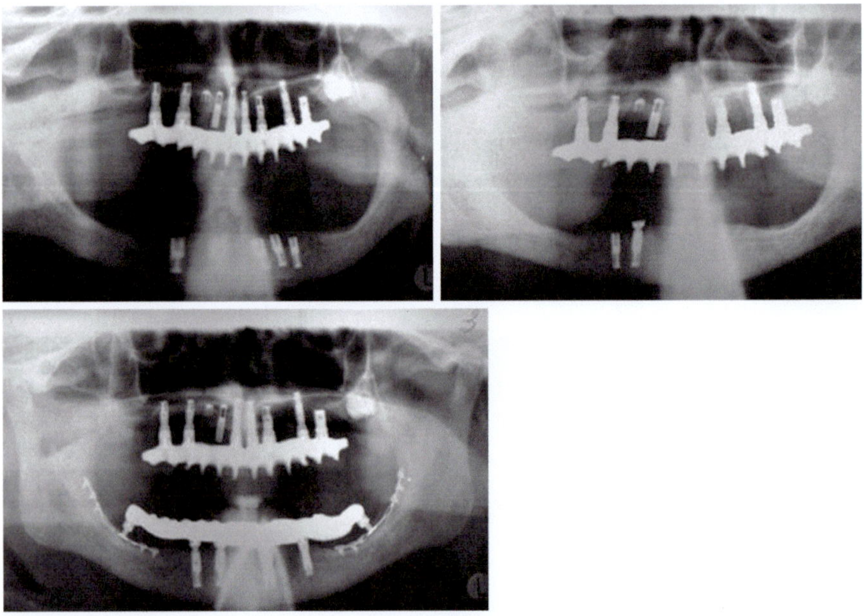

Fig. 14.52 Multiple fractures of root-form implants in the mental area due to a cantilever. The patient was rehabilitated by placing a plate-form Diskimplant® on each side

fractured Diskimplant® left in place. Copious spray and lateral irrigation are mandatory. Once the track is completed with the carbide bur, use the corresponding titanium cutter to finish the osteotomy, and insert a new Diskimplant®.

(d) Alternately, the axial shaft of a fractured Diskimplant® can be eliminated with a carbide bur, after which the perforations in the disk are connected and enlarged with appropriate drills allowing passage of a root-form implant through the Diskimplant® base. In certain situations, the existing fixed prosthesis can be reutilized after modification.

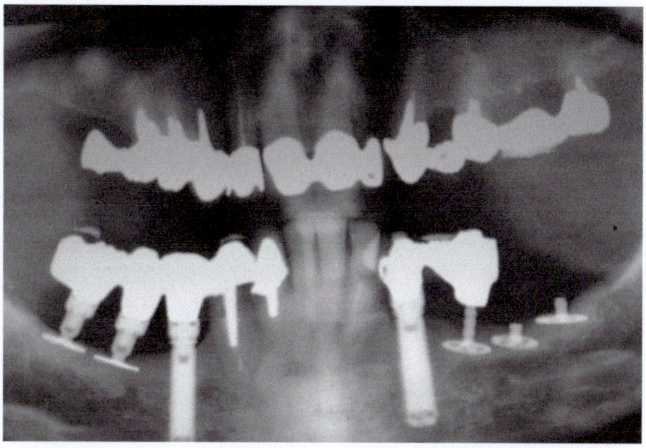

Fig. 14.53 Panoramic radiograph (1998): fracture of three early-generation Diskimplants® installed 12 years earlier, in 1986. The third implant in the second premolar position had not yet fractured. Bone height above the disk ranged from 0.8 to 2 mm

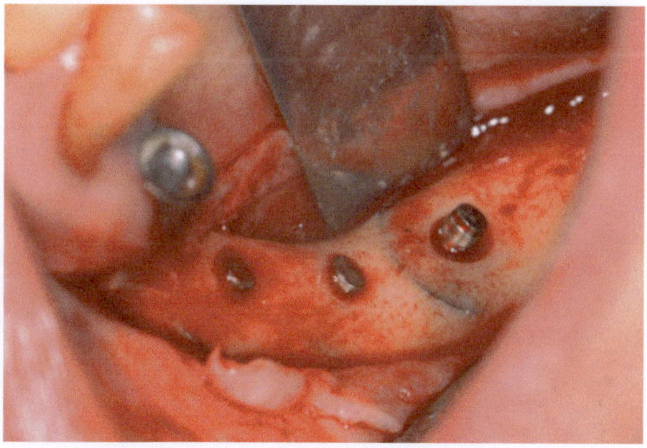

Fig. 14.54 At bridge retrieval, the shaft of the third Diskimplant® had fractured. Bone completely covered the disk, placed at a depth of 2 mm. The well-osseointegrated distal disk can been seen by transparency under the bone. No sign of peri-implantitis after 12 years of service (same patient as Fig. 14.53)

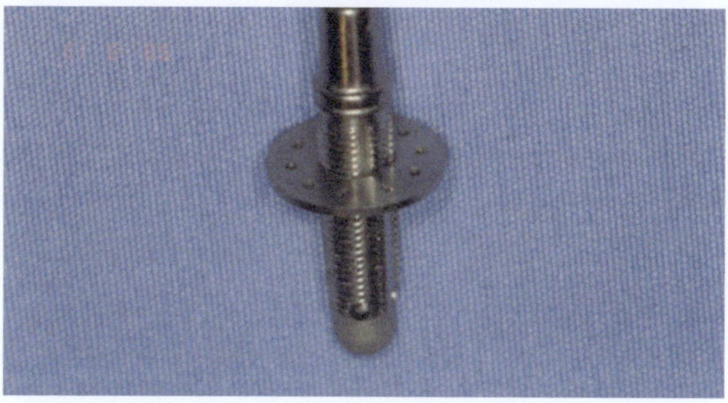

Fig. 14.55 Three microthreaded, root-form implants were placed after the openings in the basal disk had been enlarged using a carbide bur, then a diamond bur, an axial dense bone drill, and a metal tap

(e) A Diskimplant® can be removed using a titanium cutter, a carbide bur, and a sharp bone chisel to free the base. A piezotome can also be used (Fig. 14.57). Grasp the base with a dental rongeur and gently rotate it out. Install another Diskimplant® with a larger base. Wait 6 months for healing before loading.

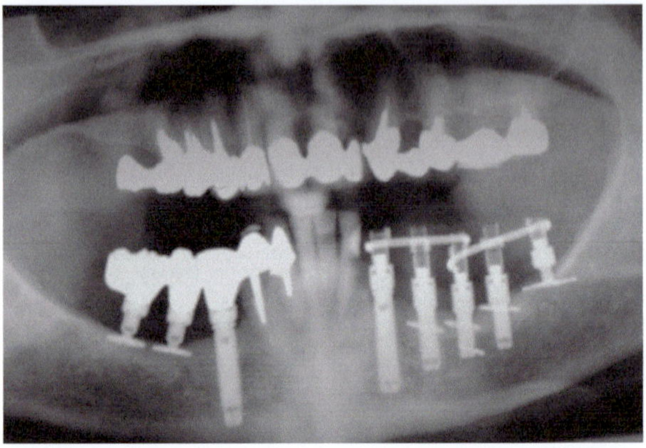

Fig. 14.56 A temporary, screw-secured titanium bridge was installed 24 h post-op (same patient as Figs. 14.53, 14.54 and 14.55)

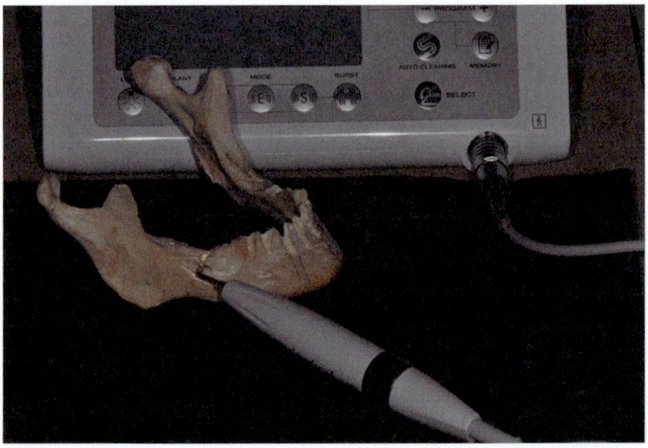

Fig. 14.57 Lateral access for the piezotome in the posterior mandible for retrieval of a fractured disk when necessary. A piezotome can also be used for Diskimplant® placement

14.8 Salvage Procedures for Complete Implant Failures

Clinical Case No. 1 (Figs. 14.58, 14.59, 14.60, 14.61, and 14.62)
This patient received root-form implants that all failed. Revision and correction were possible with basal implants. An immediate fixed, screw-secured prosthesis was installed 48 h post-op.

Clinical Case No. 2 (Figs. 14.63, 14.64, and 14.65)
Following accidental trauma, this patient lost her fixed, basal implant-supported prosthesis and had to wear a transitional full denture for 6 months. Revision and correction were performed with an immediate, fixed functional loading procedure (the prosthesis was screw-secured to basal and root-form implants).

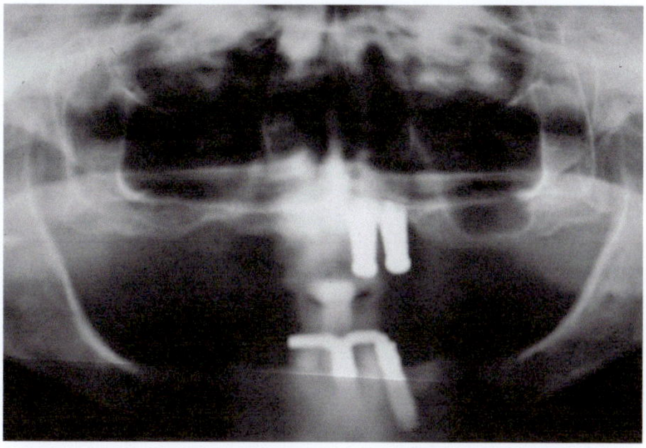

Fig. 14.58 Two root-form implants affected by peri-implantitis were mobile under a removable full denture with ball attachments. The bar attached to two root-form implants in the lower jaw was also mobile

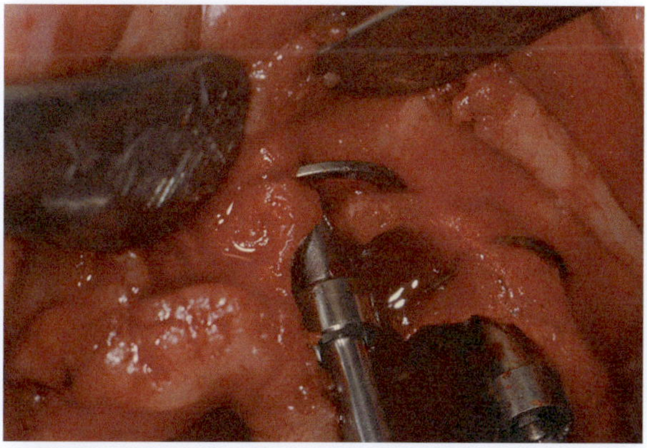

Fig. 14.59 Extensive bone loss: 9 mm diameter basal implants were installed through the palatal aspect (lateral palatal bone cut seen from the buccal aspect)

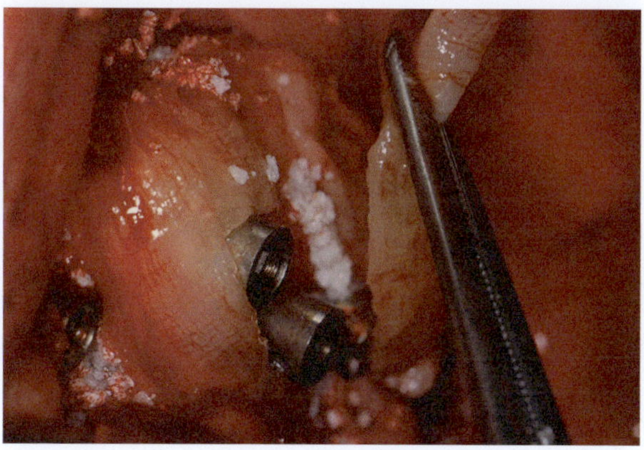

Fig. 14.60 Guided bone regeneration with bone substitute material and PRF

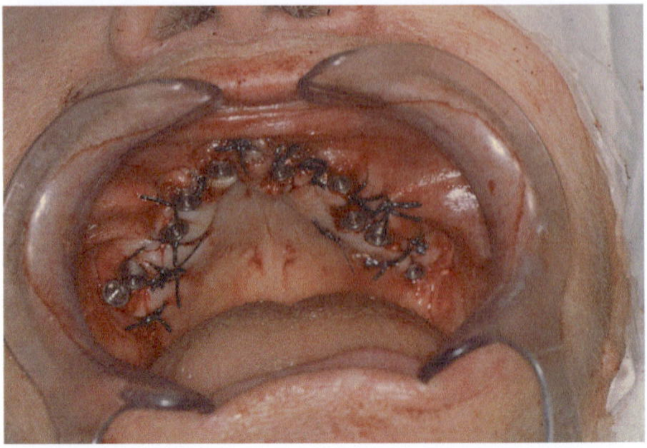

Fig. 14.61 Intraoral view of full-thickness flap sutures

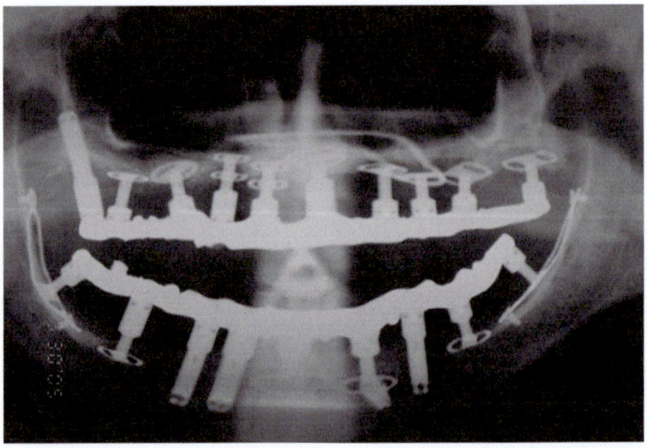

Fig. 14.62 Panoramic view after 18 years of service (same patient as Fig. 14.58)

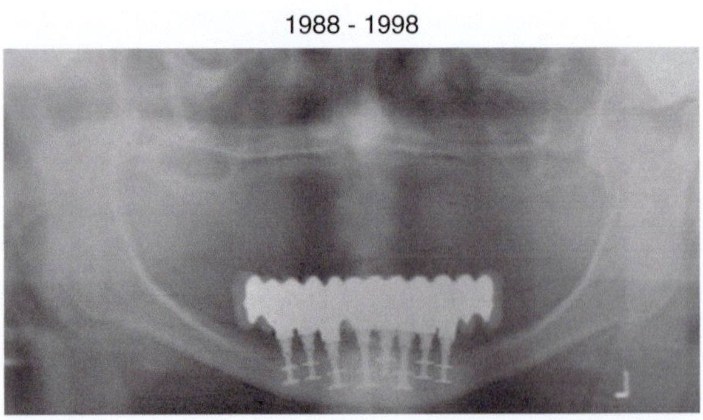

Fig. 14.63 Basal implants in the intraforaminal region of a knife-ridge after 10 years of service

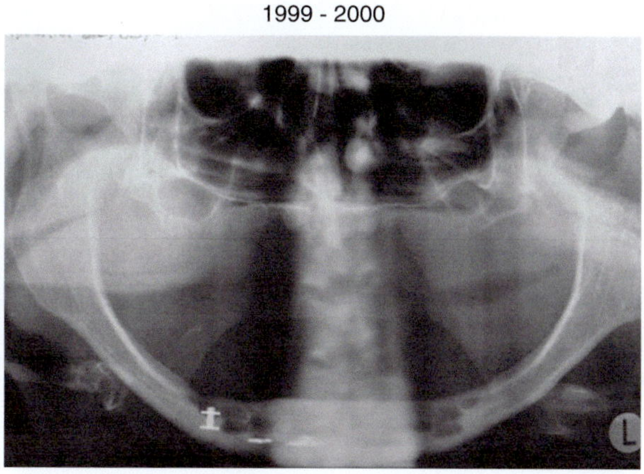

Fig. 14.64 This patient fell on a hard surface and broke the fixed mandibular rehabilitation. A removable denture was worn for 6 months (same patient as Fig. 14.63)

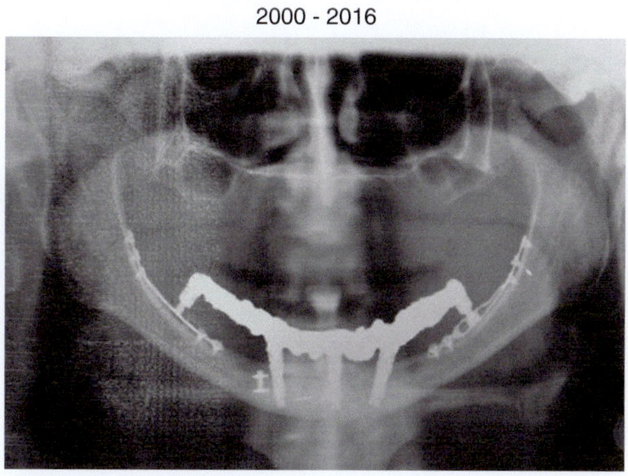

Fig. 14.65 After 6 months, five new implants were installed (immediate functional loading procedure). Plate-form basal Diskimplants® were placed on both sides in the posterior mandible. Panoramic radiograph after 8 years (2016) (same patient as Figs. 14.63, 14.64)

14.9 Prevention of Potential Problems Related to General Anesthesia (Figs. 14.66, 14.67, 14.68, 14.69, and 14.70)

Extremely atrophic maxillae are eggshell-like bony structures. Such situations can be a risk when patients must undergo extraoral surgery under general anesthesia. The implant surgeon should prepare a palatal silicone ball chairside to prevent a LeFort fracture during forced mouth opening by the anesthetist.

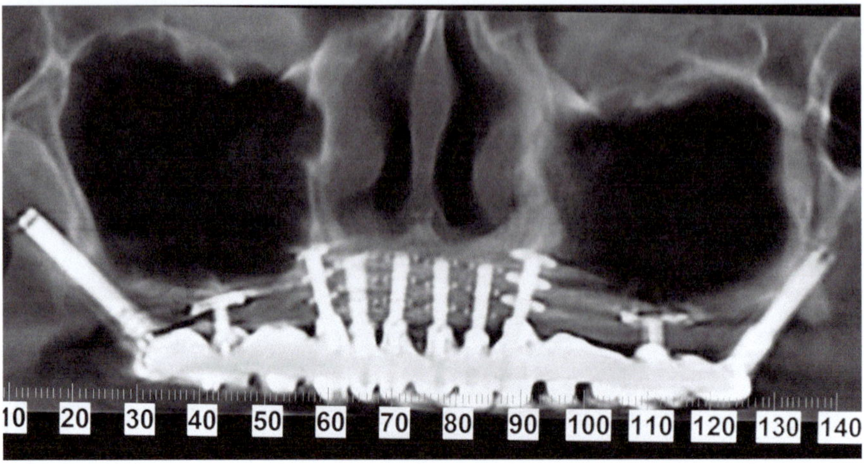

Fig. 14.66 Panoramic radiograph with the rehabilitation in place (14 years of service). Eggshell maxilla managed with a "zygomadisk"

Fig. 14.67 Intraoral view (same patient as Fig. 14.66)

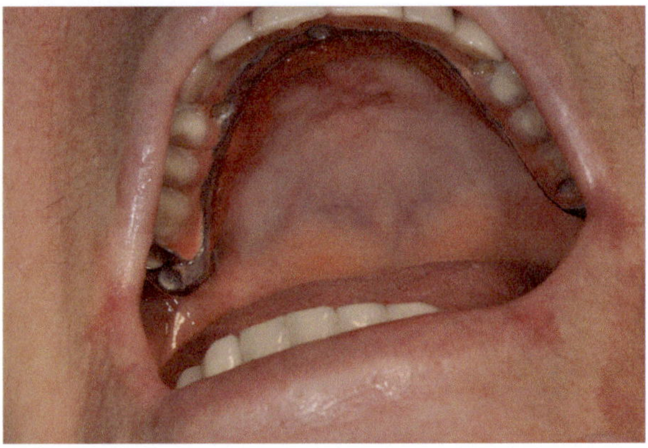

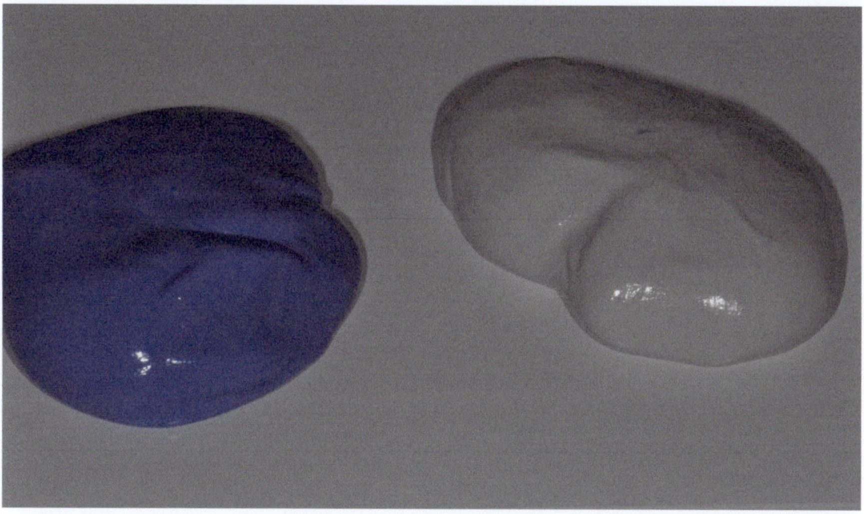

Fig. 14.68 Complications can be prevented by placing a silicone ball in the mouth

Fig. 14.69 Silicone ball in place

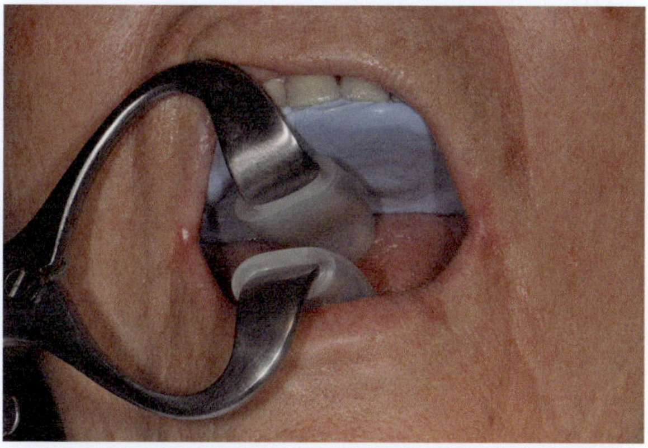

Fig. 14.70 Patients who require an extraoral surgical procedure under general anesthesia are given a silicone ball in order to prevent an iatrogenic LeFort fracture of the upper maxilla during intubation

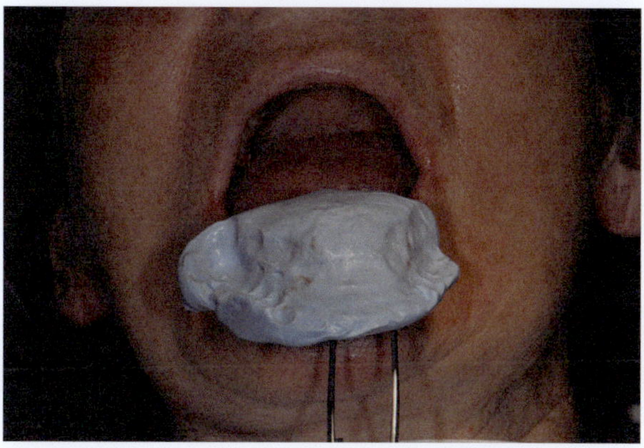

Table 14.1 Maintenance of peri-implant health and management of complications

Successful basal implant maintenance
– Oral hygiene instructions and recall
– Mechanical maintenance of prosthetic components (screw retightening, recementing, closure of screw access holes)
– Occlusion/night guard
Reversible problems
– Minor mechanical problems (screw loosening, fracture of resin or ceramics, screw fracture)
– Peri-implant mucositis, calculus removal
– Laser therapies
– Traumatic occlusion—correction
– Replacement of a fractured element (ceramic, resin, prosthetic retaining screw, titanium abutment screw, etc.)
Compromised osseointegrated basal dental implants
– Oral hygiene instructions/reinforcement
– Stop smoking
– Check the occlusion—night guard
– Shorter maintenance intervals
– Antimicrobial mouthwash and/or irrigation
– Laser therapies
– Change the transgingival abutment (in case of a fistula or fracture)
– Systemic antibiotics selected according to susceptibility test
– Nonsteroidal anti-inflammatory drugs
– Tetracycline
– Drugs to enhance bone reconstruction and mineralization
– Minor surgical treatment
– New prosthesis when prosthetic misfit is identified at implant interface
– Removal of the protruding metallic portion (disk) of an osseointegrated basal implant with a diamond or carbide bur under copious irrigation
– Placement of an additional transparietal orthopedic screw (5–6 mm) against the base of the compromised Diskimplant® with the screw-retained bridge in place.
– Addition of new implants if necessary and possible
Irreversible problems
– Major esthetic, speech, or functional problems
– Major biological or mechanical problems (implant or jaw fracture)
– Peri-implantitis associated with pain and implant mobility
– Acute neuralgia/severe psychological problems
– Complete bone breakdown and basal implant mobility/pain/infection
Failed basal implant
– Implant removal—correction of the bone defect with biomaterials and membranes
– Bone grafting (1 or 2 sessions; bone matrix cell activation with an osseotensor mandatory 60 to 90 days before surgery)
– Major surgical treatment, including closure of any oro-antral communication; return to a conventional partial or complete denture
– New implant placed after a waiting period (at least 1 year for extremely atrophic edentulous jaws)
– New basal implant-supported prosthesis

14.10 Maintenance (Table 14.1)

Follow-Up and Postoperative Care

During the immediate postoperative period, patients are instructed to refrain from brushing the surgical site. Mouthwashes are also prohibited for 48 h after surgery. The preventive program for patients with partial or full restorations on osseointegrated basal implants should include specific oral hygiene instructions and regular professional checkups. Primary and secondary prevention techniques are aimed at plaque control by the patient and the dental hygienist or dentist. For daily home care, oral hygiene can be ensured with standard Waterpik®-type appliances and superfloss and/or special peri-implant care using 3% hydrogen peroxide and disposable cotton swabs, depending on the patient's individual situation. Toothbrushes become contaminated by bacteria and should be used to clean only artificial teeth and peri-implant areas where there are at least 2 mm of peri-implant attached gingiva. In regions with no or very little attached gingiva, disposable cotton swabs with 3% hydrogen peroxide diluted in hot water should be used for daily cleaning of implant emergence profiles. Dakin Cooper solution or 2% chlorhexidine on a disposable cotton swab (never as a mouth wash) is also helpful to prevent local inflammation of the mucosa around basal implants.

Annual verification of well-balanced occlusal status is necessary to reduce or avoid mechanical problems.

Conflict of interest statement Gérard M. Scortecci is the inventor of the Diskimplant and holder of several associated patents that are exploited by the Victory company. He is an unpaid consultant to this firm and a minority shareholder in the company. No money was received from any of the companies mentioned in the book or from any of the companies whose products are mentioned.

Recommended Reading

1. Resnik RR, Misch CE. Avoiding complications in oral implantology. St. Louis, MO: Elsevier; 2017.
2. Ucer C, Yilmaz Z, Scher E, Suzuki J, Renton T. A survey of the opinion and experience of UK dentists. Part 3: An evidence-based protocol of surgical risk management strategies in the mandible. Implant Dent. 2017;26(4):532–40.
3. Lekholm U, Adell R, Brånemark PI. Chap. 14: Complications. In: Brånemark PI, Zarb GA, Albrektsson T, editors. Tissue-integrated prostheses. Osseointegration in clinical dentistry. Chicago, IL: Quintessence; 1985. p. 233–40.
4. Jordana F, Susbielles L, Colat-Parros J. Periimplantitis and implant body roughness. Implant Dent. 2018;27(6):672–81.

Postimplantation Neuropathies 15

Gérard M. Scortecci, Patrick Missika, and Alp Alantar

15.1 Terminology

Major medical terms necessary for a clinical approach to neurological involvement in the context of implant surgery include:

- Neuropathy: a general term indicating a disorder of the peripheral nerves [1].
- Postimplantation neuropathy: a relatively recent term referring to any neurological disorder induced by the placement of implants; usually of immediate onset, it may be transient or become chronic.
- Allodynia: pain caused by a normally non-painful stimulus, corresponding to a lowering of the pain threshold [2]; identification of the triggering stimulus is essential, because not all types of stimuli cause pain in all patients (mechano-induced allodynia, thermo-induced allodynia, etc.) [3].
- Painful anesthesia: pain felt in a hypoesthetic area [2].
- Paresthesia: any abnormal sensation, usually characterized by a reduction in cutaneous sensitivity (hypoesthesia or anesthesia) [4].

G. M. Scortecci (✉)
University of Nice-Sophia Antipolis Medical School, Nice, France

New York University, New York, NY, USA

University of Southern California, Los Angeles, CA, USA

Private practice, Nice, France
e-mail: scortecci@wanadoo.fr

P. Missika
University Paris 7 and Private Practice, Paris, France
e-mail: pmissika@wanadoo.fr

A. Alantar
Private Practice, Paris, France
e-mail: alpalantar@wanadoo.fr

© Springer Nature Switzerland AG 2019

G. M. Scortecci (ed.), *Basal Implantology*, https://doi.org/10.1007/978-3-319-44873-2_15

- Dysesthesia: any painful abnormal sensation unrelated to a stimulus [2]; dysesthesia thus differs from paresthesia by its painful nature.
- Hyperalgesia: exaggerated response to painful stimuli [2].
- Hyperesthesia: exaggerated perception of sensations [2].
- Neuropathic pain: neuropathic pain is defined by the International Association for the Study of Pain (IASP) as pain arising as a direct consequence of an injury or disease affecting the somatosensory system. The term "pain" encompasses a very broad group of syndromes that differ by their pathogenesis, symptoms, and treatment; the generally accepted classification is based on the site of neural involvement [5]:
  - Peripheral neuropathy (painful polyneuropathy, lancinating neuralgia, phantom pain, nerve compression, neurinoma).
  - Central neuropathy (central pain).
  - Mixed neuropathy (postherpetic neuralgia).

In this review, the term "neuropathic pain" denotes chronic pain syndromes attributable to a postimplantation lesion of the mandibular branch of the trigeminal nerve (cranial nerve V3). Pain syndromes resulting from central nervous system injuries and pain caused by physiological activation of the nociceptors that innervate the neural sheaths (e.g., inflammation, tumor invasion, etc.) are thus excluded.

15.2 Diagnosis

Positive Diagnosis

Positive diagnosis is based on subjective clinical symptoms sought during a careful clinical history and objective clinical signs detected during physical examination, completed by radiologic studies.

Clinical Assessment

Clinical assessment of orofacial neuropathies must be preceded by a careful clinical history to elicit any complaints of pain and/or discomfort. Differentiation of dysesthesia and paresthesia is the first step in such evaluation. The following questions allow distinction:

1. Do you have any abnormal sensations in the skin, lips, tongue, nose, or cheek?
2. Do you have any abnormal sensations on the right or left side?
3. How do you describe the sensation? Is it spontaneous, or does it occur only when you touch the zone, chew, or talk?
4. Do you experience pain? if so, where? Is it continuous (burning) or intermittent (lightning-like)? Is it spontaneous or triggered by touch, mastication, or speech?
5. How long does it last?
6. What exacerbates this pain? What alleviates it? [4].

Out of the 266 patients investigated by Ellies [6], 80% claimed that they had no problems during daily activities. Among those with complaints, the most commonly altered functions were speech, mastication, and ability to drink fluids. In practice, it is important to differentiate paresthesia and dysesthesia and to determine whether the pain and discomfort are stimulus-generated or spontaneous [4]. Diagnosis of neuropathic pain can be confirmed by using the "DN4 Questionnaire" (sensitivity, 83%; specificity, 90%) [7]. The first seven items relate to the following sensations: burning, painful cold, electrical shocks, tingling, pins and needles, numbness, and itching. The last three items assess hypoesthesia to touch and prick and allodynia to light brush.

Intraoral clinical examination follows the same principles as those for cutaneous neurological examination, i.e., sensitivity to light touch, pinprick, cold, and heat, existence of allodynia, and hyperesthesia, and should be extended from the gums to the mucosa of the vestibules and cheeks. Early diagnosis of pain or discomfort is essential for at least two reasons:

1. These patients must be evaluated and treated differently from those with a non-painful paresthesia.
2. Evaluation of the pain or discomfort depends entirely upon subjective patient responses, not on the objective signs sought by neurological tests [4].

15.3 Physical Examination

Clinical evaluation is based on techniques to map the distribution of defects and tests of primary sensation and discrimination.

15.4 Mapping (Fig. 15.1)

The technique for mapping postimplantation labiomental neuropathies is not specific to implantology but can usefully be applied to this discipline [8]. The main steps in the technique proposed by Essick [9], which can easily be performed during consultations for implant surgery, are described hereafter.

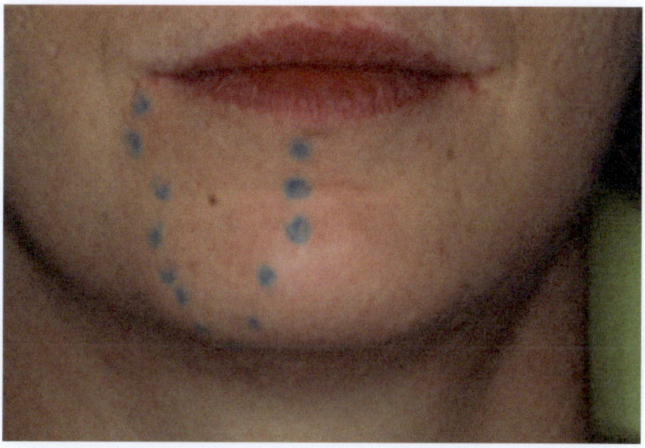

Fig. 15.1 Trigeminal neuralgia: the zone of paresthesia is delimited by a mapping procedure

In an initial step, patients are requested to circumscribe the periphery of the involved zone with their index finger. In a second step, stimulation is performed with a dental probe equipped with an endodontic stop. This permits the patient to memorize a pricking sensation in an uninvolved control zone innervated by the contralateral mental nerve (or infraorbital nerve in case of bilateral involvement). Patients are then requested to close their eyes, and stimulations (duration of 1 second) are applied along a linear axis starting 15 mm from the periphery and directed toward the center of the involved zone. Patients are asked to raise their hand each time the sensation feels "different," and a mark is made at this point with a dermatological marker. Connection of the various marks delimits the zone of paresthesia. Although mapping does not allow objective measurement of sensory capacity, it permits:

1. Identification of the affected area and evaluation of the severity of the subjective sensation
2. Follow-up of the affected area and severity of involvement over a period of time
3. Selection of a site for objective sensory tests [9]
4. Documentation of the progressive or regressive nature of the neuropathy for medicolegal purposes

15.5 Neurosensory Tests

Evaluation of postimplantation neuropathies makes use of the same procedures as those utilized after extraction of wisdom teeth or orthognathic surgery. The main examinations are tests of thermal sensation, soft touch, brush stoke direction, two-point discrimination thresholds, perception of pain, and perception of pressure [10]. These tests are generally performed in a Neurology Department. However, brush stoke direction and two-point discrimination thresholds can be tested in the dental office during a consultation for implants. When preliminary explorations suggest severe involvement, patients should be addressed to a Neurology Department.

The brush stroke direction test, which evaluates the α fibers and partially the δ fibers, allows simultaneous evaluation of touch localization. A brush (von Frey fibers or a toothbrush) is used to apply light pressure on the skin of a healthy control site innervated by the contralateral mental nerve or, in case of bilateral involvement, by the infraorbital nerve. The site being tested is first stroked from top to bottom and then from bottom to top. Before each series of stimulations, the practitioner says "first series" or "second series." The patient is then asked to indicate during which series the brush had been moved from top to bottom [11]. Described by Sekular et al. [12], this forced choice between two alternatives eliminates any biases related to the patient (loss of attention, fatigue, emotion, etc.), who might be tempted to consider that "yes" is a correct response during an interrogation based on a "yes-no" mode.

15.6 Two-Point Discrimination Thresholds

This test permits exploration of the large-diameter myelin fibers (alpha fibers) by evaluating the patient's capacity to discriminate contact at two points on the tongue or the lip. It is particularly indicated for assessment of neuropathies consecutive to inferior alveolar nerve repositioning because it is selective for the α fibers that are sensitive to traction and pressure [13]. The test is performed on patients with their eyes closed using special calipers and a ruler graduated in millimeters [9]. The caliper is first applied closed and then progressively set apart, 1 mm at a time, until the patient can distinguish two points. The minimum distance separating two points that the patient can distinguish is recorded. The two points of the caliper must be applied simultaneously to the site being tested. Each site is tested five times and the values are averaged. For the lower lip, the mean acceptable threshold is 8 mm [14, 15]. A discrimination capacity of less than 14 mm is considered normal [13, 16], while values between 14 and 20 mm are considered indicative of an "altered" discrimination capacity [14, 15]. A threshold over 20 mm is abnormal [15, 16], and the discrimination capacity of such patients is considered null [13]. Owing to the existence of wide interindividual variations [17], these absolute values must, however, be used with caution. Comparison with a control site is thus essential. For Bailey and Bays [11], mean distances – greater or less than 2 mm compared with the control value for the same side – are arbitrarily considered abnormal.

15.7 Radiographic Examination

A suspected nerve injury or a patient presenting with numbness following an implant procedure is an indication for an early radiographic exam in order to facilitate the choice between (1) temporization with medical treatment followed by clinical control and (2) removal of the implant. Radiographic examination should be performed perioperatively when a patient relates acute pain during a surgical procedure. Periapical and panoramic radiographs will be completed by CT scans in complex cases (e.g., morphology of the body of the mandible and/or atypical symptoms and/or multiple implants, etc.).

Radiographically, compression is suggested when the apex of the implant is contiguous with the superior lamina dura of the mandibular canal, without interruption of the canal (Fig. 15.2), or when only a thin band of medullary bone (less than 2 mm) is seen between these two elements. Penetration of the canal (Figs. 15.3 and 15.4) is visualized as an interruption of the superior lamina dura, with the apex of the implant superimposed over a variable height of the canal. Section of the nerve is seen as superposition of the implant over the entire height of the canal and sometimes even beyond. CT is indicated for patients with atypical symptoms such as lingual involvement. Berberi et al. [18], for example, reported a case of paresthesia of the anterior two-thirds of the tongue visualized on coronal CT scans by the lingual position of two implants plunging into the floor of the mouth.

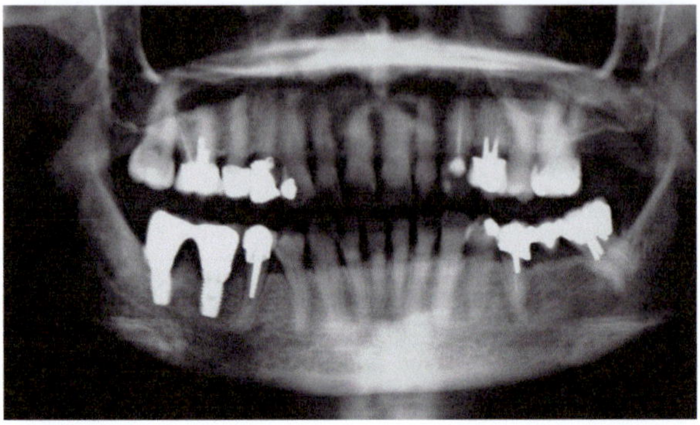

Fig. 15.2 Panoramic view showing implant-induced canal compression

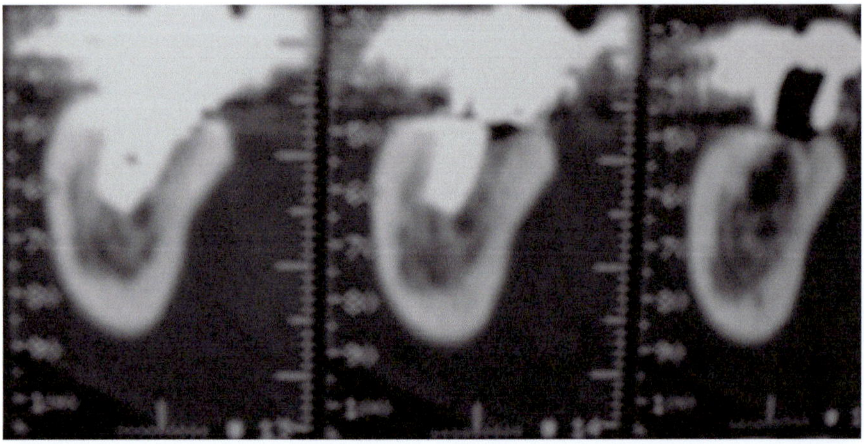

Fig. 15.3 Coronal CT scans revealing effraction of the canal. The implant must be removed

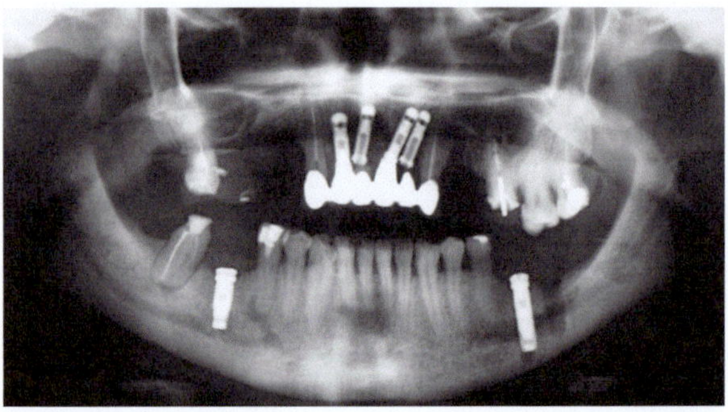

Fig. 15.4 Panoramic view showing implant-induced canal compression and nerve transfixation by implants in positions 36 and 37, both of which must be removed

15.8 Etiology

Transient or permanent anesthesia, paresthesia, or dysesthesia may result from displacement, compression, or injury of the inferior alveolar nerve [19].

Compression

The dental nerve runs throughout the posterior mandible to its foramina and can be injured during drilling or screwing of the implant. Neuropathic pain can be secondary to compression or laceration [20]. For Bert [21], transient paresthesia is more a sign of compression of the nerve fibers by an internal hematoma than penetration of the nerve trunk.

Penetration of the Mandibular Canal

The frequency of neuropathies is not significantly different between implants placed anterior to the mental foramen and those installed posterior to it. Implants placed behind the foramen are, however, associated with a higher rate of persistent lesions (longer than 6 months) than those placed in front of the foramen (50% versus 30%) [6]. Shulman and Shepherd [19] described a patient with neurological complications after placement of implants in the premolar sector. In that case, penetration of the left and right mandibular canals with perforation and displacement of the mandibular nerves resulted in immediate anesthesia and severe dysesthesia in one site and chronic paresthesia in the other.

Lesions Resulting from Traction on the Inferior Alveolar Nerve

Sunderland [22] demonstrated that stretching of a nerve, especially when performed rapidly, can rupture the endoneurium and the perineurium, leading to fibrotic modifications in the nerve and the loss of axonal guidance. For Jensen and Nock [23], excessively brutal manipulation of a nerve can sever the perineural vascularization; in such cases, recovery may be only partial and result in a permanent deficit. The rate of neuropathies following nerve repositioning depends on the technique and the number of implants placed. In a series of ten patients, Smiler [24] reported one case of minor unilateral neurapraxia that disappeared after 3 weeks. Guedj [25, 26] described minor permanent dysesthesia in one out of eight patients. Rosenquist [16] observed neurosensory loss 1 week after implant surgery in 47 out of 100 patients. For Jensen and Nock [23], complications vary with the number of implants placed. These authors reported a higher frequency of neurosensory dysfunction in sites where three implants had been placed compared with sites where two implants had been installed.

Lesions Resulting from Mental Bone Sampling for Grafting

Jensen et al. [27] reported dysesthesia in 5% of their patients who underwent mental bone sampling. All patients eventually recovered normal sensation. In the series of 121 cases reported by Antoun et al. [28], sequelae of injury to the mental nerve and the incisive nerve were always minimal and transient. The mental hematoma may explain transient paresthesia of the skin of the chin. However, this etiology can no longer reasonably be incriminated when paresthesia persists for more than 1 week; injury to the most medial inferior labial branches during incision is a more likely cause in such cases. Similar lesions can also occur during flap elevation.

15.9 Predisposing Medical Factors

As reported by Ellies [6] in his study of 266 patients, diabetic individuals show a significantly higher incidence of neuropathies. Other risk factors include immunodeficiency, delayed cicatrization, and a predisposition for microangiopathies, neuropathies, and arteriosclerosis [29].

15.10 Differential Diagnosis

The major differential diagnosis is implant-related psychalgia. For Shulman and Shepherd [19], emotional disorders are not in themselves a contraindication for the placement of implants. For these authors, implant therapy may actually help certain patients with depression. However, another category of emotionally disturbed patients demands the removal of dental implants and then subsequently requests repeat placement. Persuaded that their facial pain is of dental origin, these patients often give a history of multiple dental extractions that have never given conclusive results. When requesting that their implants be removed, they frequently complain of pain equivalent to that which had prompted the earlier dental extractions.

Anesthesia diagnosis can be used to test for implant psychalgia: locoregional anesthesia of the involved nerve trunk, which should suppress the sensation in case of iatrogenic dysesthesia, does not suppress the dysesthesia in case of psychalgia [30]. Confirmation that psychological disorders can be a cause for implant removal was made in the study of Albrektsson et al. [31]. In their series of 400 patients, three required implant removal (total number of implants removed was ten). One of the three, a 60-year-old female psychiatric patient, required removal of seven screw-type maxillary implants supporting a bridge after 30 months of function.

15.11 Treatment

A literature search retrieved very few data with a high level of evidence concerning the treatment of orofacial neuropathic pain after dental implant placement [20].

Pharmacological treatment

Drugs should be administered as early as possible to avoid pain chronicization [32–34]. Indeed, the efficacy of an appropriate treatment can be significantly reduced if treatment initiation is delayed by 9 months or more [35, 36]. An initial treatment with high-dose oral steroids (dexamethasone, 1 mg/kg) is recommended [37, 38]. However, in the context of neuropathic pain, the most frequently used drugs are anticonvulsants and antidepressants [33, 39–42]. Oxcarbazepine, an anticonvulsant which is better tolerated than carbamazepine, with less drug interaction [43, 44], is considered the first therapeutic option for various forms of orofacial paroxysmal neuropathic pain [45]. However, the proposal of considering oxcarbazepine as the first-line drug treatment in the context of dental implant-induced neuropathic pain, especially including paroxysms, remains to be confirmed by prospective controlled studies. The dose regimen should be refined depending on the frequency of paroxysms, which may coexist with permanent neuropathic pain. A number of controlled studies also illustrate the efficacy of gabapentinoid molecules (gabapentin and pregabalin) or antidepressants (tricyclics or other compounds) in various types of neuropathic pain [46–48].

Regarding gabapentin, Park et al. [33] analyzed the efficacy of this medication administered for more than 12 weeks for the treatment of dental implant-induced neuropathic pain in 47 patients. The dosage was gradually increased from 300 mg/d up to 1800–2400 mg/d. After 1 month of treatment, patients who developed side effects or reported inefficacity with gabapentin were prescribed a tricyclic antidepressant for the next 2 months. Overall, 46% reduction of pain intensity was obtained with the use of gabapentin.

The results obtained with pregabalin for treatment of postoperative pain may be more variable [49]. In case of cutaneous allodynia, oral medication can be associated with topical application of local anesthetics, such as 5% lidocaine [41, 42, 50].

Surgical Treatment

The indication for early implant removal (full or partial) depends on clinical features and the distance between the implant and the dental nerve canal, objectively estimated on panoramic views and, in case of superimposition between the implant and the nerve canal, on CBCT exams [51]. On clinical grounds, full removal of the implant should be performed in case of neuropathic pain with allodynia, if possible within the first 2–4 days after surgery. Early removal (within 36 hours after implant placement) significantly improves the clinical prognosis [38]. In any case, an implant should be removed within 21 days following surgery, during the osseous catabolic phase. If implant removal is performed later, it can induce bone trauma and worsen nerve injury [52]. On the other hand, microsurgical nerve repair cannot be routinely recommended because of inconsistent results [53].

In conclusion, when a patient presents with post-implant neuropathic pain, a detailed assessment should be immediately conducted, including at least orthopantomography. If the implant is distant from the canal, early pharmacological treatment and regular clinical follow-up are recommended, as in the first scenario. If there is a simple contact between the implant and the canal wall, the implant should be unscrewed to maintain a distance of at least 2 mm from the canal. If there is a breach in the integrity of the dental canal, complete removal of the implant is mandatory, especially if there is allodynia. The suggested treatment regimen consists of oral steroids, 1–2 mg/kg for 10 days, and anticonvulsants, 300 or 600 mg/day initially for oxcarbazepine or gabapentin, respectively, and then gradually increased in a month up to 1800 to 2400 mg/day before reevaluation.

15.12 Prognosis

Posterior Implants

Paresthesia is usually transient. The affected area decreases in size spontaneously, without removal of the implant, over approximately 3 months, and paresthesia disappears completely in 6 to 8–12 months [54, 55]. Penetration of the mandibular canal is associated with more prolonged involvement. For Ellies [6], the mean duration of long-term paresthesia is 4.5 years (range 6 months–11 years).

Inferior Alveolar Nerve Transposition

The prognosis depends on the technique used. For Rosenquist [13], neurologic disorders were frequent (seven out of ten cases) and sometimes persisted for nearly 6 months (two out of ten cases). However, in that study, all cases had resolved after 1 year. In the series of seven patients (14 nerves transpositioned) treated by Sethi [55] using the technique of Tatum [56], 50% presented hyperesthesia 24 hours after surgery. Complete recovery occurred in all patients within 6 months. Smiler [24], who transpositioned ten nerves but did not displace the mental nerve, did not observe any durable neurologic sequelae, although two patients presented moderate unilateral neurapraxia that disappeared in under 3 weeks.

Prevention

- *Anterior implants*: Considering the risk of a prominent anterior loop, a safety distance of 4 mm should be respected between the posterior aspect of the implant and the mental foramen [57–59].
- *Posterior implants*: To prevent any nerve lesion after dental implant placement in the posterior mandible, a safety distance of 2 mm should be respected between the implant and the mandibular canal [51, 60, 61]. Only reconstructed sagittal views of the mandible using standard CT or CBCT are acceptable for this purpose [62–68]. In any case, drill stops are useful surgical tools [51].

15.13 Conclusion

Preliminary evaluation of implant-related neuropathies can be accomplished by mapping the involved cutaneous zone (in cases of extensive involvement), a careful clinical history, and objective tests, such as the direction of movement, and touch localization. Severely affected patients such as those with allodynia or anesthesia, who have a poor prognosis, should be treated early with high-dose oral steroids associated with anticonvulsants and addressed to a Neurology Department. The accuracy and comprehensive nature of the information provided by the dental practitioner constitutes a valuable element for optimum management of these patients.

Key Points

- A suspected nerve injury or a patient presenting with numbness following an implant procedure necessitates an early radiographic and clinical exam in order to facilitate the choice between (i) temporization with medical treatment followed by clinical control and (ii) removal of the implant.
- A radiographic examination should be performed perioperatively when the patient relates acute pain during a surgical procedure. Periapical and panoramic radiographs will be completed by CT scans in complex cases (e.g., morphology of the body of the mandible and/or atypical symptoms and/or multiple implants, etc.).
- Radiographically, compression is suggested when the apex of the implant is contiguous with the superior lamina dura of the mandibular canal, without interruption of the canal (Fig. 15.3), or when only a thin band of medullary bone (less than 2 mm) is seen between these two elements.
- Penetration of the canal is visualized as an interruption of the superior lamina dura, with the apex of the implant superimposed over a variable height of the canal.
- Section of the nerve is seen as superposition of the implant over the entire height of the canal and sometimes even beyond. CT is indicated for patients with atypical symptoms such as lingual involvement.
- An initial treatment with high-dose oral steroids (dexamethasone, 1 mg/kg) is recommended. However, in the context of neuropathic pain, the most commonly used drugs are anticonvulsants and antidepressants. Oxcarbazepine, an anticonvulsant which is better tolerated than carbamazepine, with less drug-interaction, is considered the first therapeutic option for various forms of orofacial paroxysmal neuropathic pain.
- In case of cutaneous allodynia, oral medication can be associated with topical application of local anesthetics, such as 5% lidocaine.

Conflict of interest statement Gérard M. Scortecci is the inventor of the Diskimplant and holder of several associated patents that are exploited by the Victory company. He is an unpaid consultant to this firm and a minority shareholder in the company. No money was received from any of the companies mentioned in the book or from any of the companies whose products are mentioned.

Recommended Reading

1. Garnier M, Delamare V. Dictionnaire des Termes Techniques de Médecine. Paris: Maloine; 1969. p. 688.
2. Cesaro P. Petit glossaire de la douleur. Rev Prat. 1994;44:18–66.
3. Bennett GJ. Evidence from animal models on the pathogenesis of painful peripheral neuropathy: relevance for pharmacology. In: Basbaum AI, Besson JM, editors. Towards a new pharmacotherapy of pain. Chichester: Wiley-Interscience Publication; 1991. p. 365–79.
4. Zuniga JR, Essick GK. Contemporary approach to the clinical evaluation of trigeminal injuries. Oral Maxillofac Surg Clin North Am. 1992;4:353–67.
5. Portenoy PK. Issues in the management of neuropathic pain. In: Basbaum AI, Besson JM, editors. Towards a new pharmacotherapy of pain. Chichester: Wiley-Interscience Publication; 1991. p. 393–414.
6. Ellies LG. Altered sensation following mandibular implant surgery: a retrospective study. J Prosthet Dentistry. 1992;68(4):664–71.
7. Bouhassira D, Attal N, Alchaar H, Boureau F, Brochet B, Bruxelle J, Cunin G, Fermanian J, Ginies P, Grun-Overdyking A, Jafari-Schluep H, Lanteri-Minet M, Laurent B, Mick G, Serrie A, Valade D, Vicaut E. Comparison of pain syndromes associated with nervous or somatic lesions and development of a new neuropathic pain diagnostic questionnaire (DN4). Pain. 2005;114:29–36.
8. Alantar A, Béatrix JC, Gaudy A, Misipo E, Roche Y. Utilisation de la technique de cartographie des paresthésies labio-mentonnières dans les neuropathies post-implantaires. Med Bucc Chir Bucc. 1998;4:17–21.
9. Essick GK. Comprehensive evaluation of perioral sensory function. Oral Maxillofac Surg Clin North Am. 1992;4(2):503–5.
10. Hillerup S. Iatrogenic injury to the inferior alveolar nerve: etiology, signs and symptoms, and observations on recovery. Int J Oral Maxillofac Surg. 2008;37:704–9.
11. Bailey PH, Bays RA. Evaluation of long-term sensory changes following mandibular augmentation procedures. J Oral Maxillofac Surg. 1984;42(11):722–7.
12. Sekular R, Nash D, Armstrong R. Sensitive, objective procedure for evaluation of response to light touch. Neurolog. 1973;23:1282.
13. Rosenquist B. Fixture placement posterior to the mental foramen with transpositioning of the inferior alveolar nerve. Int J Oral Maxillofac Implants. 1991;7(1):45–50.
14. Van Sickels JE, Zysset M, Nishioka GJ, Thrash WJ. A comparative study of normal sensibility of the inferior alveolar nerve and the infraorbital nerve. Oral Surg Oral Med Oral Pathol. 1989;67:255–7.
15. Pogrel MA, Thamby S. Permanent nerve involvement resulting from inferior alveolar nerve blocks. J Am Dent Assoc. 2000;131:901–7.
16. Rosenquist B. Implant placement in combination with nerve transpositioning: experiences with the first 100 cases. Int J Oral Maxillofac Implants. 1994;9(3):522–31.
17. Karas ND, Boyd SB, Sinn DP. Recovery of neurosensory function following orthognathic surgery. Oral Maxillofac Surg. 1990;48:124–34.
18. Berberi A, Le Breton G, Mani J, Woimant H, Nasseh I. Lingual paresthesia following surgical placement of implants: report of a case. Int J Oral Maxillofac Implants. 1993;8:580–2.
19. Shulman LB, Shepherd NJ. Complications of dental implants. Trigeminal nerve injury: diagnosis and management. Oral Maxillofac Surg Clin North Am. 1990;2(3):499–513.
20. Shavit I, Juodzbalys G. Inferior alveolar nerve injuries following implant placement -Importance of early diagnosis and treatment: a systematic review. J Oral Maxillofac Res. 2014;5(4):1–13.

21. Bert M. Complications et Echecs en Implantologie. Paris: CDP; 1994. p. 24–6.
22. Sunderland. A classification of peripheral nerve injuries producing loss of function. Brain. 1951;74:491–516.
23. Jensen O, Nock D. Inferior alveolar nerve repositioning in conjunction with placement of osseointegrated implants: a case report. Oral Surg Oral med Oral Pathol. 1987;63(3):263–8.
24. Smiler DG. Repositioning of the inferior alveolar nerve for placement of endosseous implants: technical note. Int J Oral Maxillofac Implants. 1993;8(2):145–50.
25. Guedj P. Le repositionnement du nerf dentaire inférieur en chirurgie implantaire orale. Cahier Stomato. 1992;5:13–7.
26. Guedj P. A propos d'un cas de repositionnement du nerf dentaire inférieur en chirurgie implantaire orale. Inform Dent. 1993;25:1817–20.
27. Jensen J, Sindet-Pedersen S, Oliver AL. Varying treatment strategies for reconstruction of maxillary atrophy with implants: results in 98 patients. J Oral Maxillofac Surg. 1994;52:210–6.
28. Antoun H, Misch C, Dietsh F, Feghali MA. Augmentation de crête par greffe osseuse prélevée à la symphyse mentonnière. J Parodontol Implantol Orale. 1994;14(3):285–94.
29. Little JW, Falace DA. Therapeutic considerations in special patients. Dent Clin North Am. 1984;28(3):455–69.
30. Zarb GA, Schmitt A. The longitudinal clinical effectiveness of osseointegrated dental implants: the Toronto study. Part III: problems and complications encountered. J Prosthet Dentistry. 1990;64(2):185–94.
31. Albrektsson T, Zarb G, Worthington P, Eriksson AR. The long-term efficacy of currently used dental implants: a review and proposed criteria of success. Int J Oral Maxillofac Implants. 1986;1(1):11–25.
32. Harden RN. Chronic neuropathic pain. Mechanisms, diagnosis, and treatment. Neurologist. 2005;11:111–22.
33. Park JH, Lee SH, Kim ST. Pharmacologic management of trigeminal nerve injury pain after dental implant surgery. Int J Prosthodont. 2010;23(4):342–6.
34. Li H, Xie W, Strong JA, Zhang JM. Systemic antiinflammatory corticosteroid reduces mechanical pain behavior, sympathetic sprouting, and elevation of proinflammatory cytokines in a rat model of neuropathic pain. Anesthesiology. 2007;107(3):371–3.
35. Clark GT. Persistent orodental pain, atypical odontalgia, and phantom tooth pain: when are they neuropathic disorders? J Calif Dent Assoc. 2006;34:599–609.
36. Kim YT, Pang KM, Jung HJ, Kim SM, Kim MJ, Lee JH. Clinical outcome of conservative treatment of injured inferior alveolar nerve during dental implant placement. J Korean Assoc Oral Maxillofac Surg. 2013;39(3):127–33.
37. Gregg JM. Neuropathic complications of mandibular implant surgery: review and case presentations. Ann R Australas Coll Dent Surg. 2000;15:176–80.
38. Khawaja N, Renton T. Case studies on implant removal influencing the resolution of inferior alveolar nerve injury. Br Dent J. 2009;206(7):365–70.
39. Finnerup NB, Otto M, McQuay HJ, Jensen TS, Sindrup SH. Algorithm for neuropathic pain treatment: An evidence-based proposal. Pain. 2005;118:89–305.
40. Finnerup NB, Sindrup SH, Otto M, Jensen TS. The evidence for pharmacological treatment of neuropathic pain. Pain. 2010;150:573–81.
41. Zakrzewska JM. Medical management of trigeminal neuropathic pains. Expert Opin Pharmacother. 2010;11:1239–54.
42. Attal N, Cruccu G, Baron R, Haanpää M, Hansson P, Jensen TS, Nurmikko T. EFNS guidelines on the pharmacological treatment of neuropathic pain: 2010 revision. Eur J Neurol. 2010;17(9):1113–e88.
43. Stefano GD, La Cesa S, Cruccu T, Cruccu G. Natural history and outcome of 200 outpatients with classical trigeminal neuralgia treated with carbamazepine or oxcarbazepine in a tertiary centre for neuropathic pain. J Headache Pain. 2014;15(34):1–5.
44. Zhou M, Chen N, He L, Yang M, Zhu C, Wu F. Oxcarbazepine for neuropathic pain. Cochrane Database Syst Rev. 2013;(3):CD007963.
45. Demant DT, Lund K, Vollert J, Maier C, Seger M, Finnerup N, Jensen TS, Sindrup SH. The effect of oxcarbazepine in peripheral neuropathic pain depends on pain phenotype: a randomised, double-blind, placebo-controlled phenotype-stratified study. Pain. 2014;155:2263–73.

46. Argyriou AA, Bruna J, Marmiroli P, Cavaletti G. Chemotherapy-induced peripheral neurotoxicity (CIPN): an update. Crit Rev Oncol Hematol. 2012;82:51–77.
47. Kautio AL. Chemotherapy-induced neuropathy:prevention and treatment. Finland: Academic dissertation, Department of Oncology, Helsinki University Central Hospital, University of Helsinki. 2017. [Accessed November 22, 2017]. https://helda.helsinki.fi/bitstream/handle/10138/32955/chemothe.pdf?sequence=1.
48. Pachman DR, Barton DL, Watson JC, Loprinzi CL. Chemotherapy-induced peripheral neuropathy: prevention and treatment. Clin Pharmacol Therap. 2011;90(3):377–87.
49. Eipe N, Penning J, Yazdi F, Mallick R, Turner L, Ahmadzai N, Ansari MT. Perioperative use of pregabaline for acute pain—a systematic review and meta-analysis. Pain. 2015;156(7):1284–300.
50. Sindrup SH. Tailored treatment of peripheral neuropathic pain. Pain. 2012;153:1781–2.
51. Bagheri SC, Meyer RA. Management of mandibular nerve injuries from dental implants. Atlas Oral Maxillofac Surg Clin North Am. 2011;19:47–61.
52. Sebaoun JD, Kantarci A, Turner JW, Carvalho RS, Van Dyke TE, Ferguson DJ. Modeling of trabecular bone and lamina dura following selective alveolar decortication in rats. J Periodontol. 2008;79(9):1679–88.
53. Wessberg GA, Wolford LM, Epker BN. Experiences with microsurgical reconstruction of the inferior alveolar nerve. J Oral Maxillofac Surg. 1982;40(10):651–5.
54. Jemt T, Lindén B, Lekholm U. Failures and complications in 127 consecutively placed fixed partial prostheses supported by Branemark implants: from prosthetic treatment to first annual checkup. J Oral Maxillofac Implants. 1992;7:40–4.
55. Sethi A. Repositionnement du nerf dentaire mandibulaire en dentisterie implantaire : rapport préliminaire. Int J Periodontics Restorative Dent. 1995;15(7):475–81.
56. Tatum OH. Advanced surgical techniques Communication, Association of Dental Implantology Symposium. London, 26-29 May, 1988.
57. Filo K, Schneider T, Locher MC, Kruse AL, Lubbers HT. The inferior alveolar nerve's loop at the mental foramen and its implications for surgery. J Am Dent Assoc. 2014;145:260–9.
58. Mardinger O, Chaushu G, Arensburg B, Taicher S, Kaffe I. Anterior loop of the mental canal: an anatomical-radiologic study. Implant Dent. 2000;9:120–5.
59. Bavitz JB, Harn SD, Hansen CA, Lang M. An anatomical study of mental neurovascular bundle-implant relationships. Int J Oral Maxillofac Implants. 1993;8:563–7.
60. Bartling R, Freeman K, Kraut RA. The incidence of altered sensation of the mental nerve after mandibular implant placement. J Oral Maxillofac Surg. 1999;57:1408–10.
61. Greenstein G, Tarnow D. The mental foramen and nerve: clinical and anatomical factors related to dental implant placement: a literature review. J Periodontol. 2006;77:1933–43.
62. Al-Ouf K, Salti L. Post-insertion pain in the region of mandibular dental implants: a case report. Implant Dent. 2001;20(1):27–31.
63. Bellaïche N, Missika P. La tomodensitométrie dans le bilan préopératoire en implantologie orale. Inf Dent. 1996;32:2681–9.
64. Walton JN. Altered sensation associated with implants in the anterior mandible: a prospective study. J Prosthet Dentistry. 2000;83:443–9.
65. Cruccu G, Gronseth G, Alksne J, Argoff C, Brainin M, Burchiel K, Nurmikko T, Zakrzewska JM. American Academy of Neurology Society, European Federation of Neurological Society. AAN-EFNS guidelines on trigeminal neuralgia management. Eur J Neurol. 2008;15:1013–28.
66. Essick G, Franzen O, Whitsel B, Finnerup NB, Otto M, McQuay H, Jensen S, Sindrup S. Discrimination and scaling of velocity of stimulus motion across the skin; Algorithm for neuropathic pain treatment: An evidence-based proposal. Pain. 2005;102:289–305.
67. Missika P, Alantar AA. Postimplantation neuropathies. In: Scortecci G, Misch CE, Benner KU, editors. Implants and restorative dentistry. London: Martin Dunitz; 2001. p. 403–10.
68. Treede RD, Jensen TS, Campbell JN, Cruccu G, Dostrovsky JO, Griffin JW, Hansson P, Hughes R, Nurmikko T, Serra J. Neuropathic pain: redefinition and a grading system for clinical and research purposes. Neurology. 2008;70:1630–5.

Correction to: Basal Implantology

Gérard M. Scortecci

Correction to:
G. M. Scortecci (ed.), *Basal Implantology*, https://doi.org/10.1007/978-3-319-44873-2

The original version of this book was revised to include the "Conflict of interest statement" in all chapters. The erratum to this book can be found at https://doi.org/10.1007/978-3-319-44873-2_16

Conflict of interest statement
Gérard M. Scortecci is the inventor of the Diskimplant and holder of several associated patents that are exploited by the Victory company. He is an unpaid consultant to this firm and a minority shareholder in the company. No money was received from any of the companies mentioned in the book or from any of the companies whose products are mentioned.

The updated online version of this book can be found at
https://doi.org/10.1007/978-3-319-44873-2

© Springer Nature Switzerland AG 2019

G. M. Scortecci (ed.), *Basal Implantology*, https://doi.org/10.1007/978-3-319-44873-2_16

MIX
Papier aus verantwortungsvollen Quellen
Paper from responsible sources
FSC® C105338

If you have any concerns about our products,
you can contact us on
ProductSafety@springernature.com

In case Publisher is established outside the EU,
the EU authorized representative is:
Springer Nature Customer Service Center GmbH
Europaplatz 3, 69115 Heidelberg, Germany

Printed by Libri Plureos GmbH
in Hamburg, Germany